HOT
SEX

HOT
SEX
HOW TO DO IT

TRACEY COX

BANTAM BOOKS

New York   Toronto   London   Sydney   Auckland

In memory of James Rupert Murdoch
1988–1989

HOT SEX

A Bantam Book / published by arrangement with Bantam Books, a division of
Transworld Publishers Pty Limited.

PUBLISHING HISTORY

Bantam Books Australian edition published 1998
Bantam Books U.S. edition / May 1999

Library of Congress Cataloging-in-Publication Data
Cox, Tracey.
     Hot sex : how to do it / Tracey Cox.
         p.   cm.
     Includes index.
     Cover title: Ultimate bedside companion packed with
practical yet erotic tips for men and women alike.
     ISBN 0-553-38032-X
     1. Sex.   2. Sexual excitement.   I. Title.   II. Title:
Ultimate bedside companion packed with practical yet erotic
tips for men and women alike.
HQ31.C924   1999
613.9'6—dc21   98-43546
                                                        CIP

Published simultaneously in the United States and Canada

Bantam Books are published by Bantam Books, a division of
Random House, Inc. Its trademark, consisting of the words
"Bantam Books" and the portrayal of a rooster, is Registered in
U.S. Patent and Trademark Office and in other countries.
Marca Registrada. Bantam Books, 1540 Broadway, New York,
New York 10036.

Printed in the United States of America

QBP   10

Contents

· ·

Acknowledgments

· ·

Many people have contributed to this book, both with information and moral support. At the risk of sounding like an Oscar winner, I really would like to thank my family (Shirley, Terry, Patrick, Maureen, Nigel, Deborah, Doug, Charles, and Madeleine) and *all* my friends and work colleagues who supported and encouraged me when I needed it most.

Special thanks go to: Deborah Murdoch, my clever sister, for casting an experienced medical eye over the technical chapters and so generously sharing her expertise; Nigel Cox, my brother, for bravely providing an intimate male perspective without ever telling me to mind my own business; Ute Junker, for reading every word of the manuscript, ever so tactfully pointing out my errors, and putting up with the anxiety attacks; Janet Muggivan, for her inspired publicity and marketing ideas and unwavering belief in both the project and me; Pat Ingram, the best editor in the business, who took me under her wing and taught me so much about journalism and life; Eric Fleming, Janet Hall, and Grant Brecht, three of Australia's most respected psychologists, who've cheerfully given up so much of their time to teach me about sex and relationships; Shona Martyn, Jude McGee, and Jane Bowring for having faith in the idea and guiding me through my introduction to book publishing with such good humor and style; Edith Weisberg, from Family Planning, who lent her formidable expertise to Chapter 6; Di Palmer, manager of Sydney's Club Femme, for making sense of all the weird and wonderful contraptions she sells in her erotica store; Amanda Dwyer, owner/operator of Salon Kitty's, who shared her sex secrets; Gerard Webster, a psychologist specialising in sexual abuse, who contributed immensely to several chapters in the book; Fiona Lecren, from Australian Birth Control, and Genevieve Graham, from the Child Protection Enforcement Agency, for advising on serious sex-related issues.

A huge thank-you also to everyone who bared their souls anonymously and contributed real-life quotes and advice throughout the book; and the sex diary authors and the sex workers, Olivia and David, for their wonderfully frank guides in the foreplay chapter.

Thanks to the various magazines who allowed me to use some small sections from my previously published stories. Some of the information contained in this book originally appeared in:

Cosmopolitan: "Blow Him Away," October 1996; "The Top 10 Lies About Sex," February 1995; "The 50 Most Intimate Things to Do With a Man," November 1994; "The New Sex Rules," April 1995; *Australian Women's Forum*: "Masturbation: At Your Fingertips," May 1996; "The Sex Diaries," March 1995; *marie claire*: "Complete Guide to Contraception," February 1996.

Introduction

A nyone can be good in bed. Genital size doesn't matter. Looks don't matter. You don't have to have legs up to your chin, arms like Schwarzenegger, drive a sports car, or be rolling in it to be the best lover your partner's ever had. But you *do* need a good, working knowledge of your subject. And that's easier said than done.

Nearly everyone talks about sex. We're always boasting about how *fabulous* so-and-so is in bed and hinting at the real reason why we look so tired at work (nudge, nudge, wink, wink). But it's a rare person who'll confess details or talk specifics. Jane might well confide that Brad gives the best oral sex she's ever had, but she doesn't launch into a lick-by-lick analysis of *why*—and I bet you don't ask for one.

That's why we buy sex books—to find out the nitty-gritty details about things we're too embarrassed to ask friends or lovers. Trouble is, few deliver what we really want to know. Sex manuals tend to gloss over the practical bread-and-butter stuff and, instead, talk in generalities—like how women need clitoral stimulation and men's butts are a veritable hot spot. Great advice but, if you haven't got the foggiest of what to do with it, useless.

This is where *Hot Sex* is different. Instead of assuming you know everything, I've assumed you know nothing and have dished up *all* the gory details in an easy-to-follow, step-by-step format. The only way I could have been more explicit and specific is to be there in the bedroom with you, guiding your hands and whatever else you're using (and, to tell the truth, I'd really rather not).

That's not to say the book *only* deals with the basics. Experienced lovers will get loads out of *Hot Sex* because there are enough advanced tips, tricks, and techniques to keep even Annie

Sprinkle happy. But I *do* suggest everyone read the introductory chapters. Very often it's the people who *think* they know what they're doing who need educating the most. Sex is a bit like typing. You can get by using two fingers, but you'll never be as good as someone who did the secretarial course and practiced every night. Going back to the grassroots level, even if it's just to check you're on the right track, isn't a bad idea for all of us. Don't let anyone tell you otherwise: sex skills can be learned and we can *all* improve on them.

I've written the book using everyday language for similar reasons. The correct, technical terms sound terribly authoritative but if *you* don't know that a wet dream is actually called a nocturnal emission, you wouldn't have a clue what I was talking about if I used this term. Sometimes, the words I use aren't even accurate. Most people say sperm when they actually mean semen, for instance. But, hey, if that's what you call it, that's what I've called it a lot of the time because I want you to relate to what I'm saying.

I'm also guilty of making some broad generalizations about sex. Hopefully, there aren't too many, but if you read something that you personally don't agree with, forgive me. If I covered every single individual preference, research finding, exception, and extreme, I'd still be madly typing away at my computer!

Hot Sex is designed to be read cover to cover but it is equally useful if you dip into it for inspiration when the mood strikes. Because good sex is only possible if *both* the people having it are committed to making it great, I've included guides for him and her wherever possible. *Hot Sex* isn't ageist either. There's info on all the different stages of our sexual lives: everything from first-time masturbation and losing your virginity to having sex when you're pregnant and taking the monotony out of monogamy. Add hints on ditching those inhibitions, tips on building effective communication skills, and loads of relationship advice, and you really can't help but shred the sheets!

HOT
SEX

1

Masturbation

The first, most important, skip-it-and-you're-doomed step to becoming a sexpert

● ●

Human beings are funny creatures. We'll chortle over whether to swallow or not swallow and turn that disastrous attempt at a new intercourse position into dinner party fodder, but when it comes to the most innocent, basic sexual act of all, we're about as likely to fess up as the guy in the corner suffering silently from an attack of hemorrhoids. We might well be the most sexually uninhibited generation so far, but masturbation—particularly female masturbation—still has a dirty name.

Even my friends, used to me blurting out all sorts of bizarre sex statistics, aren't comfortable with it.

"What do you do to break the boredom of sitting behind a computer for hours on end?" a girlfriend asked me recently, during lunch with a group of friends.

"Drink coffee mostly," I answered. "Oh—and I masturbate. It's a little treat that breaks up the day and perks me up to no end."

There was a deathly silence. Knives and forks paused midair; someone choked on a mouthful of wine. *"Excuse me?"* my friend sputtered, redder than the beets on her plate.

"I said I take masturbation breaks," I repeated lamely. And even *I* started to feel a tad embarrassed.

The fact is, although everybody does it (and if they don't, they should), few admit it and *no one* discusses it freely. Masturbation remains one of the few sex subjects that can make the most liberated person blush. The same girl who'll cheerfully masturbate when she's between partners feels guilty if she continues when she's getting regular sex. Lots of people still view masturbation as something you do when "you can't get any," fearing that if they're "reduced" to masturbating, they're not sexually desirable enough to score "the real thing."

In reality, the more sexually active you are, the more likely you are to masturbate, regardless of whether you do or don't have a partner. Kinsey, the world's best known sex expert, found that women who have a history of masturbating are more likely to easily experience orgasm later in life with a partner. They also tend to have fewer sexual problems than women who don't indulge.[1]

This is one area where men are ahead. Most women masturbate about once a week, often not doing it regularly until their late teens. Most men masturbate at least twice as often, and started doing so around twelve or thirteen years of age. Of the women who have discovered its joys, virtually all can masturbate to orgasm—95 percent of us, in fact (and some researchers put that figure even higher). On the opposite side, if you're a female who has never masturbated, statistics indicate it's quite likely you've never had an orgasm in your life. Pretty strong support for solo sex!

The truth is good girls *do* do it and if you never have and won't try, give up now on ever having a fulfilling sex life. Masturbation is a sure way (often the only way) to discover what turns you on sexually, and unless you know how to excite yourself, you've got zero chance of telling your partner how to. Few of us are lucky enough to start our sexual lives with a lover who's so patient and skilled he can teach us about our own body. Besides, masturbating is good for you. It releases tension, frees inhibitions, is gloriously liberating—and beats the hell out of counting sheep if you're having trouble dropping off!

Convinced but have no idea how it's done? It takes a brave person (and a few million drinks) to ask even your closest friend to tell you stroke-by-stroke how to do it. Luckily, you don't need to. In this chapter, you'll find no-nonsense, no-holds-barred, practical information on everything you ever wanted and needed to know about solo sex.

A BIOLOGY LESSON THEY DIDN'T GIVE YOU AT SCHOOL

Sex is an acquired skill and you need to do your homework to become an expert. You'll never master the guitar without finding out where to put your fingers to play a chord, and sex is no different: you need to know some basic anatomy. Surprisingly few people take time out to discover how their body's sexual response system works. For men, this isn't too much of a problem. The penis is easy to study—all he has to do is look down and play around a little. Women's parts aren't in view, and it's for that reason

"The first time I masturbated, I was riddled with guilt. I'd heard horrible things about it: it was socially unacceptable, something you shouldn't do, it was dirty and messy. The general impression was only dirty old men do it. I now consider masturbating extremely healthy but while no one now denies doing it, no one really admits it either. My fantasies usually revolve around the person I'm with. I'll deliberately watch her face and her movements while we're making love, then replay them as I masturbate. I relive the sensations and try to copy the same technique she used on me to add reality. I love going down on her and most of my fantasies revolve around giving her oral sex. Sometimes, I'll catch myself moving my tongue as I'm masturbating, I'm so far into the fantasy."

Tim, 32, sales representative

I've directed both of the following biological body tours to females. Out of the two of you, you probably know least about his and your own genitals. Combine this with some "field research"—touching and testing the areas that are meant to feel good when stimulated—and you're well on the way to becoming a sexpert.

It's best if you work through the anatomy and masturbation exercises solo first, before repeating the exercise with your partner. Learn how to give *yourself* maximum pleasure and you'll have more chance of successfully passing this knowledge on. Follow the directions faithfully and by the end of the chapter, you should both know your own and each other's hot spots. There's no exam. I'm not suggesting either of you learn the correct technical terms for every part of each other's genitals by heart. "Darling, do you like it when I touch you there?" is just as effective (if not as impressive) as "Would you like extra pressure on your frenulum while I simultaneously stimulate the perineum?" But a little knowledge really does go a long way—especially in the bedroom.

> **❗ There are about 200 million sperm in each ejaculation. In just 10 ejaculations a man produces enough sperm to fertilize each of the world's two billion reproductively mature women.[2]**

How the penis works

You'll benefit more from this section if you have a real live specimen in front of you. Yes, I'm serious! Gather your courage and ask your partner to model for you—it's much easier to identify the parts we'll be talking about by looking at the real thing. Explain to him that you're giving yourself a lesson on how his penis works so you can be better in bed. Assuming it's not your first date, he's unlikely to turn down the invitation. Just remember that the penis you're studying intently is still attached to a body. Your boyfriend will probably feel a little strange and shy to begin with and may be concerned he won't "measure up." Allay his fears by talking to him as you're examining and turn it into a lesson for two. Of course he knows which parts feel good when rubbed and which don't, but chances are he doesn't know the proper terms for them either!

Think of his penis in four parts: the *head* or *glans* (the mushroom-shaped top of his penis); the *urethra* (the tiny slit at the top from which he urinates and ejaculates); the *shaft* (the length of his penis); and the *frenulum* (the small piece of skin where the head meets the shaft). Your partner may or may not have a foreskin (loose skin which covers the head of the penis). If he has been circumcised, this skin was probably removed when he was a baby. If he has not, the foreskin naturally pulls back to expose the head during intercourse, giving him the same sensations as a circumcised guy. Approach the foreskin with care: don't yank it back enthusiastically to see what's underneath. Use lubrication and ease it back gently—ask him to show you how he does it.

> "I'll masturbate about four or five times a week on average, every day if I'm horny. No matter how sick or down I am, I still do it a minimum of once or twice a week—I've never been *that* sick that sex fades totally from my mind. It's no big deal really because it only takes a few minutes. I go into the bathroom and imagine some girl I've seen that day and thought was hot. Usually I come when I'm at the part in the fantasy where she's giving me a blow job. Her masturbating herself in front of me is another favorite."
>
> John, 22, student

As a general rule of thumb, the shaft of the penis is the least sensitive part and the head the most. The head is extremely sensitive to stimulation because it contains numerous nerve endings that are close to the surface of the skin. In other words, he'll feel your touch here more than anywhere else. Even more sensitive is the frenulum. It's on the underside of his penis (the side closest to his testicles rather than his stomach). Find where the head meets the shaft and you'll see what looks like a puckering of skin in the middle. That's the frenulum—something you'll become very familiar with if you're interested in giving him pleasure!

Penises vary in size but the average flaccid penis (not erect) is around 3.75 inches long and 1.5 inches in width. When he's aroused, the erectile tissues in his penis fill with blood and it grows and becomes firm. During *orgasm* ("coming"), he'll usually *ejaculate*, that is, propel semen (or sperm) out of his penis through a series of muscular contractions. Contrary to popular belief, orgasm and ejaculation are two separate processes that don't necessarily occur at the same time. Orgasm is the sensation; ejaculation is the discharge of sperm. He can ejaculate without having an orgasm, or have an orgasm without ejaculating. So he can fake it too!

The *scrotum* is the pouch of skin at the bottom of his penis that holds the *testes* or *testicles* (balls). They have two functions: to produce sperm and to produce male hormones like testosterone. Some men like their scrotum licked, held, or gently massaged during sex. His anal region is also extremely sensitive but, again, some men like you to pay attention to it, some don't. The *perineum* is the area between the testes and the anus: it's rich in nerve endings and also responds to being stroked or licked.

> ❗ Gay and bisexual men masturbate the most—once or twice a day or more.[3]

The *male G-spot*, (see page 106 for more on this), now identified as the *prostate gland*, is found around the urethra at the neck of the bladder. I wouldn't advise cheerfully prodding the prostate gland during this exercise (unless, of course, he's aroused)—he's liable to shoot through the roof rather than find it a turn-on. Explore it during sex by inserting a well-lubricated finger gently into his anus and pressing against the front wall—it feels like a firm mass about the size of a walnut. Massage it firmly or stroke it in a downward direction during oral sex or intercourse, preferably just before he orgasms.

How the vagina works

He's been looking at his penis ever since his eyes were able to focus: your genitals are hidden from view. Just about every woman has given in to curiosity at some stage and looked at their vagina in a hand mirror, but even if you're as familiar with your genitals as he is his, you'll get a lot more out of this exercise if you look at and identify each part. Choose a private place with good lighting where you won't be disturbed. I'd suggest going through this exercise yourself first, before repeating it with your partner. Sure, you'll feel a little uncomfortable with him "down there," staring at something that's rarely exposed. But if you're seriously interested in good sex, it's a must! Common sense should tell you that if he's never even set eyes on your vagina, he's got little chance of discovering exactly how to pleasure you. Genitals are individual and vary greatly from person to person. Your clitoris isn't in exactly the same spot as his last girlfriend's was and fumbling around in the dark isn't the best way for him to find it.

> "I guess I'm pretty matter-of-fact about it all. I'll get the urge, go into the bedroom and remove my underpants. I sit on the bed with my back against the wall, legs apart and feet pressed together. I've got both the Nancy Friday fantasy books and I've marked all my favorite fantasies, so I flip through, decide which one excites me today, apply some lubricant and off I go. I can be in and out of there in the time it takes to make a cup of coffee!"
>
> Fiona, 22, receptionist

The female sex organs are highly complex but, like his, basically divide into different sections. The external organs—everything you can see outside—are collectively known as the *vulva*. The *mons pubis* is the fleshy mound covered with pubic hair, forming a V, that you can see when you stand in front of a mirror. This acts as a "cushion" during intercourse. Sit or lie with your legs comfortably apart and the first thing you'll see are folds of skin covered with pubic hair. These are called the *labia majora*. Open them and you'll expose the inner "lips," called the *labia minora*. The size and shape of both lips vary greatly. Usually, the outside lips cover the inside but it's quite normal if your inner lips protrude. The labia minora contain glands that secrete sebum, the fluid that lubricates the vagina. When you become excited, the lips become engorged with blood (just like his penis), increase in thickness, and become redder.

If you're a virgin, you may have a *hymen*, a thin membrane

that covers the opening to the vagina. If it's still intact, it usually has holes in it that allow menstrual blood to escape. Don't panic if you haven't had sex but it doesn't appear to be there. Usually it's torn during childhood through activities like horseback riding and gymnastics or from using tampons.

Between the vaginal opening and your anus is a small area of smooth skin called the *perineum*. This area is highly sensitive to sexual stimulation. Like men, some women like a finger inserted into their *anus* on orgasm, though this is individual and depends very much on the woman (and the man who's doing it).

Just above your vaginal opening, you'll see the tiny hole that you urinate from. This is called the *urethra*. The *clitoris*, the most sensitive organ, is found at the top of the vagina (the end closest to your belly button) and looks like a tiny pea covered by a protective hood of skin. The bit of the clitoris that you can see protruding is actually part of a much larger organ that extends inside. In total, the clitoris is about four inches long and when the tip is stimulated (usually with his fingers, tongue, or the head of his erect penis), the entire thing engorges and becomes firm and sensitive. The clitoris shares the same components as the penis, they're just hidden from view. Men have what amounts to a clitoris along the upper side of their penis but it's completely covered by skin while the tip of ours protrudes. So while we think of women's genitals as being "inside" and men's "outside," the part of women that is the most sexually sensitive of all is well and truly "out there." His penis is used for other things (the transfer of sperm and urine); our clitoris is exposed for no other reason than to give us pleasure. It's the only organ that acts solely to receive and transmit sexual stimulation. So forget penis envy— he's the one who should be jealous!

Find your *G-spot* by inserting your fingers and pressing upward on the front wall of the vagina (the side closest to your front rather than your back). It's a small lump on the front wall that feels spongy (see page 104 for more details).

The *vagina* itself is a muscular tube about 3 inches long that, when adequately stimulated, expands to fit any size penis with ease. When your partner initially penetrates you, the muscles of the vagina contract and grip the penis. As you continue intercourse and become more turned-on, the vagina expands even further—

sometimes so much so, you can't feel his penis inside you no matter how large it is. This explains why, for both partners, the initial few thrusts are sometimes the most pleasurable because the vagina feels tighter.

For most women, stimulation of the clitoris is necessary to *orgasm*. Intercourse can indirectly stimulate the clitoris through thrusting but more direct touching with fingers or a tongue is usually more effective. When you do orgasm, your vaginal walls contract strongly and rhythmically, usually about three to five times, causing intense pleasure.

A HANDS-ON GUIDE TO SOLO SEX

The secret to sexual pleasure is at your fingertips. Literally. You've done your homework on the basic biology of how your body works, now we're going to study how your body responds to touch by masturbating. A lot more fun, believe me!

Ⓕ   FOR HER

If this is your first attempt at masturbation, it's essential you choose a place and time where you won't be interrupted. Hearing your mother's voice on the answering machine is a tad off-putting when you're hovering on the brink of your first orgasm, so take the phone off the hook for a start. If you have roommates, lock your door. Pull the curtains if you want to and do whatever it takes to feel comfortable.

Most women don't remove all their clothes to masturbate, but for this first time, do. Look at your genitals in a mirror and reacquaint yourself with your clitoris. Remember, it's usually at the top of your vagina and looks like a tiny pea covered by a hood of skin. Stimulating the clitoris is what will give you an orgasm.

Before you start, grab a tube of personal lubricant from the bathroom. You can buy K-Y or something similar from drugstores and supermarkets, and it's better to use that than Vaseline or baby oil, which alters the delicate pH balance of the vagina and can trigger things like thrush. You will also need some massaging oil or moisturizer.

Start getting in the mood by massaging the oil into your breasts, arms, all over your body, being consciously alert to what strokes feel good, what don't. It may help if you read an erotic book or watch a video while you're masturbating; alternatively, think sexy thoughts—fantasize about past or present lovers, someone you'd like to have sex with, or a scenario that excites you.

Lie in a comfortable position on the bed with your legs relaxed and apart. When you feel ready, begin to explore your outer genitals with your fingers—rubbing, stroking, applying pressure, experimenting until you find the techniques that feel the most pleasurable. Now apply some lubricant to the inner lips or lick your fingers and use saliva.

Start concentrating your movements around or directly on the clitoris. This will feel more sensitive than the rest of your vagina so start by gently stroking it while it's still covered by the hood of skin. Keep up a steady rhythm with whatever stroke you've chosen. As you get more excited, the hood will retract. Stroking the clitoris directly may feel even better. Experiment with hard strokes and soft, circular and back-and-forth strokes to find out what feels best.

After a while, those pleasurable sensations will build and seem to center around the clitoris. At this point you may want to increase the rhythm or pressure of your strokes or simply continue what you've been doing. You'll know when you orgasm. You'll feel an unmistakable surge of pleasure—a "climax" of the feelings you've been enjoying—and your vagina will go into a series of wavelike spasms. You may feel your vaginal muscles contracting. Usually, direct contact with the clitoris is painful immediately after orgasm, so don't be alarmed if it hurts if you continue to stimulate it.

If you're hung up about it

Talk to any good sex therapist about improving your love life and the first thing they'll tell you is this: if you haven't masturbated yourself to orgasm, you haven't even reached first base yet. Sensible advice. But if you come from a strict religious background or had parents who told you touching yourself was dirty and deviant, it's not so easy to shrug off those deep-rooted attitudes, no matter how silly they are. By the time we reach our twenties, most of us have figured out that masturbation (a) won't make us blind and

(b) doesn't make us perverts. But while most people, particularly women, recognize this *intellectually*, emotionally it's a different story. If you're having problems even reading this chapter, it's probably worth making an appointment with a sex therapist to work through your feelings.

Feeling okay but just a little bit squeamish? Try . . .

Calling it by a different name

Even though we talk about sex as a natural, normal thing to do, it's still not something we do in public. It wouldn't occur to most of us to screw our partners on the living room floor in the middle of a dinner party with friends, or even sneak off into their bedroom for that matter, just because we felt like it. For various reasons—some good, some bad—sex is hidden. And the message that sends to some people is that it's not okay.

Masturbation is even more shrouded in mystery. While we're used to seeing couples thrashing about in the bedroom in movies and on TV, masturbation is still primarily reserved for porn films, reinforcing its "dirty" image and leaving some people with the impression that it's still not right to touch ourselves "down there." Even the word "masturbation" throws up lots of prohibitions for many women. So, for a start, try calling it something else: pleasing yourself, tension release, your sleeping pill. By normalizing it and using a word or expression your brain doesn't instantly associate with "bad" thoughts, it will seem less threatening. Sounds simple, but sex therapists swear it's an important step in the right direction.

Taking your time and giving yourself permission to enjoy

When we masturbate, we tend to do it very quickly and get it over with because when we first started, we were worried we'd get caught. Also, a lot of people only masturbate when the sexual tension builds so high, they *have* to get rid of it.

Turn it around from something you only do when you have to and learn to view it as a "treat." One way of doing this is to use it as a reward—start masturbating after good things have happened to you. It's fat-free (unlike that bar of chocolate), great for your health (unlike a drink or cigarette), and won't cost you a cent (shopaholics take note). Soon you'll start to associate it with good things, and the whole process will become more positive.

Upping the pleasure principle

Tried masturbating but it didn't do a thing for you? I'll bet you didn't use lubricant. Rub away all you like but if you're dry, it'll feel irritating not pleasurable. Personal lubricants (like K-Y) keep the whole genital area wet and make almost any touch feel sensational. Lubricate your mind as well with sound and pictures. Put a sexy CD on the stereo and hang an erotic print in your bedroom. Alternatively, look at a snapshot of your adored, hunky boyfriend. Make sure your surroundings are as sexy as you want to feel.

Her four most popular techniques

1. Sitting up or lying down with legs apart

This is the most popular and traditional way to masturbate, which is why it's nicknamed the "masturbation missionary position" by some sexperts.[4]

Position: Lie on the bed with your knees up and legs apart or sit up, cross-legged, with your back against the headboard or wall. Try pressing the soles of your feet together to increase tension in the groin. You might like to read an erotic book or magazine while masturbating even if you discard it and let your imagination take over once you're close to climaxing.

Technique: There's no right or wrong way to touch yourself, but most of us use our fingers. Some women are so sensitive, they'll stroke themselves through their panties; some like direct clitoral stimulation, others indirect. All but 1.8 percent of women (according to the sexperts) use some kind of clitoral stimulation to climax.[5] The middle right-hand finger is often a favorite. Experiment with an up-and-down movement on the clitoris or do slow circles around the edge if it feels too sensitive. Start by stroking lightly, though you might want to increase the pressure later. Alternatively, you can rub side to side or "flick" the clitoris, strumming it the way you would a guitar.

The rhythm varies—most women prefer it be steady, though a few stop and start. Try slow and light or fast and heavy to find the rhythm that you decide is most pleasurable. Most settle on a rhythm and continue right through their orgasm, others bring themselves to the brink and then wait a few moments before recommencing. Some start off slow, then build up to their previous speed, others simply continue what they were doing before they paused. Another popular technique is to simply place one finger on either side of the clitoris and move against them.

Comparatively few women insert things into their vagina, for good reason! The clitoris, which gives us orgasms, is outside the vagina. However, it's a good idea to include the odd "dipping" movement inside, not just because it feels good, but because it helps transfer your natural lubrication from the vagina to the clitoris. The clitoris gets dry very easily, so apply more lubricant as you go along or lick your fingers regularly.

Stimulating the same area constantly can make your clitoris feel numb, so shift your hand slightly now and then to a different area to maintain the feeling and restore sensitivity. If your clitoris starts to feel irritated, stop direct stroking and instead manipulate the little hood of skin that protects the organ. Most women do this naturally anyway since the clitoris is extremely sensitive.

Timing: There's no "normal" time span to reach orgasm; it depends strongly on your mood, stress level, and how turned on you are. Sometimes you'll find yourself climaxing within a few minutes; other times it might take fifteen.

The climax: As you approach orgasm, press the heels of your feet together to increase the tension in the groin. You could also try squeezing your vaginal muscles in and out or deliberately clenching your buttocks to create pressure. Some women find moving sensually or moaning helps push them over the brink; others will sit or lie perfectly still without uttering a sound.

Few of us reach orgasm without fantasy, so let your imagination go wild! Relive a particularly hot session with your boyfriend, what you'd like to do with another person—conjure up a sexual scenario that turns you on. Don't get hung up about your fantasy;

> "I lie down on the bed and keep my legs tight together so my hand is crunched in between my legs. I don't use lubricant—I'm usually pretty wet, especially if I'm horny enough to want to masturbate. I rub directly on the clitoris but very lightly and keep the same rhythm all the way through. I don't put my hands inside myself, but sometimes I'll squeeze my nipples really hard. Occasionally, I'll put a pillow between my legs and grind against that to come. I don't fantasize, but concentrate really hard on getting off, the sensations I'm giving myself. No man has ever been able to masturbate me better than I can do it myself—they're too heavy-handed."
>
> Anna, 25, bank manager

it doesn't mean you're odd, gay, or secretly want to be raped. Most women fantasize about things they wouldn't dream of doing in real life—that's why we call them fantasies!

2. Rubbing against something

This is the second favorite masturbatory position. Instead of applying direct stimulation to the clitoris with your fingers, you rub against something, using the effect of pressure and friction to climax.

Position: Most women who masturbate this way lie on their stomach with their genitals pressed firmly into the bed with a pillow or cushion between their legs to rub against. Others lie on their backs with a blanket or pillow between their legs and use their hands to hold either side of the pillow to keep the pressure firm. One woman I know thrusts against a rolled up sock, another the arm of her teddy bear. Some women still use their fingers but use a pillow or crunch their legs tightly together to increase the pressure. You can also sit on the floor and thrust against the leg of a chair.

Technique: Remember when you were too young to go "all the way" but used to hump against your boyfriend's leg and hip for stimulation? This is the same technique. Generally, you hold the object still and move against it, rather than the other way round, though some women will pull a sheet or blanket through their legs rhythmically. Again, you'll need to experiment and maybe "arrange" your genitals so the thrusting feels pleasurable. Most women thrust quite hard, keeping up a steady rhythm until they climax. Placing a cupped hand over the entire genital area and moving it while you're pushing against the pillow is also popular.

Timing: Again, there's no "norm." Lots of women start with this technique, then move on to direct clitoral stimulation with their hands to finish themselves off.

The climax: Increase the pressure as you approach orgasm by clenching your thigh and bottom muscles. Most women also do Kegel exercises (rhythmically squeezing the same vaginal muscle that you'd use to stop yourself urinating) as they continue thrusting. Again, fantasy plays a large part and because you're thrusting against an object, it's relatively easy to imagine the object is the person you're fantasizing about!

3. Using a vibrator and/or a dildo

Roughly 15 percent of women who masturbate use dildos or insert objects. But a huge majority of us have tried, or own, vibrators.[6] Orgasming with a vibrator requires little effort: hold it firmly against the genital area and most of us will climax within minutes! For this reason, many sex therapists recommend you don't use a vibrator to masturbate *every single time*. For a start, it's restrictive, since you won't always have it with you. Second, it doesn't teach you any of the sexual skills you can use readily with a partner. At least try to masturbate to orgasm by rubbing or using your fingers, even if you use the vibrator most of the time.

Having said that, vibrators are a terrific, quick, and convenient way to orgasm if you're tired or don't have much time. Contrary to what the porn industry believes, most women don't use

> ❗ *Women with the highest education are more likely to masturbate. Forty-one percent of women who completed high school never masturbate, but only 7 percent of postgraduates don't indulge in solo sex.[7]*

> "When I was about 13, I put a finger inside me while lying in bed and waited for the fireworks to go off. Not surprisingly, nothing happened. I actually didn't have an orgasm until I was about 22 when I found my roommate's vibrator. Over the next year or so, I experimented with it: moved it in a circular motion, teased myself, tried different pressure. But the problem with vibrators is that you don't really discover how to give yourself pleasure because the machine does it for you. After I moved out, I deliberately didn't buy one and taught myself to masturbate with my fingers. It took a while, but now I can orgasm within about five minutes."
>
> Jennifer, 32, journalist

vibrators inside their vaginas but use them outside to stimulate the clitoris. Even if you've got a penis-shaped vibrator, chances are you use the tip rather than insert it. The most effective vibrators are sold in department stores as body massagers. They work well because they have a flat surface that stimulates the clitoral area effectively—they're also a lot less embarrassing to buy if you're a little shy! (While we're on the subject, don't relegate your vibrator to the back of the closet when your boyfriend's around; he'll love using it on you and will also enjoy the vibratory sensation on his genitals.)

Position and technique: If you're using a dildo, you can sit or lie while inserting it or hold it firmly at the base and lower yourself on top—the positions are as varied as they are for intercourse. If you don't have a dildo but would like to insert something, try a not-too-ripe peeled banana; they seem to simulate the hard but soft feeling of a penis and are totally harmless to insert. Since clitoral stimulation is usually necessary to orgasm, you'll also probably need to use your hands to stimulate the clitoral area directly, using any of the techniques listed above.

Positions and techniques with a vibrator are limited only by your imagination. The standard technique is to press it firmly against the closed labia (lips of the vagina) and hold it there, varying the pressure, until you orgasm. Try it standing up, sitting with legs apart, or lying down. Another technique is to stand with your legs apart, hold the vibrator still in front of your genitals and move backward and forward, grinding against it. Moving it in a circular motion is also popular as well as kneeling on the floor and squatting over it.

Timing: If you've only got two minutes to spare, masturbating with a vibrator is the technique for you! Unless they deliberately "tease" themselves and hold off, most women can orgasm with a vibrator within sixty seconds to three minutes. To make it last longer, try setting it on the lowest vibration speed, applying pressure and moving it in a circular motion, lifting it away if you feel yourself too close to climaxing.

The climax: If you're using a dildo, inserting it right before you're about to orgasm may be the most satisfying. It gives your vaginal muscles something to contract around and makes you feel "filled up." You might want to thrust deeper or faster when you feel yourself about to orgasm.

4. In the shower

It's soapy, slippery, wet, and totally private, which is probably why the shower is the place where many women either masturbate or at least get the urge to!

Position and technique: Unless you have a detachable hand-held shower hose, you probably won't masturbate to climax in the shower, though lots of women will stimulate themselves while soaping their genitals to get in the mood. If you do have a hand-held shower, try sitting in the tub or kneeling (if the tub's full, make sure your genitals are above water level), then turning the shower to maximum pressure and directing the jet so it runs over the clitoral area. You might want to use your hands as well. One word of caution: it's fine to use soap as a lubricant outside the vagina but don't push soapy fingers inside (again, it can lead to an imbalance and cause things like thrush and cystitis). If you're lucky enough to have a Jacuzzi (or access to one), you'll no doubt have discovered the pleasure of positioning yourself so a strong jet of water stimulates the clitoris.

> ❗ *Twenty-six percent of women (aged 18–35) have used a vibrator at least once.*[8]

Timing and climax: Some women can climax using their hand-held showers but most use it more as preparation, to get themselves in the mood, rather than to actually bring themselves to orgasm. Many switch to one, or several, of the other three techniques to finish the job.

Why not try . . .

- **Masturbating in semipublic:** want the added spice of danger? Try masturbating in the bathroom at work, on a plane, or at a party. Do it while you're driving or under a blanket on a long, boring plane flight. One girl I know can bring herself to orgasm (and continue a conversation) by sitting on the floor with her legs tucked under her, heel pressed firmly against her clitoris.
- **Watching yourself in a mirror:** you'll see how you look when you're turned-on, the sexy expressions you make while you orgasm.
- **Caressing more than just your genitals:** try rubbing or pinching your nipples or stroking your tummy just above your pubic hair as you're about to orgasm.
- **Leaving your underpants on:** instead, slip your fingers around the sides—it'll bring back memories of those first forbidden touches!
- **Masturbating while sitting in a chair with your legs over the side:** it's gloriously wanton.
- **Doing it from behind:** lie on your bed on your stomach with a pillow under your hips, masturbating from behind.
- **Standing up or leaning against a wall.**
- **Squatting Indian style!**

TEN GOOD REASONS TO MASTURBATE

1. It feels great.
2. It teaches us about our own body: what turns us on, what doesn't. Masturbation helps you identify what your basic sexual needs are and how best to satisfy them. Pass this on to your partner and you have a solid basis for a sizzling sex life.

3. It releases tension and helps us sleep—a secret sleeping pill without any side effects!

4. It teaches us to separate love from sex. We're more able to distinguish sex affairs from love affairs because we realize having an orgasm doesn't mean we're in love.

5. If you're single, it stops you climbing the walls or sleeping with the first guy or girl you meet.

6. It's totally safe.

7. It's a great beauty treatment. Orgasm improves circulation, combats the effects of stress, makes skin glow!

8. You can concentrate purely on your own pleasure without worrying about someone else's.

9. The more you masturbate, the more orgasms you'll be capable of having both with and without your partner. The more you do it, the easier they are to reach!

10. Being able to give yourself an orgasm is true sexual independence.

 FOR HIM

The first time

If you're male and old enough to read, you'd probably die laughing at the suggestion that you might need advice in this area. While some women don't start masturbating until their late teens or even late twenties, most men are quite good at it by age twelve or thirteen. But even if you've brought yourself to orgasm a thousand times, don't smile smugly and flip the page just yet. The *way* you masturbate could be causing problems in your sex life with your partner.

Because of our illogical but pervasive perceptions about masturbation—that it's "naughty" and something "dirty old men do"—your first masturbatory experiences as a boy were probably furtive and riddled with guilt. "Playing with yourself" was something you got over with as quickly as possible—fabulous when you've only got three minutes before Aunt Gertrude comes knocking, not so fabulous when you're with a partner later on. If it still only takes you a few seconds or minutes to masturbate yourself to orgasm, you're probably intimately familiar with the term *premature ejaculation* (orgasming too soon, before you or your partner is satisfied). In effect, from a very early age you've "programmed" your penis to ejaculate quickly by ensuring orgasm follows mere minutes (or seconds) after direct stimulation.

As they get older, most men relax into masturbation. They have more privacy, no longer feel guilty, and start experimenting with different techniques and varying sensations. The more you "hold off" your orgasm when masturbating yourself, the better you'll be at delaying it during sex with someone else. If you're still using the same technique you applied when you were thirteen, it's time to try something new!

Humor me. Pretend this is the first time you've pleasured yourself. Pick a time and a place where you won't be interrupted, don't set any time limits, and try one, or all, of the techniques listed below. The aim isn't to see which technique brings you to orgasm the quickest but to experience (and get your penis used to) different sensations. Masturbation isn't and shouldn't be something you do simply to ease tension. It's an experience that should be enjoyed for its own merits.

His three most popular techniques

Contrary to popular perception, most men don't read "girlie" magazines while masturbating. The men I interviewed weren't too enthusiastic about watching porn videos, either ("How often do you get the whole place to yourself to do that?"). Simply fantasizing—forming visual images in your head—is the most popular accompaniment to solo sex.

Unlike women, who often have two or three favorite fantasies that guarantee them orgasm, yours vary depending on what's happening in your life, even on that day. You'll build a fantasy around seeing a flash of lingerie on a train, replay a recent and particularly hot encounter with your girlfriend, or fantasize about what you'd like to do with the girl you took out for the first time the night before. Some men up the fantasy factor by sitting on their hands before masturbating to make them go numb. The idea is that if you can't feel your own hand, it feels like someone else is touching you.

1. Making a fist

Making a loose fist and running it up and down the penis is the most common way men masturbate, varying the tightness of the grip, speed of the strokes, and length of the movement to suit individual preferences. Like women, men discover what feels best through experimentation.

Position: Most of the men I interviewed said about the only prerequisite for where they masturbated was privacy. If your roommate or girlfriend is away for the weekend, you'll do it while lounging on the couch watching a video. Standing in front of a mirror is also a common turn-on. However, the most usual place is lying on the bed, legs slightly apart.

Technique: Most of you reach for some sort of lubricant first, and you aren't too fussy about what you use—soap, shampoo, baby oil, hand cream, Vaseline, your girl-friend's super-expensive face cream (thanks, guys!)—whatever you can lay your hands on. Personal lubricants like K-Y aren't popular, though once used, men tend to stick with them. While the penis isn't as sensitive to products as the vagina, a personal lubricant works more effectively.

The usual method is to make a loose fist, palm facing the side of the penis, starting at the top and moving down in a pumping motion that runs up and down the length of the penis. Some men go right to the bottom of the shaft, others concentrate more on the head. Most men prefer to increase the tightness of the grip as their hands move over the head, others find their glans too sensitive and

> "It's totally normal to continue masturbating even if you're living with a girl and have a fantastic sex life. Masturbation is one form of sex. It provides different feelings than sex with another person, so even if you're getting heaps of it with her, you still crave that different sensation. The only problem usually is opportunity. My (now ex) wife once caught me masturbating in the shower and was horrified. I thought at the time it was because she thought masturbating was dirty but I realize now it was because I wasn't having sex with her. She couldn't understand why I'd prefer to do it myself when she was lying in the next room."
>
> Gary, 25, lawyer

do the opposite. Rhythm is most important. No matter what stroke is used, keeping up a steady, constant rhythm is what builds sexual tension.

You might like to stroke, massage, or hold your testicles with the other hand or rub the perineum, the area between your testicles and your anus. Some men also like to touch or pinch their nipples.

In the same way that women tend to concentrate on their clitoris, most men eventually focus on the frenulum. The shaft is relatively insensitive and serves more to let your hand move up and down rhythmically. As your hand moves up and over the frenulum, try using a rolling action with your fingers and palm, manipulating the area firmly but not too vigorously. (One man confessed he ended up with a friction lesion on his frenulum during a particularly frequent and enthusiastic masturbation period in his life. The pain was secondary only to the embarrassment of being told what had caused it by his family doctor.) You could also try squeezing the base of the shaft to increase sensitivity and maintain the erection.

As an alternative, use your fingers to gently stroke the penis and testicles until you achieve an erection, then use two or three fingers and your thumb instead of your whole fist to slide up and down. Or try holding a finger still over the frenulum and moving your other fingers and thumb over the front of the penis in a smaller movement.

Timing: Like women, how soon you reach orgasm depends on how horny you are and how vivid the fantasy, but it also depends on factors like whether you feel stressed or tired. Most men reach orgasm fairly quickly—usually within two to five minutes—and deliberately slow it down or stop and start if they want to delay the inevitable. Try reversing your hand movement as you feel orgasm approach. Bend your wrist toward you so your fist is twisted and your palm now faces the opposite side of your penis. This shifts the stimulation to different areas.

The climax: When they feel they're about to come, most men increase their stroke so they're moving up and down the shaft as rapidly as possible. Some grab hold of their testicles as they are ejaculating, claiming it makes the orgasm last longer; others grasp the bottom of the shaft for the same reason. Once the orgasm starts, almost all men either slow down dramatically or stop stimulation completely. This is because the penis, particularly the head, is incredibly sensitive just after ejaculation (something girlfriends often don't understand because lots of women like to be stimulated right through to the last spasm of their orgasm).

What do you do with the little pile of semen you've created? Most men either ejaculate straight into a towel or over their bodies, wiping it off with a tissue afterward.

2. Using a pillow

Rubbing against stockings or something silky is often how young boys first discover they can make themselves orgasm. While The Fist technique is certainly more popular, particularly if you're *dying* for it, many men said they rubbed against a pillow when they were in a more mellow, sensual mood.

Position: Most men either stand or kneel with a pillow, folded over, in front of them. They then rub the penis in the fold and simulate intercourse. Others stand, place a pillow at groin level, and move their penis and testicles over the top in a back-and-forth motion.

> **❗** *Once every 5 minutes—that's the number of times the average 12-to-19-year-old guy thinks about sex.[9]*

Just as some women swear they can orgasm simply by squeezing their thighs together, several men I interviewed said they'd been able to mentally will themselves to a climax in certain situations (and they were proud of it too—"Look, Mom, no hands!") After traveling for a week on the road with his friends (with no opportunity to masturbate), one man said he put a pillow over his lap, squeezed his thighs together, sat on his hand so he could massage his testicles, and orgasmed simply by the pressure of his erect penis straining against his (by now rather tight) jeans. Now there's a challenge for the guy who believes he's tried everything!

Technique: You don't need to be a Masters and Johnson pupil to figure this one out. Either pretend to have intercourse with the pillow, rubbing your penis in and out of the fold you've created, or rub your penis back and forth across the top. Use your hands to hold the pillow in place.

Timing: Some men use the pillow technique in much the same way as couples do foreplay, switching to The Fist or more direct stimulation once they approach orgasm. If they don't switch to something else, the thrusting speeds up, just as it does during real intercourse.

The climax: Some men clench their buttocks together as they continue thrusting but most use fantasy to push themselves over the edge. In that instant, the pillow becomes almost lifelike—you'd swear it grows a set of breasts in that crucial moment!

3. In the shower

Masturbating in the shower is more common with younger men, probably because it's the one place you're guaranteed some sort of privacy as a teen. But even if you live by yourself, all that warm water gushing gently over your genitals, soaped-up, slippery hands washing your penis—the resulting sensations have made many a man forget about problems at work and focus on more pleasurable thoughts.

Position: Most men stand, usually facing away from the door (old habits die hard); others find it more comfortable to sit down. While soap is the classic lubricant, others find it irritating and use hair conditioner instead.

Technique: While with other masturbatory techniques most of you went straight for the goodies, the shower was one place where the rest of the body came into play. Some men started by soaping themselves all over ("like a lover would"), and nearly all soaped and massaged their anus, perineum, scrotum, and testicles before even touching their penis. From there, most moved into The Fist technique.

Timing and climax: Possibly because they didn't concentrate exclusively on the penis or head immediately, most men said they took a little longer to reach orgasm this way. Another very obvious benefit? Cleaning up afterward is a cinch!

HOW MASTURBATING CAN MAKE YOU A BETTER LOVER

If you have trouble reaching orgasm with your partner or if you're a premature ejaculator, masturbation can help. For men, it's invaluable for gaining control over your orgasms. For women, it's about the only way you'll discover what your partner can do to turn you on. Here's how to make it work for you.

> "We used to have a 'jerk-off room' in the house that I shared with my friends which had a stack of pornography, which we called 'jerking-off books,' by the door. When we felt horny we'd grab one from the pile, tell the others 'I'm going into the jerk-off room' and that was that. Most of the time, no one even looked up from watching TV. We were all very open about it, so much so that when friends came over to our place, they'd do the same thing. In my circle, masturbation is seen as normal as breathing. But I think we're the exceptions rather than the rule."
>
> Dean, 20, plumber

F FOR HER

- **Don't use the same method constantly.** Many women can happily give themselves an orgasm but rarely climax with their partners. Assuming your relationship is healthy and you don't have any psychological hang-ups about sex, this usually means you haven't shown him how you masturbate yourself (see "Why you should do it in front of each other" page 27) or the method you use to masturbate isn't one that's easily transferred to couple sex. For example, he can't turn himself into a human vibrator and give you the same sensation it does. So if that's the only way you can climax, you've got two choices: use the vibrator when you're with him or learn a more couple-friendly technique. Practice until you can masturbate yourself to orgasm with your fingers and try as many variants as possible. If you can only orgasm one way, you're restricting yourself sexually. The more techniques you experiment and are successful with, the more chance you'll have of re-creating them with a partner.

- **Play games with yourself.** Practice control over your orgasms. Set a timer and don't allow yourself to orgasm for five minutes; the next time try and orgasm within one. Read the section in Chapter 4 that talks about the G-spot (page 104) and set some time aside to find it. Practice Kegel exercises (see page 86 for more details). Pull in your vaginal muscles to the count of three, push out for three. Try masturbating while tensing your muscles; do the same while relaxed.

"I used to work on a magazine and one of my jobs was to edit an excerpt from an erotic novel. I was stuck reading the book for hours and could feel myself getting all hot and bothered. In the end, I just had to relieve myself so I went to the bathroom, locked myself in, and masturbated for ages. I could hear my workmates chatting a few feet away and that turned me on even more. Since then, I've masturbated in various bathrooms, once standing up in a dark corner at a party where everyone was out of it but me. The more chance I have of being caught, the better."

Debbie, 23, writer

Ⓜ FOR HIM

- **Do it more often.** If you ejaculate prematurely—you have an orgasm before either you or your partner is ready—masturbate more frequently. The more you masturbate, the less sensitive your penis will be to stimulation. Haven't seen your girlfriend in a week and feeling paranoid that the sex session you've been dreaming about will be all over in three minutes flat? Masturbate at least twice during the day you'll see her, if possible an hour before you have intercourse. This will help delay ejaculation.

- **Time yourself.** Try counting backward as you're masturbating. The aim is to take your mind off what you're doing. Start with a high number, like 500—the higher the number, the more your brain has to focus on counting. The first time you might only make it to 488. The next, aim to get down to 450, then 400, etc. You can use the same technique during intercourse.

WHY YOU SHOULD DO IT IN FRONT OF EACH OTHER

Partners can't read minds. So get rid of that "If he/she truly loved me, they'd know what turns me on" stuff right now. Body language can speak volumes and talking to each other is essential but, as the saying goes, a picture is worth a thousand words. Watching each other masturbate, you see firsthand what technique you each use—the pressure and speed, how you speed it up or slow it down on approach to orgasm, how you stimulate yourself (or not) while you're actually having an orgasm, and what you do with your spare hand. All you need do then is copy each other.

Generally, men are more comfortable masturbating than women are. If your girlfriend's the I'm-game-for-anything type, doing it in front of her may simply be a matter of taking a hold of yourself during foreplay. Chances are, she'll sit back and watch—lots of women are *fascinated*. If she ignores what you're doing, simply say, "I've had fantasies about masturbating in front of you. This feels great." If she still doesn't get the hint add, "This is how I do it when you're not around. Watch." If you want her to imitate your technique, get her to put her hand over yours so she can feel the pressure and rhythm you're using. Ask her to copy you and give lots of positive feedback—"Wow! You're

> **❗ Number of women who masturbate: 70 percent or more.**
> **Number of men: 94 percent—but they usually do it twice as often as women.**
> **Number of men who continue masturbating after marriage: 72 percent.**
> **Number of women who do the same: 69 percent.[10]**

better at it than I am." Uninhibited women can easily apply the same principles.

Your partner's a little shy and so are you? Talk about it first. Say you watched a show/a friend told you/you read about how watching each other masturbate will improve your sex life immeasurably. Ask if your partner agrees and suggest that the next time you make love, you try it. Don't be concerned if it all seems a bit serious and uncomfortable the first time round. Start by showing one technique you use: come on—that's a mere second or two of embarrassment! And get them to do the same. Later, when you both feel more comfortable, you'll be more confident and relaxed about bringing yourself to an actual orgasm. Masturbating in front of your partner or watching them masturbate has always been up there with the most popular male sex fantasies—and the new breed of sexually liberated females are adding it to *their* list.

2

Foreplay

Not just the appetizer, it can be the main course (and dessert) as well!

• •

Foreplay?" joked a male acquaintance (note, not a *friend*) of mine. "Isn't that when she says yes?"

Tragically, he's not the only guy to think that way. It takes the average man two to three minutes of direct sexual stimulation with a partner to orgasm. It takes the average woman twenty to thirty—which goes a long way to explain why women are a lot keener on foreplay than men. Unless you're talking fellatio, of course—there's no such thing as a bad blow job. What are the three things men want more of in bed? Oral sex, oral sex, oral sex.

Okay, we've got the message already—only problem is, men don't seem to have gotten ours. Let me put it very clearly. MOST WOMEN WANT MORE FOREPLAY. Some women would be grateful for any at all. But like everything else attached to sex, there are some outdated attitudes about it that seem to be clinging on for dear life.

Despite the name, foreplay isn't necessarily something you do *before* sex. Stop thinking of it as an appetizer that's to be raced through to get to a "main course" of intercourse and you're halfway to becoming a better lover already. If you're both really aroused, foreplay might be something you do *after* penetration, when you've taken the edge off. Experienced couples do it *during* intercourse—

they'll take a break for some oral sex or masturbation to keep the mood hot and heavy for longer. The most inventive lovers of all do nothing *but* foreplay the entire sex session. Not every time, just sometimes. Orgasms through mutual masturbation and oral sex are often more intense for both sexes; for some women it's the *only* way they climax.

Foreplay isn't a luxury to indulge in when you've "got time," especially if you are planning to have intercourse. It's necessary for the woman's vagina to physically prepare for penetration; without it, she'll be left dry but not high. And even men who can get an erection by inserting a coin in a slot machine can't deny that a good, slow, erotic "tease" dramatically heightens the sensations of intercourse.

Just one tip before you go gleefully poring through this chapter, eager to try out every suggestion: don't try to do everything at once. One of my girlfriends, who'd complained to her lover that she was bored with sex, had ice dripped over her breasts (and up her nose), (prickly) feathers stroked all over her body, and a (rather too ripe) banana shoved you-know-where, all while she was blindfolded and tied to the bed, all at once. Full marks for effort but the shuddering climax he'd hoped for didn't happen. She felt shuddery all right—like she'd just been put through the spin cycle of a washing machine.

If there's one rule about foreplay it's this: savor each experience, relax into it and take your time. Anticipation is one of the biggest turn-ons of all. Herein lies the secret of being a truly good lover—and truly hot sex.

WHAT EVERYONE WANTS MORE OF— MASSAGES!

In an ideal world, we'd all have two professional massages a week. Unfortunately, few of us have the time (let alone the cash), so that leaves . . . our partners, right? While no one particularly wants to start every romp around the bedroom with a leisurely massage, once a month is something all of us can aspire to. By all means take turns massaging each other, but not in the same session. There's nothing worse than having to put all those sensual feelings on hold if you have to reciprocate the minute your partner's hands leave your body!

A sensual massage

Schedule it for a Saturday or Sunday afternoon when you have hours to while away. Take the phone off the hook, put something slow and sexy on the stereo, and make sure the room is warm. It's more pleasurable for both of you if you're *both* undressed—though he's probably better off keeping his underwear on if it's his turn to play masseur (an erect penis tends to get bumped around a bit). If you really want to make his day, leave one thing on (like a pair of sexy panties or high heels) while you're massaging him. Aim to spend at least an hour sensuously plying him with your hands.

I've written this for a woman to follow, but the same technique will work for him, too.

Get him to lie facedown and cover all the bits you're not massaging with towels. Start by warming some scented oil or baby oil between your palms. (Don't drop it directly onto his skin—it's cold!) Now gently stroke along his back. Skim your fingertips very lightly over the skin to make it supersensitive (this is the part where he gets goosebumps) before moving onto firmer strokes. You don't need to be a professional because almost any-

> "My first husband was so predictable with foreplay, I could not only tell you exactly what he'd do, but what order and how long he'd spend on each bit. First he'd kiss me on the mouth, fondling my breasts at the same time. About one minute later, his hand would go straight to my genitals, he'd put a finger inside me and move it in and out a few times, then climb on top. He refused to talk to me about sex and denied there was a problem (he told me I'd been reading 'too many books' if I expected more). No wonder I left him."
>
> Rachel, 32, gym instructor

thing feels good, but you could try some or all of the following strokes.

- **Circling:** make firm circular movements with the hands, working outward and away from the backbone (the hand movements mirror each other).
- **Gliding:** put your hands on the lowest part of his buttocks, palms flat and fingers pointing toward his head. Use the weight of your body and push both hands up along the spine.
- **Thumbstrokes:** use your thumbs in a circular motion to ease muscular tension, particularly in tight areas. Similarly, try running your knuckles along either side of his spine for a blissful sensation. Generally, you should always work upward and away from the spine.

Make sure you pay attention to every (nongenital at this point) part of his body during the massage; massage his back and front including his hands, feet, bottom, and chest. For the first half hour, make it more relaxing than sexy—for the last, tease him mercilessly! Run your hands between his buttocks and penis, rub his inner thighs and lower stomach, but don't touch his penis, no matter how much it strains toward you. After at least forty-five minutes of stroking and kneading, he's ready for the pièce de résistance: an erotic genital massage!

> ❗ *Around 28 percent of women aren't happy with the amount of foreplay they're getting, yet almost all of us need it to allow penetration and achieve orgasm.[1]*

The knock-their-socks-off erotic version

Genital massage has been around for thousands of years, but has only recently been discovered by Western society—and westernized, of course! The true, unadulterated version draws heavily on the *Kama Sutra* and Tantric sex and is preceded by all sorts of bizarre, complicated rituals. But for our purposes (and because, to be honest, I've never found things like breathing in each other's breath terribly sexy), we'll skip straight to the nitty-gritty. You'll chuckle over the names but these explicit techniques are easy to learn and can transform the most mediocre lover into a wow-honey-that-was-*incredible* lay overnight. You may need to have the book beside you the first couple of times to follow the instructions, but once you've mastered it . . . well, your lovers won't forget *you* in a hurry!

Ⓕ FOR HER

Most men assume the "power position" during sex, so erotic massage will be especially pleasurable for him because it's a totally different sensation. Instead of you lying back and him doing all the work, he gets to relax and experience the sensation of touch while *you* take control.

Most of these techniques work best with him lying on his back on the bed, legs comfortably apart, and you kneeling between them. You'll need lots of oil; a water-based one, sold at most sex shops, is ideal, but unscented massage oil or baby oil will do the trick. Ask him to give you feedback all the way through the massage, saying which strokes and pressure he prefers. Watch his face and read his body language for clues. The idea isn't for him to orgasm quickly but to immerse himself in the concept of receiving pleasure. If it seems like he's losing control, stop what you're doing and lay both hands on top of his penis. Hold still, maintaining a firm but not heavy pressure, for about thirty seconds to calm him down. If you want him to orgasm, speed up the strokes.

The roll
Once he's lying on his back, kneel between his legs. Hold his testicles between your fingers and thumb and roll them gently, slowly, and lightly using the pads of your fingertips.

After a few minutes, change into a tickling stroke: put your hands underneath his testicles so they're resting gently on your fingertips and, using the pads of your fingers, tickle them. The lighter the pressure, the more exquisite the sensation.

Spiraling the stalk
This is great to use if he's having trouble getting an erection.

Hold the base of the penis with one hand and take a firm hold of it with your other. Start at the bottom and slide to the top using a circular, twisting motion as you wind toward the head. Picture a corkscrew—that's the sort of movement you're imitating.

When you get to the head of the penis, use the palm of your

hand to caress the entire surface. Only work upward.

The 12 o'clock stroke

Save this one until he's aroused and has a full erection. It's called "12 o'clock" because you're moving directly upward in a straight line.

Open your hand so your thumb and fingers are separated to make an L-shaped space. Slide your hand underneath the testicles until they rest between that space (if you're using your left hand, your fingers would be on the left-hand side of the testicles, thumb on the right). Push up a little so you're lifting them slightly.

With your palm down separate the first two fingers of your other hand to make a V and slide the penis between them working upward from the testicles to the head and tilting your hand so the flat of your hand brushes up against the shaft of the penis. Only work upward with this stroke. When you reach the head, remove your hand and start from the bottom again. Don't just slide up the middle; try sliding up the sides as well.

Making fire

This is the final technique because he's almost certain to orgasm.

Imagine you have a stick between your hands and are trying to start a fire by rolling it. Hold the palms of your hands straight, facing either side of his penis.

Using a rolling/rubbing motion, start at the bottom of his penis and slide upward, then down again, keeping the motion consistent and rhythmic. His penis will sit naturally between your palms. Start slowly, then build pressure and speed when he approaches orgasm.

> "My girlfriend puts a hell of an effort into our sex life. Each time we have sex, she'll introduce something new—whether it's a position, a technique, or a location. It used to freak me out. I couldn't help obsessing that she'd done all this with someone else (or was doing it on the side and picking up tricks that way). Then I figured she just had a vivid imagination and was really into sex. She drives me nuts outside the bedroom, but there's no way I'm letting go of her."
>
> Neil, 19, mechanic

Ⓜ FOR HIM

Rather than foreplay, think of her erotic massage as a sensual gift. It may lead to intercourse, but she's far more likely to enjoy it if there's no pressure to have sex at the end. As with the male massage, most of these techniques work best if she's lying on her back with her legs apart and you're kneeling between them. Put pillows under her knees and let her legs fall open naturally: it's more comfortable and she'll feel less vulnerable and exposed.

Don't use oil on her vagina; use a thin, liquid lubricant. K-Y is too heavy. Try Astroglide, Glyde, or Sylk (available at pharmacies and sex shops). Warm the lubricant by rubbing it between your fingers.

Ask her to tell you which strokes feel best, whether she prefers a firm or gentle touch. If you're unsure, err on the too gentle side; she'll probably push against your hand if she wants more pressure. Keep the rhythm regular and don't chop and change techniques too much. Watch her face—if it's relaxed, so is her body.

Remember, erotic massage isn't meant to replace foreplay. Use these techniques every single time you make love and sex will, once more, become routine and predictable. Instead, adapt the strokes to suit her individual preferences, combine techniques, invent some of your own—then transport her to orgasmic heaven!

Stroking the thighs
Perform this first to relax and arouse her.

Alternating between using the flat of your palms and your fingertips, lightly brush up the inside of her thigh. Then do the whole length of her body. Start at the ankles, brushing over the genitals and pubic hair, then move up to the breasts, circling around them. Repeat several times.

Focusing on the genitals, stroke the pubic hair and genital area using soft, gentle motions. Use your fingers to gently stroke and "tap" the outer labia (the outside lips), keeping up a regular, consistent rhythm.

Awakening the clitoris
Lie next to her or kneel between her legs. Using the knuckles of your first two fingers, knead the outer labia lips, moving backward

and forward while massaging. Make sure you're kneading, not pinching. Working downward, massage the whole labia with a firm but gentle pressure. Move downward toward the anus, then lift your hand and start at the top again. Alternatively, you can use your thumb and first finger if that feels more comfortable.

The two-finger stroke
Nicknamed the "bread and butter" stroke, this technique is the easiest and simplest way of giving her pleasure.

Rest your thumb and index finger at the top of the vagina (the end where the clitoris is), on the inside lips. Rotate your fingers around the top of the clitoris, then move your fingers downward. Massage and roll evenly, rubbing up and down on either side of the vagina, settling into an even rhythm.

She's ready for more direct clitoral stimulation when she opens her legs wider, pushes against your hand, or raises her pelvis off the bed.

Rock around the clock
It's extremely useful to imagine a clock dial surrounding the vaginal area, the top (near her pubic hair) being the 12 o'clock position and the lowest point (near the vaginal opening) being 6 o'clock. If she tells you what feels good, you can memorize the position (3 o'clock, 9 o'clock) for next time. Plus she can direct you more accurately. This technique was adapted from the Tantric original by the outrageous (but ever inventive) sex guru Annie Sprinkle.

Using the tip of your finger, move around the clitoris in a circular motion. Using bigger circles continue the circular motion down the entire length of the vagina, alternating with stroking, teasing caresses with your fingertips.

Now move back to the clitoris and circle directly over it with a fingertip. Some women don't like direct clitoral stimulation, so check with her which area feels best when stimulated, using the "clock" as a guide.

Try "pulling" the clitoris between two fingers. It's not actually possible to get a grip on it, but the pulling motion feels fabulous!

Entering the garden

This is a double-action stroke that works on the G-spot and clitoris simultaneously to bring most women to orgasm.

Insert a finger (or two) into her well-lubricated vagina, curving them so you're working on the front wall (imagine you're aiming upward to her stomach). Hold your finger still for a few seconds; she may move against it, but don't apply pressure until she feels comfortable.

The G-spot feels like a small, textured lump. When aroused, it engorges with blood and becomes more sensitive. Once you've found it, move into a "come here" motion, like you're beckoning someone with your finger. Don't press hard or constantly; a gentle, stroking motion is usually far more pleasurable. Try a "zig-zag" motion so your fingers are passing over the G-spot without concentrating on it too directly.

With your other hand, "rock around the clock," circling the clitoris with your finger, thumb, or a flat-surfaced vibrator. Also try moving directly back and forth over it as she's about to orgasm.

ABOVE THE BELT: A GUIDE TO STIMULATING HER (AND HIS) BREASTS

If you're a DD cup, encouraging him to pay attention to your breasts usually isn't a problem (getting him to pay attention to anything else probably is). But for those of us whose grandmothers don't even notice when we go without a bra, our breasts are often bypassed on the way to what men perceive to be the real goodies, the genitals. Yet for most women—and lots of men—the breast area is highly erotic, playing a vital part in sexual excitement.

As with the rest of our bodies, what we like, when, and how we want you to touch them is all individual. As a general rule, start off gently and slowly, increasing the pressure in line with your partner's arousal. Watch their body language carefully to see how they respond to different touches—and make sure it's desire that's making the nipples erect, not the cold breeze drifting in through the open window!

Ⓜ️ **FOR HIM**

Try sucking, nibbling, licking, stroking, or gently squeezing the entire area. The nipples and areola (the pinky brown area around the nipples) are sensitive but so is the area underneath. Some women feel zilch when you directly touch their nipples, but stroke underneath and, *hey presto*, they'll stiffen immediately. Use your tongue, fingers, whole hand, lips, and the head of your erect penis to stimulate the entire area.

❗ *Men are more likely to reach orgasm during intercourse while feeling your breasts than you are from having them felt.[2]*

Some women like their nipples flicked, pinched hard, or bitten. But this very much depends not only on personal taste, her mood, and how many glasses of wine she's had, but where she is in her menstrual cycle. Sometimes, even your fingers might feel too rough; other times, what seems like a fierce bite to you might not be hard enough for her. There's no magic way of telling what she'll want on a particular day—just ask her what feels good.

Ⓕ **FOR HER**

Some men's nipples seem to be directly linked to their penis. Suck, stroke, or tweak them and they'll get an instant erection. Other men are lukewarm to the idea—play all you like, but he'll still look about as excited as someone sitting in the dentist's waiting room. Again, there's only two ways to find out which category he fits into. Open your mouth and apply it to a nipple to see how he responds, or ask him directly.

Use the same techniques he uses on you (or that you'd like him to)—nibbling, stroking, sucking the nipples gently to begin with, upping the pressure if he seems to enjoy it.

Try a Tantric technique. Put a glass of water with ice cubes in it by the bed. Rub an ice cube on his nipples to make them stand up and get the blood flowing to that area. Now use your fingertips to make a circular motion around the nipple, alternating occasionally with a little pinch. Pull at the nipples to draw them out, watching his face to see which motion arouses him most.

DELICIOUS DETOURS

"Happiness isn't a destination; it's a means of traveling." This old saying can be applied to foreplay. Rush through the "traveling" and you might find the destination isn't quite as exciting as you'd expected. Lavish attention on the *whole body* and you can't help but take your time.

Erogenous zones are areas on our bodies that create intense sexual arousal when stimulated. Apart from the obvious parts that we all share (like the penis and the clitoris), each of us has our own secret area that sends frantic YES! YES! messages to all the right places. For some, it's being bitten in the small of their neck. Others go crazy when someone strokes their buttocks. But what works for one lover won't necessarily work on the next, so consider each new lover unexplored territory. There are few places on our bodies that we don't like being touched. Why restrict foreplay to the breasts and genitals when the entire body is itching for attention?

- **Take a body tour.** When you get to a new city, you often take an orientation tour to get your bearings, right? Then what's stopping you doing the same with your new lover's body? You can go all out here and even use a few props. Make him lie down naked on his stomach and close his eyes—make sure the room you're in is private and warm—then trail a scarf slowly and tantalizingly across his naked bottom and back. Then turn him over and stroke a feather around his penis and scrotum. You can then move on to using your hands, hair, breasts, and mouth on his nipples and genital area, creating different sensations as you search for his ultimate pleasure zones.
- **Try stroking her face,** the back of her neck, her back. Play with her hair, lift it up from her neck and stroke underneath, slide your palms up and down her arms—and this is just while you're watching TV together. Don't even make it to the bedroom.
- **Massage his feet,** kiss his toes, massage his hands, then take each finger into your mouth and suck it, pretending it's his penis.
- **Don't dive straight for his penis during foreplay.** Use long, sensual strokes up his inner thighs until he's *trembling* with desire.

- **Bottoms up!** Both your bottoms are an arousable area. Try massaging them, stroking, even gentle slapping. Don't neglect the perineum (the area between your genitals and your anus). Press firmly and massage with two fingers, gently stroking along the entire length; use your tongue to do the same.
- **Use your fingers to rub along the outline of his lips,** then insert a finger into his mouth for him to suck. Do the same with your nipples. He can do the same with his penis.
- **Get into neck nibbling.** Do you know anyone who doesn't enjoy having their neck kissed or gently nibbled? (If you do, they're either incredibly ticklish or totally uptight.) It's a sadly ignored area that can produce amazing results.
- **Suck her toes,** slide your tongue into her belly button (try diving on her after a shower if you're paranoid about lint)—have fun with foreplay! It really doesn't matter if she laughs instead of sighs—she's still complimented that you find *all* of her sexy, not just "the good parts."
- **Kiss all over his body,** not just on his mouth and genitals.
- **Use your whole body to massage his.** Lie on top of him when he's lying on his back or front, gyrate slowly and revel in the simple sensation of skin against skin.

And for my next trick . . .

- **Tie him up.** We've all seen it done in the movies. You don't need to pop down to a sex shop and buy one of those leather numbers to slip on (unless you want to, of course) or crack a whip (ditto) to play the dominatrix. But you *do* need a bedpost (or chair) to tie him to, a couple of long scarves (some old stockings or a few of his ties will do), and a nasty smile on your face. Once he's comfortably trussed (don't cut off the circulation, you need the blood flowing for him to get an erection, let alone keep his heart pumping), you can try out a number of erotic scenarios, like . . .
- **Masturbate for him.** Watching you give yourself pleasure will give him a big kick. The effect will be even more spectacular if you masturbate loudly and theatrically while he's tied up and is utterly helpless. If you want to get him *really* worked up, simply leave him tied up and then . . .
- **Blindfold him.** Even a see-through chiffon scarf can increase the sexual tension tenfold. It also makes you less inhibited

about what you do to him because he can't see you. Tie the scarf across his eyes then build the anticipation by withdrawing completely for a few seconds, then caressing him in his favorite places, and a few he's not expecting. This also lets his imagination run wild—you could be a provocative French maid, slave girl . . . you get the picture.

- **Undress each other.** Don't just fling your clothes in a corner and hop into bed naked; let him undress you and vice versa. Stop along the way to lick and caress the body part that's just been exposed.

- **Play the vamp.** Thought the only time you'd use those long, black gloves was on black tie occasions? Put them on now and start masturbating him. Yes, it does come out in the wash.

> **❗ Ninety percent of women would pick cuddles over orgasms if they had to choose between the two for the rest of their lives.[3]**

- **Make it good enough to eat.** Whipped cream, bananas, and berries aren't just good for fruit salads. Take them out of the kitchen or, better still, stay there and satisfy two appetites at once. Having a feast off each other's bodies is silly more than anything else, but even if it simply makes sex more fun, it's worth the experiment. Unless you're talking hot and spicy foods, it's safe to smother or insert most foods in and around the genitals for both of you to devour. While you're at it, grab some ice cubes from the freezer, put them into your mouth, then suck his penis.

- **Drop it.** Leave the sisterhood stuff outside the bedroom door. If he fantasizes about you dressing up as a waitress, serving him exactly what he hungers for, he *is* treating you like a sex object—but isn't that the point?

- **Go for the cliché**—most men love it. Invest in some sexy black underwear. After a night out, take off your clothes to reveal stockings and garters. (Even better, flash him a glimpse *while* you're out.)

- **Tease, tickle, and titillate.** Brush your lips over his mouth but don't let him kiss back. Put his penis momentarily in your mouth, then withdraw and start kissing his neck. Sit on top of him and let him partially penetrate you, then get up and walk away. The trick is to keep him unbelievably aroused rather than frustrated. At some point, though, you have to put him out of his misery by bringing things (and him) to a fabulous finale!

THE LONG, SLOW STRIP

You probably can't equal (but then again, who knows?) the hot little strip that Kim Basinger did for Mickey Rourke in *9½ Weeks*. But you can certainly make up in enthusiasm whatever you lack in professional technique. Here's a wiggle-by-wiggle guide to taking it all off and really turning him on.

- You absolutely must wear stockings and garters and sexy underwear. Add a silky, short slip (à la Kim).
- Put on some music. Anything you like to dance to will do (though heavy metal possibly won't create the atmosphere you're aiming for). Try some Barry White or Prince; if you have the original Joe Cocker song "You Can Leave Your Hat On," put it on and hit the play button!
- Gulp some champagne for courage, sit your partner in the living room, and tell him if he laughs you'll not only kill him, you'll stop immediately. (He won't even smile!)
- Start by rubbing your hands over your body, letting the slip ride up your thighs and the straps slide down off your shoulders. It's best if you have a slip you can step out of, rather than one you have to pull over your head (and end up getting stuck in).
- Removing your stockings is next. Really work this one, rolling the stockings down seductively, leaving your garter belt on.
- To begin with, play it coy and keep your eyes modestly lowered, so he gets the impression you're undressing privately and he's not supposed to be looking. As you get to your garter belt, move into a more dominant role—fling yourself and it around a bit like professional strippers do. (Practice this in front of a mirror first and keep your distance. Flicking him in the face with the belt will ruin the mood—and he needs two eyes to watch you.)
- Remove your panties a bit at a time. Play it up a little by almost taking them off, then deciding not to. Put one leg up on the side of a chair as you push them down over your thighs, so he can see your genitals.
- Walk over to him and look him straight in the eye when you

undo the final garment (your bra) thrusting your breasts forward. That way you can also finish the show off with an extra most strippers never supply—taking *his* clothes off in the middle of a long, slow, French kiss.

TOUCH UPS

The sexperts call it "mutual masturbation," a deadly term that brings up an image of a group of people, all sitting around in a circle, playing with their own genitals. While mutual masturbation *can* mean masturbating in front of each other, it's usually used to describe your giving him a hand job and vice versa. In other words, it's "heavy petting"—what you were (probably quite rightly) accused of doing when you stayed out late with your boyfriend as a teenager.

Like every other sex skill, expertly masturbating someone else's genitals takes practice. Though it's pleasurable to be touching each other simultaneously, if you're really serious you'll take turns. It's far too easy to lose concentration and focus instead on what he/she is doing to you. This is one area where I'm pleased to be female. The great thing about penises is that they're usually happy no matter what you do to them—the very fact that your hand is "down there" stroking him, will usually be enough to get his juices flowing—unlike vaginas and clitorises, which are supersensitive, contrary creatures, highly individual and finicky.

There's another huge difference between the two sex organs. For women, gentle is nearly always best; for men, firm is invariably better. What sends you orbiting into orgasmic heaven can leave him limp; what makes him groan with pleasure can have you yelping in pain. So, if you're a female, you can probably up the pressure a bit. I'm not suggesting you wring his penis with abandon or bend it willy-nilly (it's *attached*, remember, and not made of rubber), but you can prob-

> "I swear it's true: I've never had a woman try to masturbate me to orgasm. Usually, they'll stroke and play around a bit but they've never taken a firm grip and done it the way I do. It doesn't worry me as long as they're good at oral, but I find it intriguing. Why don't they?"
>
> Shane, 36, small business owner

ably go harder than you think. If you're male, tone it down a little. She'll soon let you know if your touch is so soft she's forgotten you're even in the room.

As with any sexual technique, the best way to get good at mutual masturbation is to ask your partner to show you how *they* do it and imitate. At the very least, guide each other by saying what feels good and what doesn't. Even a "harder" or "move up a bit" is better than nothing.

Ⓕ FOR HER

Just as you hate him diving straight for the clitoris, he hates you pouncing immediately on the penis. Kiss and stroke everywhere, glide up the inside of his thighs, pay attention to his testicles and the area of his tummy his erect penis sits on.

Remember our biology lesson? (If you don't go back to page 4 and read "How the penis works" again.) The head of the penis is packed with nerve endings and so is the frenulum (the string of skin underneath the penis where the head meets the shaft). Pumping up and down the shaft alone will do little more than give you a miniworkout.

If he's uncircumcised, don't pull back the foreskin until he's well lubricated (either with preejaculatory fluid—the stuff that comes out when he's excited and looks like sperm—saliva, or personal lubricant). Even then, proceed with caution. The head of the penis is more sensitive on uncircumcised men; you're better off using the foreskin as a buffer between you and the head, and manipulating that up and down over it.

- Get into a good starting position. Chances are you're lying beside him, but while this is the most usual position, it's probably the hardest to work with. If you're serious, get him to stand in front of you or sit astride him. Want to stay lying down? At least prop yourself up on one elbow so you can work properly with one hand; better still, shift your weight so you can use both hands and still be balanced. Make sure you're on the right side (that is, if you're right-handed, that's the best hand to use). If it feels awkward for you, it's going to feel less than perfect for him.

- Start by stroking his penis until it hardens, then roll it gently between your palms before moving into the basic stroke. Make an open fist with your hand (see page 21 for more detail) and move it up and down the shaft of the penis in a regular rhythm. As you get to the head, try closing your fist and gliding over it, increasing the pressure a little.

- Ask him to put his hand over yours to show you what pace he likes. The three things to keep in mind are: smooth, firm, and consistent. Try to make one long, smooth action rather than a number of jerky movements. This shouldn't be too hard because it's a very simple movement—just close your fist as you go over the head, and open it to move down the shaft. Try long strokes taking in the whole length, or short strokes concentrating on the head.

- Start off slow and speed up as he approaches orgasm. The faster and harder you masturbate him, the quicker he'll orgasm. If you want to tease, speed up for a while, then slow down before speeding up again.

- You have two hands. Use the other one to cup the scrotum, play with his nipples, massage the perineum firmly with your fingertips.

- Some women use two hands on his penis—one holding it firmly at the base, the other moving up and down the shaft. Others prefer to make a thumb and first finger ring rather than a loose fist. (While we're on the subject of hands, change them often so they don't become numb.)

- As he's about to climax, he'll tense up and breathe heavily. If you're watching closely, you might notice the head of his penis becoming dark red and his testes lifting toward his body. Most men prefer you to be working quite fast until they start ejaculating, then to slow it right down or simply stop and hold the penis during ejaculation. Lots of men say they like less pressure on the head the closer they are to coming. It's incredibly sensitive just after ejaculation; resist the urge to do one last stroke for good luck and remove your hands gently. (This is also why he'll wince with pain if you cough while he's still inside you but has already ejaculated. Coughing involuntarily squeezes your vaginal muscles around his—ouch!—oversensitive penis.)

- As an alternative, let him masturbate his penis between your breasts. If they're little, hold them close together with your hands to create cleavage.

COMMON MISTAKES WOMEN MAKE

- You're either too hard or too soft. Getting the pressure right is simply a matter of asking him which feels best. Men with smaller penises generally like a softer touch (the nerve endings are more concentrated).
- You don't ask what he likes and use the same technique on everyone. (You ask people how they like their coffee, don't you?)
- You don't keep up a steady rhythm or do it for long enough. Many guys complain that women are jerky, stop at all the wrong times, and don't position themselves properly, so their hands go numb way too quickly.
- You don't hit the right spot. The bottom of his penis may feel wonderfully macho and hard to you, but it's stimulating the top that feels best to him.

Ⓜ FOR HIM

Just like Monopoly, you can't collect your $200 until you've passed Go. In other words, don't even think about touching her genitals until you've paid your dues on her breasts, neck, and stomach, and stroked up her thighs.

- You're probably lying beside her, hopefully with the hand you're most comfortable working with free. If she's not already wet, lubricate the area with saliva or personal lubricant. Her natural lubrication will keep the area moist once she's fully aroused.
- Start by "warming" and stimulating the whole genital area. Place your whole hand over the closed outer lips and rub in a circular motion. You'll be stimulating the clitoris by moving her lips against it.
- When she starts to become aroused, the outer lips will open naturally themselves. Gently part them a little wider and move your fingertips up and down the inner lips, in a long, slow, soft movement, grazing the clitoris—still covered by a little hood of skin—on your way up and down.
- Wait until she's well lubricated before honing in on the clitoris. Then circle around it with one fingertip several times before

sliding back down the inner lips again. Get her to guide you by putting her hand over yours to show you what speed and pressure she likes. Even lubricated, the clitoris is extremely sensitive. If you're too rough, too direct, or stimulate for too long, too soon, it gets oversensitive and feels painful. Concentrate exclusively on the clitoris only when she's close to orgasm.

> "I went out with a bodybuilder whose idea of foreplay was taking his clothes off. I guess I was supposed to get off by looking at all those muscles. It was all over in about three minutes—and he didn't know what afterplay was either."
>
> Helena, 26, journalist

- An alternative technique is to use vibration. Place your middle three fingers over the top of the vagina (where the clitoris is), press firmly (but not too hard), then vibrate your hand gently but rapidly and consistently or move it in a circular, vibratory motion.

- The three golden rules for men: gentle, slow, and regular. Keeping up a steady rhythm for a long period of time, even if your technique isn't perfect, will get you further than switching all over the place with the most adroit strokes. While she can speed up, slow down, or stop completely to tease you, you do the same and she'll end up frustrated rather than turned-on.

- Most women like to be penetrated with a finger (fingernails trimmed, please!). Use one finger to begin with, add another when she's more excited or use your thumb and press deeply. Move it in and out of the vagina, gently to start with. Some women love to be penetrated deep and quite hard but still keep it slow. She'll be wetter inside, so spread the lubrication over the clitoris. Keep stimulating the clitoris while penetrating her by keeping the flat of your hand firmly pressed against it while your fingers dip in and out.

- A lot of the time you'll have one hand working on her clitoris, the other inside her. When you've got one hand free, use it to stroke her nipples. As she's about to climax, she may clench her buttocks, tense up, hold dramatically still, and go completely quiet. (Not all women put on a Meg Ryan *When Harry Met Sally* performance.) At this point, it's crucial to keep doing whatever it is you're doing—don't stop or change *anything*.

As she's coming, slow down but keep going (gently). She'll push you away when she's had enough.

- Try rubbing her clitoris with the tip of your erect penis as a sexy alternative to using your fingers.

COMMON MISTAKES MEN MAKE

- You're too rough. This is the number one complaint of all women, regardless of age.
- You get offended if we try to guide you and don't read our body language. It doesn't matter how many lovers you've had, each female is different. We're not criticizing you when we move your hand, simply teaching you what suits us. Many women say men don't read their body language for signs. If she presses against you, she wants more pressure; if she pulls away, she wants you to be more gentle.
- You don't keep a consistent rhythm. Just as we start climbing the climax ladder, you change techniques and we slide right to the bottom again.
- You push your fingers inside too soon. Stimulate the labia and clitoris a little first.
- You stop at the crucial moment. Our orgasms often last longer than yours do (we *knew* there had to be some payoff for having to suffer through period pain). You might think she can't possibly still be having one, but she may be. If you stop what you're doing while we're still climaxing, the orgasm continues but it's not as intense and we feel horribly robbed.

BLOW THEM AWAY!

If you're not good at giving oral sex (even worse, can't be bothered learning), give up now on ever graduating from sex school. Nothing will score you more points in the bedroom than delivering mind-blowing fellatio (to him) or cunnilingus (to her).

Oral sex is the one erotic act everyone consistently reports wanting more of. Without it, many women would never orgasm with a partner. Equally adored by both genders, oral sex appears to have universal appeal. If being told "You're a great lay" is a compliment, you'll be worshiped for performing phenomenal blow-jobs.

Why the fascination? The thought of someone's tongue licking your genitals seems naughtier than intercourse; unless you're in the 69 position, it's perfectly acceptable to lie back and receive pleasure without having to reciprocate simultaneously; and tongues are usually wetter, softer, and more agile than hands and penises. They're also warm, and genitals respond to heat much more than they do cold fingers. Convinced it's a skill worth mastering? You should be. Read on . . .

Ⓕ FOR HER

Giving him mind-blowing fellatio (the fancy term for oral sex) is number one on his sex wish list, and it's the thing most women feel least confident about. Who better to ask for tips than a sex worker who specializes in it? (If you have something against taking advice from experienced, high-class prostitutes, get over it now. They make a living out of sex and are experts in their field.) I asked Olivia, a skilled fellatrix, to reveal her most intimate secrets for this no-holds-barred guide to giving him pleasure. Prepare to turn from the most nervous novice into an instant expert—and have him begging for more! This is her guide, so I'll let her tell you in her own words . . .

Ten-step guide to the best fellatio he's ever had
1. Learn to love it
"Women who love sex are good at it; it's as simple as that. If you don't like giving him oral sex, the best techniques in the world won't turn you into a skilled fellatrix. Usually it's the smell, swallowing, or gagging that women are scared of, and all are easily fixed. Turn a shower into foreplay if he's not scrupulously clean and use the soap as a lubricant to masturbate his penis (if he's uncircumcised pull the foreskin back very gently and wash underneath). Gagging isn't a problem if you use my techniques, and you don't have to swallow to be good at oral.

"Fellatio, or 'French' as we call it, is requested and enjoyed by almost all clients, regardless of the prostitute's speciality. Show him that you love doing it—make lots of noise and '*uuumms*,' compliment him on his penis—and he'll be anything *but* putty in your hands! Get to know his penis: examine it, talk about it. Be aware of his body language. Learn how to read his moods and play up to any secret fantasies."

2. Give him lots of foreplay

"Women aren't the only ones who love foreplay (even if *he* hasn't realized it yet) and your mouth shouldn't be anywhere near his penis till it's rock hard. Pamper him by giving him a massage then a 'body tease.' Oil his body and yours and lie over him, supporting your weight on your hands. Come in close and slide up and down, gyrate your pelvis against his body letting him feel how turned on you are, and push your butt in the air (especially if there's a mirror behind you). If you've got long hair, use it; lean forward and let it caress his body. Bite his nipples, and tease him by lowering yourself over his penis so your genitals are touching, but don't let him penetrate. Give him 'Spanish': put his penis between your breasts and roll and knead them around it using your hands. Stroke, lick, and nibble your way down his body while you're telling him exactly what you're about to do to him. Get feedback: ask him what *he'd* like you to do."

3. Vary the scene and stimulate all his senses

"Don't do it in the same position every time. Guys love getting a blow job just about anywhere but variety's a turn-on. Try him standing up and you kneeling or squatting in front of him; him up against a wall; a '69er'; in the car; in the park while walking home from a restaurant. Different locations add a fresh psychological kick. It doesn't matter what you're wearing but lots of men find it exciting if you're totally naked and he's fully clothed with just his fly undone; alternatively, try you fully dressed and him totally naked. Make sure he can watch. Men are erotic visualists and are primarily aroused by what they can see, one reason why they're so into porn mags. He'll want to see your face, maybe even hold your hair back. Don't close your eyes, keep them open. I hold eye contact with the man while I'm fellating him and make 'horny eyes'—narrow them sexily and make them smolder. If you're too embarrassed to look at him, look at his penis instead."

4. Don't just concentrate on his penis

"His anus, perineum, testicles—all are erogenous zones you should pay attention to before and during fellatio. Get him to lie on his back then lick and stroke him on the perineum (the area between his anus and testicles), massaging it with slight pressure. Bend his legs back and lick from the base of his anus through to the scrotum. Cradle his testicles in your hand, lick them, take one or both in your mouth. Massage near the base of his penis, one hand holding it, the other massaging."

5. Use your hands and start masturbating him

"Always use two hands during oral: one to stimulate him elsewhere (nipples, testicles, anus), the other as a guide. It gives you more control and he can't gag you. I usually keep one hand at the bottom of the shaft of his penis, then it's up to me to control how deeply I take it into my mouth. Lots of men like to put their hands on the back of your head but tell him it's hands-*off* if he won't stop pushing you deeper than you want to go. 'Deep-throating' is a head game more than anything else. If you can do it, great! If you can't or don't want to, rest assured that it doesn't necessarily feel better; it's just what he's seen in a porn film. Most feeling is at the head of his penis not the bottom. If you're really paranoid about gagging, place the penis to one side of your mouth rather than dead center."

6. Take control of his penis but handle with care

"Some women are too rough! The best way to find out how he likes being masturbated is to get him to show you how he does it himself then imitate the technique. Don't tug or yank at his foreskin if he's uncircumcised; make sure it slides up and over the penile head. Take a firm grip, then start teasing. Let him see your nice pink tongue and play up the lick movements. Do long, lollypop licks, lick up the side, around the head, cover your teeth with your lips (and keep them that way!) and do 'lip-pinches' (a biting motion without teeth involved) up and down the side of the shaft. Use lots of saliva: the more lubricated he is, the more pleasurable it will feel. Finally, take his penis right into your mouth, swirl your tongue around the head, then withdraw and give a big 'uuummm' of satisfaction!"

7. Technique is all-important

"The basic technique is to slide your hand up and down his penis (closing it when you reach the head, opening it slightly as you slide down the length) as it's moving in and out of your mouth. With your lips covering your teeth, close your mouth around the penis and encircle it so there's a firm but comfortable pressure. You're not actually sucking, more making sure your mouth is a snug fit. Practice on your finger and imagine it's his penis. What sort of sensations seem like they'd feel good? Imagine how his penis feels when it's in your vagina and try to imitate the sensation. When you're confident, move into the 'twist-and-swirl': make a gentle twisting motion with your hand as you're sliding it up and down his penis and swirl your tongue around the rim of the head, paying particular attention to the frenulum (see 'How the penis works,' on page 4). Tense your tongue and vibrate it; swirl it around the head and the base—the more tongue movements while it's in your mouth the better! As with women, a steady rhythm is important. Start off agonizingly slow, then increase the pressure and the rhythm as he approaches orgasm."

8. Tease him mercilessly

"Take him to the brink of orgasm (you'll get better at timing this with practice!) so he experiences that intensely pleasurable preorgasm wave several times, then stop fellating him and use your mouth on his testes, the perineum, and his anus before returning. Be creative and use different strokes: long slides up and down his penis, taking it deep in your mouth; shorter strokes concentrating on the head and inserting just the tip. Once he's approaching orgasm, however, stick with the same technique and rhythm."

9. Step up the stimulation just as he's about to orgasm

"The male G-spot is about 1 to 2 inches inside the anus, and by inserting a finger, you'll make his orgasm even more intense. If he enjoys anal stimulation, he'll push his butt toward you or stick it up in the air the minute you start to explore the area. Be gentle and make sure your finger is well lubricated. If you feel uncomfortable doing this, give him a stronger orgasm by pressing the perineum area firmly with your thumb as he's ejaculating."

10. Decide beforehand what you'll do when he ejaculates

"It will be obvious when he's about to orgasm: the penis starts to throb, jerk, and spasm; some men stop thrusting and stay perfectly still, others thrust harder. Some men are oversensitive when they orgasm so keep your hands away from the head of the penis and masturbate him at the bottom. If you're going to swallow his semen, do it properly. Don't make faces; simply swallow it and say 'yuuumm.' If you don't want to, don't take any sperm in your mouth; spitting it out is rude, unattractive, and insulting. Instead, withdraw when he's in the throes of orgasm and continue stimulating him with your hand. A sexy alternative to swallowing is to let him ejaculate elsewhere on your body—over your breasts or your neck. If you rub it into your body afterward, he'll know you enjoyed fellating him as much as he enjoyed receiving it!"

! *If his sperm tastes bad, it could be something he ate. What he eats and drinks hours before making love strongly affects the way he tastes. For the best flavored sperm, feed him bland foods like pasta and potatoes; for the worst, serve a curry, washed down with beer and coffee.*

Tricks of the trade

- Drink a hot drink beforehand. The sensation of a hot mouth around his penis is sensational! Smearing honey or cream over it, then licking it off, adds a fun element.
- Play up to the power fantasy. Power—having it or being completely dominated—is a common fantasy for many men. Let him call the shots and kneel before him or *you* take control and let him know you're boss!

- Brush your tongue with a toothbrush every time you brush your teeth. A healthy, pink tongue is a turn-on.
- If he goes limp, slow it down. Ask him why. Either he's stressed or tired and can't concentrate, or you're not fellating him correctly. Applying too much pressure—holding him too tightly with your hand or sucking too hard—can make him lose his erection. Also bear in mind that men are individuals with their own preferred turn-ons and techniques. Talk, start again, and slow it down.
- To make him come quickly, insert a finger into his anus or press the perineum firmly with your thumb. The more extra stimulation you give, the quicker he'll usually orgasm.
- It's what you do before your mouth even touches his penis that counts. The more foreplay and teasing he's had, the more sensitive he'll be. Just about any sensation will feel great!

HIS TOP FIVE ORAL SEX TURN-OFFS

1. **She acts like she doesn't want to be there.** A woman who's performing fellatio only because she has to was listed as the number one passion killer.
2. **She bites.** While some men actually like their penises being "nipped," most feel faint at the mere thought! Accidentally biting or scraping his penis with your teeth is an absolute no-no. Keep them covered at all times with your lips.
3. **She's too rough.** Yanking back the foreskin on uncircumcised men, holding or sucking too hard, pumping his penis "like she's trying to draw water from a dried-up well" were all top turn-offs.
4. **She's got no idea what she's doing.** "Women who do that stupid bobbing-up-and-down head motion might as well not bother," says Olivia. Not knowing how to pleasure him orally, and not bothering to find out by reading some sex books or asking him what feels good, was a common complaint.

Ⓜ FOR HIM

Cunnilingus is the rather unexotic name for you giving her oral sex, but men who master it rarely lack lovers. Trouble is, it's *dark* down there and you're often forced to rely on touch and feel rather than eyesight. Apart from eating more carrots, there's not too much you can do about the natural lighting around her vagina. But you can persuade her to let you turn the lights on because it's essential you get this technique right. With some women, oral sex is the only way you'll get her to reach orgasm; for the rest, it's often the most intense. Again, I went to an expert to find out how best to perform cunnilingus. David is a male escort and sex worker who only services women. And guess what's the most commonly requested thing on his menu? Here, in his words, are his professional tips. Don't just read this section, *study* it. If you want to make her quiver, this is how!

> **❗** *Ten percent of men and eighteen percent of women would prefer to have an orgasm through oral sex than intercourse. More than twice as many career women would prefer to climax by tongue than women who don't work.[4]*

A ten-step guide to ohmygod-don't-ever-stop oral sex for her

1. Women are slower to become aroused and slower to reach orgasm than men, so time—not rushing her—is the biggest luxury you can give a woman

"If she's stressed, relax her first by massaging or stroking her body until she starts to become aroused. Follow this with lots of kissing on the neck, and stroke and lick her breasts and nipples before moving on to her genitals. Leave her underwear on and stroke her through the fabric until she becomes wet; only then remove it."

2. *Start by running your hands up and down the outside, then the inside of her thighs and at this point, ask her how she likes oral sex: slow, fast, gentle, or hard*
"While kissing and licking down her body, pull the outer vaginal lips over the inner in a gentle, circular motion to warm the entire area."

3. *Position counts*
"If she's shy, it's best if she lies back while you're kneeling at the foot of the bed between her legs. Lots of women love being licked while they're standing and you're kneeling (it appeals to their slave fantasies, plus they can control the pressure and rhythm by holding your head) or being licked from behind. Another favorite, which gives her ultimate control: lie back on the bed while she kneels above you and lowers her genitals down to your mouth. She may put her hands flat against the wall for balance. Some women like to feel completely exposed with their legs wide open, others prefer their legs quite closely wrapped around your head. It all depends on how sensitive her clitoris is."

> "I stayed with a complete loser of a guy for six months simply because he gave the best oral sex I'd had in my life. I was addicted to it. I couldn't give him up because—and sadly, this is true so far—I knew I'd never find a tongue like that again."
>
> Mary, 24, secretary

4. *It's really important to keep her moist, so use lots of saliva to lick the entire area before concentrating on the clitoris*
"Don't tense or point your tongue; it's better to use the whole surface of the flat of your tongue rather than just the tip. That's the one thing that most men do wrong. Start with indirect stimulation, gently wiggling your tongue around and over the clitoris: it's toward the top of the vagina and feels like a tiny marble."

5. Move into longer, wet, gentle strokes with your tongue, keeping up a slow but steady rhythm

"Rhythm is really important; chopping and changing techniques and rhythm all the time doesn't work with women. Read her body language or ask her what stroke feels best, then keep on doing it. If she pulls away, you're being too rough; if she presses her vagina closer or pulls your head closer, step up the pressure slightly."

6. It's generally best to be too gentle than too rough

"Again ask her what feels best. Try shaking your head from side to side, making circles around the edge of the clitoris as well as up-and-down strokes."

"It's weird but I don't really like guys giving me head. I don't know why, I just feel uncomfortable. I'm not prudish about anything else. I've only ever liked it with one guy—and he was so good, he had a reputation for giving great oral sex. Somehow he hit all the right spots. With everyone else though, I can take it or leave it. Leave it really."

Nikki, 17, student

7. Make sure she knows how much you are enjoying yourself by making noise

"If she thinks you're enjoying it as much as she is, she relaxes and knows she can take her time. Again, you have to be prepared to settle in and keep going until she says to stop. The tongue movements are gentle and if a guy can't keep them up for at least ten to fifteen minutes, his tongue's too tense or he's doing it too fast."

8. When she's really aroused, insert a finger inside her vagina

"A lot of women like to be inserted with a finger or dildo just before they come but others find it distracting. If she's good at communicating, she'll pull your hand away if she doesn't like it; if she does, she'll usually move her hips against your hand to achieve deeper penetration. Some women like manually stimulating their own clitorises while you're performing oral; others put their fingers down to feel your tongue working on them. If she does either, lick her fingers as well."

9. When you're not manually masturbating her as well as licking, use your other hand to knead her breasts and nipples or to stroke the perineum, the area between her anus and vagina

"Some women like a lubricated finger inserted into their anus as they orgasm; try inserting the tip gently and see if she pulls away before going any deeper."

10. Her body will tense when she's closer to orgasm

"At this point, increase the pressure slightly or move a little faster. The most important thing, though, is to maintain the rhythm as best you can even if she starts moving around. As she's actually orgasming, switch back to slow, gentle strokes but make sure you cover the whole clitoral area by using the whole surface of your tongue. Most women's clitorises are unbearably sensitive immediately after an orgasm, so don't be surprised if she puts a hand down to cover it or pushes your head away."

THE FIVE THINGS MOST MEN DO WRONG

1. **You only do it if we ask and obviously find it distasteful.** A man who turns his nose up and says "it smells," even when she's fresh out of the shower, is being ridiculous. Assuming she doesn't have any infections, the natural scent of a vagina is musky and sensual. Don't blame her for swapping lovers if you can't be convinced.

2. **You're too rough.** Some women like a very firm tongue but gentle suits most of us. The clitoris is sensitive so while over-enthusiastic licking will have her squirming, it's with pain not pleasure.

3. **You don't do it for long enough.** You might be able to orgasm at the mere sight of her mouth wrapped around your penis, but she takes longer to climax. Tell her she can take as long as she wants because you *love* doing it to her, and she's yours for life.

4. **You change techniques too often.** Women need regular, consistent rhythm for an extended period in order to

orgasm. While she might be impressed with your extensive repertoire of mouth movements, stick with one or two each session. The clitoris is a funny beast—it can be terribly turned-on by one sensation but take ages to get used to another if you change.

5. **You stop at the crucial moment.** You might like stimulation to stop while you're orgasming, but we prefer it to continue, though often softer, right through to the last spasm. If you stop just as we're hovering on the brink, we often don't make it over the fence.

THE UPS AND DOWNS OF 69

Sixty-nine got its name because the numbers are head-to-toe, as you are. It simply means both of you giving each other oral sex simultaneously. The usual position is the female on top of him, her rear pointed toward his face, genitals lowered so he can lick them. Meanwhile, her mouth is positioned above his penis.

It's the idea of 69—giving pleasure to each other at the same time—which is the turn-on for most people. In reality, it's all too easy to get lazy on your end. If your partner is sending you through the roof, you'll forget about them and try to get away with a few lackluster licks; same goes for them if you're working your magic. On the upside, 69 is great for variety and works well when you're *so-o-o-o* turned-on,

> **❗** *Number of women who enjoy receiving oral sex: 73 percent. Number of women who like giving it to him: 24 percent.*[5]

just about anything will feel good. If you like the position but have trouble keeping your mind on the job, take turns. He can give her cunnilingus in that position while she uses her hand on him. She can fellate him while he uses his hand to stimulate her.

3

Intercourse

Some new angles on the old in-out, in-out

• •

It's God's fault that couples have so many problems with intercourse. If he really wanted women to enjoy it, he would have put the clitoris *inside* the vagina. I mean, what was he thinking? The only organ in the body designed exclusively for sexual pleasure and it's stuck right up there in penile no-man's land. (Did Adam have an L-shaped one, or has God got a wicked sense of humor?) This simple design fault has caused no end of problems. Because many women need clitoral stimulation along with thrusting, it's the reason why most don't orgasm during intercourse. (If you're male and absorb this point, your Filofax will never be empty again.)

> ❗ **The number of synonyms for sexual intercourse in Roget's Thesaurus: 47**

It's also responsible for the main male beef about screwing. While women mutter about a distinct lack of intercourse orgasms, men are complaining about our lack of enthusiasm. They say females very often consider intercourse to be the part where they get to relax while he does all the work. Like, why should they bother when *they're* not going to hit the jackpot?

Happily, both problems are solved with one, simple solution. Remember that dopey saying your grandmother used to spout? She was right. Busy hands *are* happy hands—and so are the genitals they're busy with.

Clitorises aside, there's a lot more to penetration than you think, and a myriad of ways to vary that one in-out movement. Intercourse is often thought of as the least creative sex act of all. I beg to differ. Hopefully, you will too when you've read through this chapter.

THE FIVE FAVORITE POSITIONS

There are more than 600 documented positions for intercourse (the *Kama Sutra* describes 529 of them). You'd be asleep within minutes if I tried to list each one and since most are variants on the five basic positions, I'll focus on these and let you use your imagination to discover the other 595![1]

Despite the endless variety possible, the average couple alternates between two or three positions, most settling on missionary, woman-on-top, and rear-entry. There's no such thing as the "best" position—it all depends on your shapes and height, your individual preferences, and mood at the time. Some positions work well if he comes too soon, side-by-side suits lazy, Sunday-morning sex, rear-entry a fast and furious "quickie."

For most men, orgasm is guaranteed in just about any (if not all) intercourse positions. For women (sigh!), as I said, it's a different story. Clitoral stimulation is pretty much an essential for most of us to come during intercourse, so I've not only addressed this section to women but included "Orgasm potential for her" under each position. Having said that, don't be too concerned if your partner's favorite position is different from yours or vice versa; take turns or do both in the same session.

Whatever you do though, do it with passion. Both of you will get a lot more out of all that humping and grinding if you thrust your hips to meet each other's, grab buttocks and pull them close to you, run your hands up and down backs, arms, and backs of thighs, and lick or bite the closest thing to your mouths. Go for it. Make so much noise, your neighbors consider double-glazing their windows.

Missionary

Rumor has it that early missionaries, sent to "civilize" the colonies, considered this the only respectable way to make love. Hence the name "missionary" position and its rather staid image.

> "I don't come during intercourse but I love it all the same. It makes me feel close to my boyfriend. Our bodies fit together, it's all wet and hard, and I feel all filled up. The initial thrust is always the best, especially if we've teased each other to the point where neither of us can wait any longer."
>
> Naomi, 25, secretary

It was probably the first position in which you had intercourse. I suspect it'll be the last (bodies aren't too agile at ninety) and, even if we hate to admit it, it's how most couples have intercourse most of the time. For good reason. The basic position—the woman lying on her back, legs apart with the man between them—requires zero imagination, little effort on her part, and is reasonably comfortable for both. It's the position you use when you're both fairly interested in sex but not spinning cartwheels over it. Ironically, it's also the first position to spring to mind when you're so eager for him to be inside you, you don't care how the hell he does it, so long as he does it *now*. Missionary also appeals to the come-on-you've-got-to-admit-I've-put-on-weight girl (that is, 99 percent of women) because of the flat-tummy thing. We lie on our backs, the flab spreads out, and we look extra thin. Bonus!

Why it feels good for her
You're face-to-face and can talk and kiss, so it can be quite romantic. But you also have less control over what's happening and basically can't move very far. Bend your knees for deeper penetration. Stimulate the clitoris more effectively by keeping your legs together (squeezing your thighs) and have his legs open, lying over the *outside* of yours.

Why it feels good for him
He basically runs the show, being in complete control of the depth of penetration, the angle, and the pace. For this reason, it's not a bad choice if he's a premature ejaculator because he can stop if he

gets too carried away. If the opposite's the problem (he's had one drink too many and is having trouble orgasming), reach down and hold back the skin on his penis, grasping at the root of the shaft with your finger and thumb, while he's moving in and out of you. There is one drawback for both of you: neither of you can see any of the real action.

Orgasm potential for her
It's not great for manual stimulation of your clitoris but it can make him last longer in intercourse if that's a problem.

How to make it even better
Put one or two hard pillows under your rear end; pull your knees up to your chest or wrap them around his back for deeper penetration; try lifting your legs high and resting one or both feet on his shoulders; lie sideways and move most of your body off the bed, head resting on a cushion on the floor (yes, the blood will rush to your head but that's the idea—some women swear this makes female orgasms scream-material).

One way to make it instantly more exciting for both of you is to put a ban on using the missionary. If you do "slip up" (and you will—anything banned becomes immediately desirable), it'll seem naughty, forbidden, and anything but boring.

How to vary it
Get him to stimulate your G-spot. Rather than thrusting in and out, you half sit up, lift your rear end, then slowly lean backward, repeating until one (or both) of you climax; let him lift your legs up and hold them; roll over completely and end up with you on top!

Comfort rating for him
His arms can get tired supporting his own weight.

Comfort rating for her
Unless he rests his weight on his elbows or hands and knees, even breathing can be difficult. If he's the size of a sumo wrestler and you're a waif, forget it.

> ❗ *Number of positions in which most couples have intercourse: 2 to 5. The favorites: missionary and woman-on-top. Number of lovers who use more than 20 positions regularly: 5 percent.*[2]

Woman-on-top

Any woman worth her stuff, in or out of bed, has to revel in this one, even if it's just for the connotations of the name. You on top, you in control—it's deliciously *liberated*, not to mention a hell of a turn-on for both of you. For best control and balance, most women sit on top of their partner, who's lying on his back, then lower themselves onto his penis, legs bent at the knees and folded backward. You can also try squatting. In the basic position, you're usually facing him. Don't try woman-on-top unless he's very hard—it's incredibly easy to bend a semierect penis and cause injury.

Why it feels good for her
It's the opposite to the missionary: instead of him calling the shots, you have complete control over the depth of penetration, angle, and speed. You're in the power position and can show off all you like. Exhibitionists don't do it any other way but even if you're not, it's still fantastic. (If you don't feel confident about showing off your body, simply lean forward.) If deep penetration sometimes hurts—if your cervix is sensitive for instance—this is one position you can relax in, without fear of pain. He can only go as deep as you let him.

Why it feels good for him
He gets off on watching your body and what's happening—this position lays it all right in front of him. He can see your body clearly and watch the expressions on your face as you approach orgasm. *You* might think breasts look ridiculous wobbling up and

down; *he* thinks they look sexy. Not only that, he gets the double bonus of watching his penis disappear into your vagina while *you* do all the work. The pressure's off. You're looking after your own pleasure (at least in terms of penetration), and he doesn't have to worry about timing or depth.

Orgasm potential for her
Both his hands are free to caress your breasts and stimulate the clitoris (lean forward and lift up a little for easier access). If you're a fan of the G-spot, this position is likely to hit it (lean backward). It's also pretty easy for you to touch your own clitoris and bring yourself to orgasm while he's inside you.

> "I hate getting on top. My legs cramp up, I feel stupid, and it hurts my back. I also hate doggie-style. It makes me feel cheap and undignified."
>
> Louise, 32, real estate agent

How to make it even better
Try moving in small circles as you're lifting yourself up and down; tease him a little (or a lot) by rubbing his erect penis over your vaginal lips, letting him enter just a fraction then denying him full penetration by lifting tantalizingly higher; turn him on by playing with your own breasts or your clitoris.

How to vary it
Face his toes instead of his head (resist the urge to do a 180-degree turn while impaled unless you warn him first); get him to hold your waist to help you move up and down; lean forward or backward to experience the sensation of stimulation on different parts of your vaginal walls; lie (instead of sitting or crouching) on top of him with your legs outside or inside his; try him sitting in a chair with you on his lap; try him sitting up with legs straight out in front of him, you lower yourself onto his penis and sit with your knees bent and feet flat on the floor.

Comfort rating for him
Ten out of 10—what's *not* to like? Women are usually lighter than men, so he's unlikely to complain about your being too heavy.

Comfort rating for her
It can be tiring if you're using your legs to move up and down but think of it this way: you can skip the squat machine at the gym the next day.

Rear-entry (or "doggie-style")

This position allows *deep* penetration and ignites the animal instinct in anyone with a libido because it's so primitive. It's a firm favorite with any couple who really get into sex, and is avoided by couples who think walking hand-in-hand along a beach is racy. A warning for women with men who come too soon: don't even let him think about this one unless you're both happy with a quickie. With the combination of deep penetration, the unleashing of the "beast" in him because he's "taking you," fantasies soaring right off the pleasure scale because he can't see your face and could be having sex with anyone . . . He'll last, *ooohh*, two seconds if you're lucky.

❗ In our moms' day, men use to initiate sex pretty much all of the time. Now only 12.2 percent of women say they never make the first move.[3]

Why it feels good for her
Uninhibited women love rear-entry—anyone with a slave fantasy can let their imagination run wild (rear-entry is him at his most dominant and you at your most submissive and vulnerable). Because you can't see him, he could be anyone (the guy on your favorite soap opera, the wonderfully *built* workman you saw on the street, your boyfriend's best friend). Your breasts are often hanging down so the blood flows to the nipples and makes them extra sensitive.

Why it feels good for him
It allows him to penetrate as deeply as he possibly can and he's visually stimulated (turned on by what he can see more than what he can feel). The sight of his penis pumping in and out of your vagina is, well . . . his idea of heaven, really. Your rear end presses against his testicles for extra stimulation and, speaking of rear ends, most men *love* being able to see yours. (No, he's not looking at how "fat" it is.)

Orgasm potential for her
Orgasms often feel more intense because he's hitting all your sensitive parts (the front wall of your vagina). His hands are totally free to stimulate your breasts or your clitoris. This is by far the best position to stimulate the G-spot, since the penis hits the front vaginal wall directly.

How to make it even better
Give in totally and let him penetrate you from behind while you're on all fours.

How to vary it
Rather than kneel: you lie facedown, flat on the bed, legs spread, he lies on top of you and penetrates from behind (great for indirectly stimulating the clitoris). Try him standing behind you, you stand then lean forward until your hands touch the floor. Attempt the "wheelbarrow": he stands behind you, then lifts and holds your straight legs like a wheelbarrow while you've got your weight supported on your elbows on the bed.

Comfort rating for him
He's a prime target for carpet burn on the knees if you're doing it on the living room floor but does he care? Nah!

Comfort rating for her
Rear-entry positions allow deep penetration—too deep sometimes, especially if he gets completely carried away and starts thrusting like he's trying to find oil. If it feels too deep, lift your rear end. Better still, simply ask him to hold back and go shallower.

Face-to-face positions while sitting or kneeling
Close and intimate, many people find these positions a relaxing variation on the norm. Positions where you're sitting on the end of the bed, he's kneeling in front of you on the floor; you sitting in his lap while he also sits up—these are all examples of what the sexperts call "face-to-face." They're good for adding variety and are relatively easy to move into from missionary or woman-on-top since most are derivatives of these anyway.

Why it feels good for her

They're versatile, there's good eye contact, and he's in the ideal position to hold his penis and use it to manually masturbate your clitoris and vaginal lips.

Why it feels good for him

You can put your hands behind him and pull him to you by grabbing his buttocks. He'll like the visual stimulation of watching your genitals do their stuff.

Orgasm potential for her

In most positions, he can see and touch the clitoris easily, making it easy for him to masturbate you to orgasm.

How to make it even better

Try rocking as you're thrusting, using your legs as leverage to maintain a steady rhythm.

How to vary it

Use it to spice up your favorites. Change into a face-to-face sitting position from woman-on-top or missionary, even if it's just for a few moments.

Humans are one of the few species to have sex in private and the only ones who have sex just for fun. Most other animals are sensibly stingy about copulating: it takes time (better spent gathering food) and it's risky (couples locked in an embrace risk being surprised or killed by predators).[4]

Comfort rating for him

Your heights and sizes can make some positions difficult, even impossible. Don't choose a position that he feels twisted in if he's got back problems or if you're a bigger person than he is.

Comfort rating for her

Some women complain of leg cramps but if you share the work—sometimes he thrusts, sometimes you do—it shouldn't be a problem.

Side-by-side

It's comfortable, cuddly, and sensual—perfect for those languid days when you're nicely turned-on but not frothing at the mouth to get it. The favorite is the Spoon (nicknamed because the shape the two of you make is like a pair of spoons nestled together). You lie on your side, he enters you from behind, arms wrapped around you. Draw your knees up to allow him to penetrate, then keep your rear end stuck out toward him and the top knee forward.

Why it feels good for her
There's lots of body contact, and both his hands are free to play with your breasts, neck, clitoris. It's very cuddly and effortless if you're tired or not feeling well.

Why it feels good for him
It's great for premature ejaculators because it's less "full-on" but also comfortable enough for him to settle in and take his time orgasming. There's maximum body contact and it's easy for her to reach behind and caress your buttocks, testicles, or perineum.

Orgasm potential for her
Hit the G-spot by getting him to lean back and away from you diagonally. It's easy for him to reach around and use his fingers to stimulate your clitoris.

How to make it even better
Turn it into an X: your heads are at opposite ends of the bed and you're making an X with your legs, he's inside you, each of you has one leg underneath each other's, one above. Clasp hands for control; this is great for slowing him down if he ejaculates too quickly.

How to vary it
Grind your rear end against his penis; bending from the waist and moving your upper torso downward. Reach around to fondle his penis while it's moving in and out of you.

Comfort rating for him
For relaxed, unhurried lovemaking, it's a winner all round.

Comfort rating for her

Ditto. It's also more comfortable than him-on-top positions if your partner is heavy. A bonus for both of you—you can fall asleep in exactly the same position you made love in.

LOSING IT: A GUIDE FOR THE FIRST TIME YOU HAVE SEX

There's a school of thought that says how and who you lose your virginity to will not only affect your sex life forever but your future relationships with the opposite sex. Heavy stuff, but quite logical when you think about it and certainly well worth bearing in mind if you are contemplating taking the plunge.

If losing your virginity is a positive experience, you're more likely to view sex as something that's healthy and enjoyable and lovers as nice people who can be trusted. The reverse happens if it's a nightmare. That clumsy, five-minute fumble can have extraordinary repercussions so *no one* should take losing their virginity lightly.

Even if it's no longer something we save for our wedding night, it's still a huge changing point in our lives. It's the initiation ceremony that we think will transform us from awkward schoolgirl to alluring woman, from gangly youth to macho man. Because of the double standard—women who lose it early are sluts, men who lose it early are studs—most women pick their first partners carefully (if not sensibly). Most guys can't *wait* to "pop their cherry" and do so with the first girl who'll say yes. Regardless, there are things both sexes can do to make the first experience more enjoyable and much less traumatic.

Ⓜ Ⓕ FOR BOTH OF YOU

Accept that practice makes perfect and your first time probably won't be all that wonderful. Most people are eager to experience what, on TV and the big screen at least, looks like damn good fun, but are horribly disappointed the first time round. It helps if you're sexually educated—have read a few good sex books, experimented with foreplay, and have a vague idea of what's going to happen—but even then you should prepare yourself for surprises. When I first had sex, I knew all about clitorises and orgasms, but boy did I get a shock when the guy actually started *moving*. Somehow, I'd imagined that once in, you both just . . . I don't know, *lay there*, clamped together!

F FOR HER

- **Don't do it until you're absolutely, 100 percent convinced you want to.** The guy who says "Unless you have sex with me, I'm not going out with you anymore" should be ditched immediately. The boyfriend who's eager but lets *you* decide when is a sensible choice.

- **Tell him you're a virgin.** It doesn't matter how old you are, it's always best to confess. The first time round, you need lots of time to get aroused and you need him to enter you gently. A good lover will do this automatically the first time you make love, but lots of guys don't fit into this category.

"I always thought it wouldn't bother me if he was a virgin but a guy asked me out recently who I was hot for. He was twenty-four, and we got along really well but when he told me he was a virgin, I just couldn't look at him the same way. I kept wondering what was wrong with him. Was he gay? He said he'd been too busy to worry about women—but seriously, for the last eight years? Come on! In the end, I just couldn't be bothered."

Deborah, 22, receptionist

- **Be prepared.** If you're both around fifteen or sixteen, you're extremely fertile. Don't kid yourself: you can get pregnant doing it "just once" if you don't use contraception. If both of you are virgins, you don't need to use a condom for sexually transmitted infection (STI) prevention, but they're often the easiest, and most accessible, method of contraception if you're not on the Pill. If you want to go on the Pill, see a doctor or go to a family planning clinic and ask for a prescription. Remember with most Pills you have to wait for a while before they start to work. (See Chapter 6 to help you decide which contraception is best for both of you.)

- **Choose the time and place as carefully as your partner.** Some women do lose their virginity while carried away in

> "I planned my first time down to the last detail. I was going out with the cutest guy in school and we had lots of foreplay. Sure, it wasn't as great as I thought it would be, but we did it again the next night and I started to see what all the fuss was about."
>
> Amelia, 30, teacher

the heat of the moment, but most plan the event. If it's at all possible, do plan it. The first time is real butterflies-in-the-stomach material. You'll not only be experiencing new physical sensations, you'll be struggling with a few psychological issues as well. Will he still like me afterward? What do I do if my parents find out? Think through all these questions beforehand and if you still want to go through with it, try to find a time and place where you can both take your time without getting interrupted. In a perfect world, you should snuggle up in each other's arms afterward and spend the night together, but this isn't always possible.

- **Don't be surprised if you're not as "turned-on" as you have been in the past.** Chances are the two of you have "heavy petted" before (he's had his fingers inside you, fondled your breasts, maybe even performed oral sex). But while previously you were nearly sliding off the couch with excitement, now nothing much is happening at all. Relax—it's normal. You're just a little tense and apprehensive. Take your time and let him know he may need to spend longer on foreplay than usual. If you find you're still not lubricating (or "getting wet"), apply some personal lubricant (you can buy things like K-Y at a pharmacy or supermarket). Don't even attempt intercourse unless you are wet—it will hurt.
- **Gently does it.** It's easiest to stick to the missionary position the first time round. That simply means he'll lie on top of you. It's a good idea if you use your hand to guide his penis into your vagina. This gives you control over when he penetrates, so it's less of a shock. You may have a hymen—a protective membrane over the opening to your vagina—but you probably won't. Things like using tampons, gym class, and riding horses usually break the hymen way before you're even *thinking* about intercourse. If it hasn't broken, him pressing his

penis gently against it will break it and allow you to have sex. When he first penetrates you, try "bearing down" slightly with your vaginal muscles (push them "out," using your tummy muscles). He should thrust very slowly and gently at first and stay shallow. He can move deeper as you both relax but it's best if he doesn't really "go for it" the first time.

- **Don't expect to have an orgasm.** He probably will, usually very quickly; you probably won't. This doesn't mean you're not capable of one, just that women usually have to "learn" how to orgasm; with men it's much more automatic. You might like to read Chapter 1 on masturbation, before or after you've had intercourse, and teach yourself to orgasm that way.

- **If he's a virgin and you're not, be a little tactful.** He'll already be feeling nervous and worried that you'll think he's hopeless (even if he is, tell him he was great). Expect him to orgasm in about one second flat and you won't be disappointed. Guide and help him along but not in an "I know what to do, you don't" way. If he wants to take control, let him. Most of all, keep in mind that even if he's an abysmal lover at first, as long as he's willing to learn, time (and you) can turn that around pretty quickly.

Ⓜ FOR HIM

- **Admit that you're a virgin even if you're embarrassed.** Be realistic: it's unlikely you're going to be the best lover she's ever had if you've never even had intercourse before.

- **Use a condom.** If you don't know her well, they're protection against sexually transmitted infections (STIs). If she's a long-time girlfriend, you're both virgins, and she's on the Pill, fine, don't use one. Just make sure she hasn't got some starry-eyed idea that it would be romantic if she got pregnant. If you have any doubts at all that she's not taking the Pill even though she says she is, use a condom.

- **Decide how "special" you want it to be.** If you really don't care who it's with, you just want to do it, then there's no

❗ *World distance record for ejaculated semen: 8.5 feet.[5]*

problem—just make sure you've always got condoms and will be able to cope emotionally if it's a horrible experience. Doing it with a girlfriend you love (and who loves you) is obviously less frightening and a lot more fulfilling, but not always possible. Don't be pushed by your friends into having sex before you're ready. For starters, you don't *know* they've already done it (often the biggest boasters haven't) and there's no magic age that you must do it by.

- **Don't freak out if it's all over quickly.** You'll feel more comfortable and confident about intercourse if you've had some experience with foreplay *before* you go barging in there, so to speak. But while it's important for female virgins to have lots of foreplay on D-Day, for you it's probably a case of the less you have, the better. Don't panic if you ejaculate before your penis even enters her, or if you thrust only once or twice then orgasm. You're as turned-on as hell at the mere *thought* of finally being able to do it and this is completely normal. If she's willing, wait for a little while then try it again—you'll last longer the second time round, even longer the third, etc.

> "I lost my virginity to a girl I loved deeply. But after we'd done it, I wanted to get out there and do it with other girls, try out what I'd learned. I was a complete bastard and did just that. I still feel ashamed about it now and that was ten years ago."
>
> Trevor, 24, shop assistant

- **If she's a virgin and you're not, recognize that it's an emotional experience for her.** While you can't wait to "get rid of" yours, she's probably thought carefully before "giving" you hers. It really is a gift she's bestowing on you and you should be incredibly complimented. Return that respect by taking it slow and easy and don't do it unless you're prepared to stick around for at least a little while afterward. If you only want sex, not a relationship, have it with someone who isn't a virgin.

PUSHING ALL THE RIGHT BUTTONS

Women can only orgasm from clitoral stimulation. Casually slip *that* statement into any conversation about sex and you're virtually guaranteed a brawl. If you think there's controversy over the G-spot, the debate over whether women can have vaginal as well as clitoral orgasms burns twice as fiercely. It didn't even occur to our parents that intercourse might not be the be-all-and-end-all when it comes to coming. But when Masters and Johnson, the highly influential sex researchers, told us *categorically* that the origin of *all* female orgasms was in the clitoris, it divided men and women—and women and women.

> "When we're doing it missionary style, I get him to move really slow and close my legs around his penis. I squeeze my vaginal muscles tight then get him to use one hand to rub my clitoris. If he's penetrating me hard and stimulating my clitoris at the same time, I climax really deeply and it seems to go on for ages."
>
> Mandy, 18, fashion student

For a start, most men are loath to give up on the myth of the almighty penis as the ultimate satisfier. A survey by sex researcher Shere Hite showed that the overwhelming majority of men would like their partners to reach orgasm from their penises alone, without additional clitoral stimulation.[6] Then there's a group of people that won't, and feel they can't, admit that clitoral stimulation is the only way they climax. These are the women who've "faked it" during intercourse for sometimes years. It's a little hard to turn around to a long-term partner and say, "Yes darling, it's true. And I've lied to you approximately 500 times over the last five years." The rest of us divide again, this time into women who've *only* had orgasms via the clitoris and will happily admit it, and those who swear on their mother's life that they've also had them vaginally.

While the hard facts of sexual research lean toward the "clitoris-only" side, there are so many personal accounts from women who say they have vaginal orgasms that sexperts are now pretty convinced that there's a kind of orgasm that originates in the vagina. Most probably, it's linked with the G-spot or the A-spot (see Chapter 4). Women who have vaginal orgasms say they're not as intense as the clitoral kind but feel "deeper," more prolonged, and appear to be accompanied by contractions of the uterus and the vagina, as clitoral orgasms are.

Regardless of what theory you believe, there's little doubt that even if you *can* have vaginal orgasms, stimulation of the clitoris during intercourse makes them even more intense. Who knows? Try the following tips and maybe you'll join the select (and small) group of lucky women who claim there's such a thing as an out-of-this-world, OHMYGOD orgasm where both vaginal and clitoral orgasms happen simultaneously!

- **Talk about it first.** Be honest with your lover. If you can only come during intercourse if he's stroking your clitoris as well, tell him. Explain that it's not his fault but that lots of women are built that way and it's a matter of biology, nothing to do with his sexual technique.

> "I can't relate to those guys who get all uptight if a girl wants you to masturbate her during intercourse. My first serious girlfriend said to me, 'You're not going to like this but it's the truth: most women fake orgasm during intercourse and the only way I'll come is if you play with my clitoris at the same time.' I assumed all women were like her and have always done it since. A lot of women have said to me, 'You know, you're the first guy that's ever done that without me having to ask.' "
>
> Peter, 36, small business owner

- **Make sure he knows where your clitoris is.** Show him and let him take a good look in daylight. Then while you're having intercourse, guide him with your hand to where it is. Different positions can make him lose his bearings.

- **Choose a position that allows easy access.** If you skim through the intercourse positions, you'll find which are best for clitoral access under the "Orgasm potential for her" section. It takes more than a few seconds of stroking, so make sure his hand's not twisted and cramped. He should be comfortable while he's doing it so it doesn't detract from *his* enjoyment. Occasionally, climax before or after intercourse instead through oral sex or masturbation.

- **Share the workload.** In other words, stimulate your clitoris yourself sometimes so he doesn't have to. Or put your hand over his while he's stroking it. You can guide his strokes better and it seems more of a together, two-way thing.

- **Tell him to be more gentle than usual.** Often the act of thrusting makes it hard for him to keep his hand movements soft.

> ❶ *Number of women who've faked an orgasm: 56 percent. Number of women who enjoy intercourse: 94.7 percent. Number of women who cannot orgasm just through penetration: over 93 percent.[7]*

ROCK'N'ROLL YOUR WAY TO ORGASM: A RADICAL NEW WAY TO HAVE INTERCOURSE

The Coital Alignment Technique (CAT) is the brainchild of American psychotherapist Edward Eichel and it's an entirely new approach to intercourse. Even the most jaded sex therapist sat up and took notice when Eichel published his findings back in the early 1990s because they were so astounding. Not only did CAT increase the chance of intercourse orgasms for women, he wrote, it upped the odds of experiencing *simultaneous* orgasms. (Despite common perception, the chances of both of you screaming "Yes! Yes!" at exactly the same time during intercourse are rare—that is unless one of you is faking.)

Eichel tested his theory on 43 men and women. Before using his technique, 23 percent of the females said they orgasmed during intercourse; this jumped to 77 percent after using CAT. Not one woman had had a simultaneous orgasm with her partner; more than one-third did after using the technique.[8]

The theory behind it is quite simple. Eichel is of the school that believes clitoral stimulation is necessary for women to orgasm. He decided the in-out motion of thrusting was pathetically hopeless at achieving this and invented an alternative "rocking and rolling" motion. CAT puts rhythmic pressure on the clitoris and keeps it there. Trouble is, it's not an easy technique for couples to master. You have to think very much "outside the box" to stop doing something that's become second nature after years, so while some devotees now don't have intercourse any other way, most go back to the old in-out-in-out simply because it's easier. Want to give it a try? Here's how to do it . . .

The position

He gets on top of you, lining up his pelvis over yours. His penis is inside you but he's riding "high" so the shaft of it is outside the vagina and pressing against your mons pubis (the fleshy mound covered with pubic hair). He rests his full weight on you and doesn't prop himself up on his elbows. His weight makes him slide forward, toward your shoulders and head. Make sure he doesn't slide back; his pelvis shouldn't slip below yours. Wrap your legs around his thighs and rest your ankles on his calves.

The movement

You're using your pelvis, not your legs and arms, to move. This is the moment you regret not enrolling in those Arthur Murray dance classes because coordination is everything. The aim is to establish an identical rhythm—both of you moving in exactly the same way at exactly the same speed.

The woman leads in the *upward* stroke: push up and forward to force his pelvis backward. He allows his pelvis to move back but continues to press against yours. The penis disappears into the vagina during the upward stroke. For the *downward* stroke, reverse the process. He forces your pelvis backward and downward. You press against him as he's doing it, pressing your clitoris against the base of his penis. During the downward stroke, his penis rocks forward and presses against the mons pubis, sliding into a shallower position inside the vagina. You're using pressure and counterpressure, not thrusting in and out.

To orgasm

Instead of speeding up, as most couples do during thrusting, the idea here is to maintain a steady, even pace. Don't speed up, don't slow down. If you've got it right, orgasm will happen naturally—for both of you.

CAN I STOP NOW? A WORD ON THRUSTING

Position isn't everything, and if you haven't gathered *that* by now, you haven't been paying attention. But quite apart from things like clitoral stimulation, you can ruin the best-laid plans for the world's greatest sex simply by thrusting incorrectly.

Thrusting—the act of his penis penetrating the vagina and moving backward and forward—seems simple enough. Just a case of put it in there, (almost) take it out again, and repeat until white stuff comes out, right? Not quite. There are some misconceptions (aren't there always with sex?) that both of you should be aware of. Since he's often the one in control of thrusting, I've directed most of my comments to the male. But that doesn't let *you* off the hook. If there's one thing you can do to make thrusting more pleasurable for him, it's to thrust back, pushing your pelvis up to meet his. Don't just lie there, do something! If you're on top, some of the comments below apply to you too, so read on . . .

- **We don't need a marathon session every single time.** Some men pride themselves on being able to have intercourse for hours on end. If by this you mean prolonging intercourse by switching positions, stopping for oral sex and mutual masturbation (maybe even a bowl of cornflakes to keep the energy level up), congratulations. But if you're boasting about thrusting, in the same position, for hours on end, well . . . it gets a bit monotonous, really. Most women I know find "will-he-ever-finish" men boring. Besides, being pumped for too long can hurt. We stop enjoying it, lubrication slows down, and our vagina gets dry. Despite this, most men I know worry themselves sick that they don't go on for long enough. Granted, it is nice if the act takes more than three minutes, but don't get *too* hung up on the time thing. Ask your partner how long she'd like you to last—you might be surprised by her answer.

- **Keep your thrusting consistent and rhythmic.** There's nothing worse than that constant stop-start technique some men use. Often it's because you're worried about coming too soon, but sometimes you think it's a turn-on for us. By all means tease—it can be exciting if you deny us the long, hard

"A girl that says, 'Harder, harder,' gets me every time. There's nothing better than letting go at the end and just going for it."

Doug, 19, laborer

thrust we're dying for—but don't do it too often or too regularly. Then it's just frustrating. Most of the time, aim for continual, regular thrusting and don't go too fast; men who thrust as fast as a jackhammer never make it onto the good-lover list.

- **Ask her how deep she wants you.** Sometimes women want their partners to thrust *very* hard and *very* deep. Other times shallow, gentle thrusts feel better. It depends not only on the position, but our mood and for some women, what stage they're at in their menstrual cycle. Here's a no-fail, magical way to find out what she's in the mood for today: ask her. You may find your girlfriend never wants deep penetration because it hurts. If even the mildest thrust sends her shooting through the roof, she needs to see her gynecologist. Otherwise, it's probably because her cervix is in a position where it's getting bumped. Try aiming to the side instead of dead center.

BOTTOMS UP! A GUIDE TO ANAL STIMULATION

Our rear ends are "forbidden" zones, so the naughty element (if-I-can't-do-it-I-must) makes anal stimulation automatically exciting for many people. Quite apart from the psychological kick, the anus and rectum in both sexes are packed with nerve endings. For some, it's their most highly charged erogenous zone.

But for every couple who adores adding anal stimulation to their lovemaking, particularly during intercourse, there's another that turns pale at the mere idea of someone touching them in their most "private" spot. For that reason, I wouldn't advise anyone to pounce on their partner, airily promising the best sensation they've ever had, without telling them exactly where they plan to stick their finger first. If your partner blanches at the prospect, that's their choice, and it's not up to you to change their mind. However you *can* gently point out that if they're worried about it being messy, they needn't be. The lower rectum is normally empty and as long as fingers are clean and well lubricated with nails trimmed, they're not going to cause any damage. (Inserting *objects* into the rectum is another story. We don't want you the laughingstock of the hospital emergency room, do we?) Washing your hands thoroughly afterward, *before* touching her vagina or his penis, protects against any transference of bacteria.

The feelings produced by anal stimulation are quite different from what you're used to, and it's great for heightening sensations you're already experiencing. Combine it with intercourse and your orgasms will feel exquisitely erotic; you can also use it during oral sex or while masturbating each other. Simultaneous clitoral and anal stimulation makes both feel even better; insert a finger during intercourse to give him an exceptional climax.

If this is your first time, I'd try the following exercise during oral sex or mutual masturbation first, then introduce it during intercourse. It's a bit hard to keep thrusting away *and* ask questions and gently explore the area at the same time. Get to know each other's "yes" and "no-thanks-very-much" spots first, then try it just as your partner approaches orgasm.

> "The first time a lover put his finger up my anus, I was absolutely horrified. He gave no warning, just shoved it up there with no lubrication. I hated it, but it's a different story with the guy I'm seeing now. He knows when and how to do it properly and now I can't orgasm unless he penetrates me anally."
>
> Sue, 26, mother

Ⓜ FOR HIM

Move from stroking and caressing her genitals and start stimulating the perineum (the smooth area between her anus and vagina). Stroke first, then use three fingers and massage firmly.

Let your fingers brush across her anus and see how she reacts. If she pulls away, or clenches her buttocks together, she's either not interested or nervous. If you haven't discussed what you want to do before now, you're playing with fire if you proceed any further!

If she lifts her buttocks or presses against your hand, that's a pretty good indication that she'd like you to continue. Before you do, you *must* apply some lubricant to your finger and her anus. Continue stroking the opening until she's relaxed, then insert the tip of a finger into her rectum. Hold still for a moment or two, then try circling or moving your finger gently in and out. Keep the heel of your hand pressed on the perineum.

Ask her if she's enjoying it before pushing your finger further inside. If you stimulate her clitoris at the same time, she'll get double the pleasure.

FOR HER

If his erection's a little halfhearted, this can firm him up in no time. Apply the same techniques listed above on him then . . .

Finger massage his entire rectum, moving in slow circles. Then insert one or two *well-lubricated* fingers about 2 inches into his rectum. Hold them still until he relaxes, then feel the front wall of the rectum until you find a firm, walnut-sized mass. That's his prostate gland and G-spot (see "How to find his" on page 106 for more detail). Stroke or press it with a downward movement, using the heel of your hand to press behind the scrotum for extra *uuummmm*.

 FOR BOTH OF YOU

If you can't have sex (don't have a condom on you, don't want to have intercourse during your period) or simply want to try something new, give gluteal sex a go. This simply means him using the valley created by her buttock cheeks as an alternative "vagina." It's different, exciting, and very easy. She clenches her buttocks together and rotates her pelvis; he thrusts between them.

A QUICK FIX

If you don't have time for a prolonged sex session or don't particularly want one, give in to the oh-so-sweet pleasures of a "quickie." A quickie is fast, hasty sex of any form. Done at the right time with the right partner, it can be equally, if not more, satisfying than those long, drawn-out sex sessions. The trick is both of you being in the same gloriously turned-on mood simultaneously. This is one instance where you can forget everything I've told you about spending time on foreplay. The whole appeal of a quickie is that it happens spontaneously and the only foreplay you need is "Let's do it." Just remember one thing: a quickie quickly turns from erotically exotic to furiously frustrating if it's the way you have sex *every* time. A quickie works best:

- When you're both semi-clothed. If you're prepared to take your clothes off, you're not impatient enough to enjoy one. *Ripping* them off is a different story.
- When they're spontaneous. Both of you have a sudden urge at the same time.
- When you're both working hard and are too tired for extended sex sessions but want to keep the fires hot.
- When the female initiates it. Men often feel like fast sex, so he'll be *excruciatingly* turned-on if you're the one to suggest it.
- If your sex life is dull and needs an instant lift.
- If one or both of you are a little anxious that you're not performing up to par. It takes the pressure off and lets animal instinct take over.
- When you're *dying* to have sex but you're in public or can't justify disappearing for a long time. You're in a park where families are playing ball not so far away? If you've got a short skirt on, pull your panties to one side, sit on his lap (he can unzip under the cover of your skirt) and give him a loving kiss. The people at the next picnic table will think you're wonderfully romantic!

Some more "quick advice":

- Try doing it in a chair—even better, his or your office chair when no one else is around (don't even think about it if there's a chance of anyone interrupting—it's not worth losing a job or reputation over). You lie back in the chair, he kneels in front of you. Wrap your legs around his rear end.

> **❗ Find sex funny? It's perfectly normal.** The sudden release of emotion and tension during or after orgasm can make us laugh. It's all part of the sexual response.

- Don't restrict "quickies" to intercourse. Give her oral sex as she's about to walk out the door to meet a girlfriend (leave her clothes on, just pull her undies to one side); give him the best fellatio he's had in the same situation.

- Start wearing stockings and garters rather than pantyhose. They look sexier and allow faster, easier access for quickies.
- Rear-entry positions require minimal undressing. You standing up, facing him, against a wall is another alternative (if your heights match up okay). Stand on one leg and hook the other around him for balance and deeper penetration.
- Give in to that *melting* desire, even if you are both dressed to go out and your friends are waiting patiently at a bar. Quickies are quick: you could have *done* it in the two minutes you spent hesitating, one hand on the doorknob.
- Try elevators, the beach, parks, planes, trains, or automobiles. The venue possibilities are endless!

SIZE *DOES* MATTER

Our genitals are as individual as every other part of our body. Take a look at how many different nose shapes and sizes there are, and you'll get a good idea of the numerous variations in vaginas and penises. As usual, what one sex wants the other doesn't. Men stress out that their penis is too small (I've yet to meet a man who worries about the opposite), women worry their vaginal canal is too big. There are ways to get around too big or small in both, but let's look at the emotional side first.

Being different from the norm in anything is difficult, but it's how you respond to the situation that counts. You can make a big deal out of it and become paranoid, or accept what nature has given you, work with it, and get on with having a good sex life. You *can* get penises enlarged and vaginas tightened through plastic surgery but it's a pretty drastic (not to mention expensive) solution. Experiment a little first with the following suggestions, and you may discover the size of your genitals isn't really that important. People don't fall in love—or lust—with body parts; it's the person they're attached to.

Ⓕ FOR HER

If sex is extremely painful or penetration impossible, you could be suffering from *vaginismus*, a condition where psychological factors cause a muscle spasm in the vagina, closing it tightly. If this is you, go straight to Chapter 7 for help.

If your vagina is too small

Women who don't have major problems but whose vaginal canals are small sometimes feel "stretched" or uncomfortable during intercourse. Fortunately (or unfortunately, since it can often go too much the other way), giving birth through natural labor usually cures this completely. But don't panic! Having a baby isn't the only option. There are other ways you can help make things more enjoyable.

- **Always use a lubricant.** I'm a strong advocate of personal lubricants, so you're probably sick of hearing me mention them, but adding extra lubrication is the single most effective thing you can do to make sex more comfortable. If you're too embarrassed to have the tube by the bed, go to the bathroom before you have sex and insert some deep into your vagina. Warmth and your natural lubrication will spread it to all the right places.

- **Don't attempt intercourse until you're really turned-on.** Explain to your partner that you need lots of foreplay for your vagina to lubricate and expand. If he still doesn't spend time stroking, arousing, and exciting you before penetration, switch partners.

- **Choose positions that allow you to spread your legs wide.** Make it easier for him to penetrate by spreading your thighs open and bending your knees. As he penetrates, bear down slightly (like you're trying to push something out of your vagina). You'll feel more in control and it loosens the vaginal muscles. Instead of penetrating in one, quick movement, ask him to slow it down and insert his penis in stages, a little at a time. You tell him when you're ready to accept deeper penetration. A sensitive lover will let you call the shots. If you trust him to wait until you're ready, you'll relax, and so will your vaginal muscles.

If your vagina is too big

Some women are just built this way, others find their vaginal muscles become slack after having babies. Either way, if you're not "gripping" his penis, the sensation is less pleasurable for both of you. Luckily, this problem's relatively easy to fix if you're prepared to do some homework.

- Do your Kegels daily. Dr. Arnold Kegel developed the following vaginal "workout" way back in the 1950s. It's a series of exercises designed to strengthen the muscles surrounding the pelvic platform, which contract during orgasm. First, you need to isolate the pubococcygeus (PC) muscle. Do this by inserting a finger into your vagina and tightening your muscles around it. It's the same muscle you use to stop peeing when there's no bathroom in sight. Got it? If you can feel your muscles squeezing your finger, you're in good shape. If you can't, you will be!

- Contract and relax the muscle, 25 times, twice a day to begin with. Start off doing it slowly and work up to the number of repetitions. When you get to the point where you can do 25 *fast*, you're ready to move on—to 50, twice a day! Mastered that? Okay, now try holding each contraction to the count of three, before releasing. Do 25 repetitions, twice a day and again, work up to 50. Once you're at this point, which should only take a few weeks, you'll notice a huge difference during intercourse. Not only will your vagina feel tighter, you can "massage" his penis by doing Kegels while he's inside of you.

- Put one or two firm pillows underneath you while he's on top. It alters the angle of the vagina, making it seem tighter. Don't open your legs wide in any intercourse position; the closer your thighs, the tighter your vaginal canal. Choose positions that "slant" your vagina—rear-entry and any position where he's entering from an angle.

Ⓜ FOR HIM

If your penis is too big

You probably feel ten feet tall when you're changing in the locker room, but not so good when new partners look frantically at the door every time you drop your trousers. The good news is the vaginal canal is elastic enough to deliver a baby, so it's totally capable of accommodating even the largest penis (90 to 95 percent measure 5 to 7 inches when erect). The trick is to:

- **Make sure she's fully aroused and her vagina is physically ready for you.** You need to spend more time on foreplay than the average guy, and use extra lubrication. Even if she's a little bit wet, it'll still hurt. Squeeze that tube of K-Y—and don't be stingy.

- **Choose a position that doesn't allow deep penetration.** Try side-by-side or one where she's in control, like woman-on-top. When you first penetrate, start by inserting a third of your penis, and get her to bear down (push her vaginal muscles "out") at the same time. Hold still until her vagina gets used to you, then you can go a little farther. Once you're fully penetrated (if you're extremely big, she might never want the full length), you can very gently start moving in and out. Deep, hard, or fast thrusting is out unless she's used to you and can cope.

If your penis is too small

You cringe every time someone makes a joke related to penis size and *hate* changing in the locker room. The first time you're with a new partner, you're terrified she'll say something like "Is that it?" when you undress or "Is it in yet?" during intercourse. But if she's got good PC muscles (encourage her to do the Kegel exercises described earlier), you can both still be a good, snug fit. Here's how to make the size of your penis irrelevant.

- **Do not make intercourse the main event.** If you've made her come three times already through oral sex, genital masturbation, or indulged her with a sensual massage, intercourse becomes part of lovemaking rather than the whole show. This takes the pressure off both of you. Most women find it difficult reaching orgasm through intercourse alone, so she'll welcome the shift in emphasis.

- **Choose deep-penetration positions or positions where her vagina is "closed."** Rear-entry, her-on-top but leaning backward, anything that alters the slant of the vagina and closes it up a little will make you feel larger to her and increase friction. During missionary, put one or two firm pillows underneath her. Rather than opening her legs wide, get her to keep her thighs pressed close together with your legs *outside* hers.

- **Thrust hard and deeply.** If your penis is smaller than average, you can usually thrust harder and deeper than usual (though still check with her to find what feels best).

- **Masturbate frequently to avoid premature ejaculation.** It's highly unfair but unfortunately true that men with small penises very often have problems coming too soon. This is because all penises have roughly the same number of nerve endings in the head. If your penis is small, they're concentrated over a smaller area, which makes you more sensitive. The more you masturbate, the less sensitive you'll become, especially if you practice controlling your orgasms while you're doing it.

SEX DURING PREGNANCY

"Oh, it's so *romantic*," people say, patting your belly and watching you and your partner exchange soppy, loving looks.

Having a baby together is romantic—and that's partly the reason why sex gets put on the back burner. Your partner loves you to death right now but he may see you differently: you're no longer his gorgeous, sexy girlfriend but a mother-to-be. You're also struggling to reconcile your "new" (more responsible) self with the "old" you (who loved hot, furious sex in the very room the crib's now in).

As one of my pregnant friends told me, "My hormones have sent my libido through the roof but every time I feel horny, I feel guilty. It's like, I'm meant to be a future mother and all I want to do is screw all the time. The two don't go together."

But they can. After the first few sickly months, a lot of women find their energy soars and that the hormones sparked by pregnancy give their libido a huge kick. If your partner is supportive, reassuring you that you don't look fat just pregnant, this can be one of the most sexual times in your relationship. Most pregnant women cram their bookshelves with texts on kids and conception so I won't go into specifics about health or harm to the baby here. But you might like to keep the following in mind.

• **How sexy you feel depends very much on your partner's reaction.** If he embraces the whole pregnancy thing and is as excited about the first kick as you are, chances are your sex life won't suffer too much. This is the time when you'll feel most vulnerable about your body. If you usually run around in sprayed-on jeans and tight sweaters, you'll start to hate anyone who still can. The perfect partner will convince you that your new look is just as erotic and you'll both revel in those nice, full breasts and that wonderfully big belly.

- **Mothers have sex, too.** Let's be honest here: motherhood doesn't have the sexiest image, and he's been as brainwashed by society as you have. If you think he's starting to treat you too much like a Madonna figure (the religious one not the singer), have a talk. Tell him as much as you love the thought of the baby growing inside you, you're the same person you were before you got pregnant. Mothers have sex. So do mothers-to-be.

- **No, the baby's not listening.** "You have this weird feeling that the baby is listening and hearing everything," said one expectant mom. It isn't. Can you remember *your* mother screaming, "Oh Harold, that's *fantastic*"?

- **Don't be surprised if your sexual tastes change.** Before getting pregnant, you loved oral sex and were so-so about straight sex. Now you hate oral sex and love screwing or vice versa. Sometimes, you won't want sex at all. Your body feels heavy and awkward, your doctor's always poking and prodding, complete strangers keep putting their hands on your stomach. Sex can feel like just another intrusion at times like this.

- **What if I feel more turned-on than ever?** It happens—a lot. Surging hormones can cause as many erotic episodes as teary ones. While your friends are obsessing about what color to paint the baby's bedroom, *you're* obsessed with what you're going to do in your own when Daddy-to-be comes home. Don't waste a second feeling guilty. Enjoy! Lots of

> "When my first wife got pregnant I hated it. She was even more uptight than she was before. She made me watch the birth and I couldn't relate to her sexually after that. Every time I thought of her vagina, I thought of the baby and all that blood coming out. With my girlfriend, it's different. We had a baby girl last year and she made me feel part of the whole thing. We had some sort of sex right up until the very end and she was happy for me to hold her hand and look at her face during the birth, rather than what was happening below."
>
> Martin, 30, plumber

women find they orgasm more quickly and more intensely than before. Delight, don't despair, when your body does all sorts of weird things—like spurt milk out of your nipples in the middle of a climax!

- **Will I hurt the baby?** This is his top concern. All that bashing around with a penis, he figures, has to push the baby all over the place. A bit of wishful thinking on his part—it's not *that* big! Your gynecologist or any good pregnancy manual will tell you which positions are safe and when it is safe to have sex when you're pregnant. Get professional advice when you first find out you're pregnant to allay all your fears.

4

Orgasm

The 30 (if you're lucky) seconds we go to *so-o-o-o* much effort for

• •

Rumor has it a group of scientists once electronically wired up a mouse so every time it pressed a lever, it triggered off an orgasm. The mouse died within twenty-four hours—from orgasm overdose. While the researchers were tucked up in their beds, he was pressing that lever over and over and over again until his little body could take no more. That's what I call dying with a smile on your face.

The first person to dream up a *human* instant orgasm trigger will shoot up and off the Forbes list within weeks. And no prizes for guessing which sex will be first in line to buy it. For him, orgasms seem to require the same amount of effort it takes to switch on the TV. *With* a remote control. For women, just learning how to have one often involves a long, laborious mission of self-discovery. And even when we do master it, the little buggers sometimes still refuse to materialize on command when we're with a partner.

Perhaps it's because, unlike men—who ejaculate life-giving semen when they orgasm—there's no obvious biological reason for women to have one. Some researchers believe they do have a role in procreation because orgasms encourage us to have sex more often (upping the chance of our eggs being fertilized). Other studies show the contractions during orgasm make the cervix "dip" into the seminal fluid, giving the sperm a leg up on the way to meet the egg. Whatever. For women, climaxing sure as hell isn't as easy as painting by numbers. Which is why it's not realistic or sensible to expect you'll both be able to tick the "Yep, I had one" box *every single time* you make love.

Sometimes he'll have one and you won't, other times you'll strike it lucky and he won't score, and on some occasions neither of you will climax. Orgasm shouldn't be the ultimate aim. Having said that, it's always rather nice if you *do* have one, which is why this chapter is entirely devoted to making both your orgasms more likely, frequent, and intense. Who knows? If you study hard enough, you might even beat the tally of one multiorgasmic woman who reputedly astonished sex researchers by having fifty orgasms in a row, stopping only when they ran out of male volunteers. (Shame the mouse wasn't around!)

> **❗ Orgasms promote cardiovascular conditioning, make the skin glow, improve overall body tone, and can cure menstrual cramps. The emotional release makes us feel less irritable and more relaxed.[1]**

WHAT DO ORGASMS FEEL LIKE?

The first time I had an orgasm I thought I'd wet myself. I was staying with my sister and discovered a personal massager, shoved in the back of a closet, while they were out. I looked at it for a while, turned it on, and watched it vibrate, then thought, "Hmmm, I wonder what would happen if I just held it pressed against here for a second. Oh! That feels great, I'll just do it for a little bit longer and . . . OH MY GOD! What the hell was *that*!" I looked down at the floor in astonishment, convinced I'd had some totally bizarre bladder attack. I had no idea I'd just orgasmed, but I knew *something* had happened.

Which is why when women ask me, "How do I know if I've had one?" my answer is always this: if you have to ask, you haven't had a *clitoral* orgasm, though you may have climaxed vaginally. Vaginal orgasms feel wonderful but they're sometimes vague and undramatic. Clitoral orgasms are peel-me-off-the-ceiling stuff. The feeling is so powerful and unmistakable, you've got as much chance of missing it as you have of not noticing a bright green alien sitting in your living room.

But even if they know they orgasm (and do so frequently), most women and men are curious about them. Do they *feel* the same for everyone? Are theirs different from other people's? Biologically, everyone moves through the same stages. We become *aroused*, then move to a *plateau* phase (highly aroused), on to *orgasm*, then *resolution* (when the body returns to normal). Psychologically, it's unlikely everyone experiences the same sensations, since orgasms appear to be as individual as the people who have them. Nevertheless, in an attempt to answer the questions, here's what one representative of each sex said when asked to describe what *their* orgasms felt like—from the very first, tentative flutter right through to the passionate finale.

> **❗ Number of women who think it's important to satisfy their partner during sex: 34 percent. Number who think it's important to satisfy themselves: 50 percent.[2]**

What she feels

"Sex with someone new, that I'm crazy about but haven't slept with yet, is different from sex with a long-term boyfriend. I'm usually wet the whole time I'm around a new guy—sometimes even thinking about him makes me lubricate. I'm more turned-on but, ironically, I'm often *too* turned-on to orgasm clitorally because when we finally get down to it, all I really want is penetration. I have a dull, aching feeling in my lower belly and a need to be 'filled up.'

"No matter where he touches, it all seems directly linked to my vagina, making it throb until I can't wait for him to be inside. Inevitably, the initial thrust is the best because it satisfies that need immediately.

"If he's big and thrusts long and hard, the aching feeling builds and then peaks, spreading into mild, pleasurable waves which I feel deep inside. My vagina seems to spasm, but less fiercely than with a clitoral orgasm. Vaginal orgasms affect a larger area—like waves of pleasure are crashing all over my body. Clitoral orgasms all radiate from the clitoris. They're more a euphoric explosion, an eruption.

"I can masturbate to a clitoral orgasm within a few minutes but I need to know and relax with a partner before he can give me one. That's because I have to concentrate, block him out of the picture and focus entirely on the sensation. In other words, I have to think about me, not him. Oral sex orgasms are the best—really intense, strong, and powerful. When he starts, I feel incredibly sensitive and everything feels great. That sensation then becomes sharper and isolates around the clitoris. It's weird, but sometimes it feels as though the rest of my body disappears and all that's left is that tiny little area. If someone chopped my arm off at that point, I wouldn't know; all I'm aware of is what's happening to that inch or less of flesh.

"At that point, I deliberately tense up the muscles in my legs and buttocks. I start to feel really hot, almost like I'm burning up, then, as I climax, my vagina starts jerking and pulsating and there's a few seconds of exquisite sensation. Even if I don't make any noise, I can't help breathing heavily and faster. Sometimes, I'll have three or four intense spasms, then nothing. Other times, especially if he continues licking softly, they're followed by smaller waves, spaced less closely. Sometimes I'll ejaculate fluid—or at least it feels like I do but I've masturbated and checked the sheets and there's nothing there. After orgasm, I push him away immediately—I'm way too sensitive to be touched. The orgasm itself lasts about ten seconds but it feels much longer. I'm completely exhausted afterward and don't want him anywhere near me. I feel a bit faint, so lie back for a minute or two. I guess that's why French women nickname orgasm *le petit mort,* the little death.

"I don't think most women have orgasms. Lots of women think they have them because sensations build then ebb away but that's not an orgasm, that's just desire. In some ways, I'd like to be a male because it seems so easy for them. Men try to put off

Men aren't the only ones who have "wet dreams." Up to 40 percent of women have woken in the throes of orgasm.[3]

their orgasms for as long as possible but women are always trying to induce theirs. I don't know any woman who, when she feels an orgasm coming, tries to stop it. Why would she? Women have to be in a certain head space to come; they're not that easy to achieve. I guess the equalizer is men's orgasms seems quicker than ours and they can't have them as often."

What he feels

"Penises have a mind of their own. If I'm seeing a girl that night and know I'll be having sex, I'll look down during the day and find I've got an erection even though I'm not aware of it. Obviously my subconscious is having a heyday.

"Despite what women think, the more teasing and foreplay the better. The feeling of your penis filling up with blood and becoming erect is fantastic. It happens really quickly—one minute it's flaccid, the next ready for action. I'm not conscious of my nipples becoming erect or anything but I feel tingly everywhere. I'll put off the moment of penetration for as long as possible—the anticipation is almost as good as the real thing.

"Girls, if you're with a guy who's trying to rush things at this point, you can bet he's trying to hurry everything up in case you change your mind! Spontaneous, fast sex is great but usually, the more touching and caressing she does the better.

"Just before I climax, I can feel the sperm traveling up the shaft in a rush of fluid. Once you feel that happening, ejaculation is inevitable. If I try and stop it because I want it to last longer, the sperm still comes out but it feels all rushed and I don't feel fulfilled. It's a bit like being fed chocolate cake intravenously: the end result is the same but there's no pleasure in it. My brain has to be conscious of me having an orgasm before it registers the nice part; your body and mind have to be in tune.

"Orgasm is a release. It feels like you've been holding on to something forever and are then allowed to let go. The sperm pumps out in jerky spasms and you feel this body-shattering intense pleasure. My orgasm seems to last about six seconds though my friends have told me theirs last only two to three. I'm either lucky or my sense of timing is shot!

"If I haven't had sex with a girl for a while, it's best if I masturbate a few times first, otherwise I come too quickly and it doesn't feel as good. I think most men are always trying to think of ways to make their orgasms last longer because they're usually so short. They feel different when she fellates me, more acute and protracted. I'd never knock a blow job, but there's something about being inside her that I prefer.

"Sperm is such an integral part of coming yet most women say they can't feel it shooting into them. That's kind of disappointing for men.

"I lose my erection within seconds when my penis is removed from the vagina and hits cold air; once I've come, it's like *all* over, that's it. Then I need quiet time to chill out, even though I do feel close to my partner if I love her. Unlike women, our orgasms don't seem to vary as dramatically in a physical sense, but some do feel different than others. What makes them stand out isn't what's happening to your body but your head and your heart. If you're with someone you want to snuggle with afterward, that's what makes them special."

FAKING IT

If the Oscar judges were serious about finding award-winning acting performances, they'd look to the bedroom rather than the big screen—there's some pretty convincing acting going on out there! Most all of us have faked an orgasm at some point and if *you* never, ever have, you're in the minority (or lying).

Why aren't we more honest? Sometimes, it's just *easier* to go with the flow. Did cavewomen enjoy being hit on the head and pulled around by their hair? Hardly. They simply figured it was easier to placate their partner than be eaten by another, more dangerous, wild beast. In the superstressed, super-fast-paced 90s, both women *and* men resort to playacting. We're not only too tired to have orgasms, who's got the energy to go through the hassle of explaining why we didn't?

Why women fake
Because we don't want to hurt him and it's easy to get away with
Men rarely notice when we fake it. Whether this is because we are really good actors or because the female orgasm is so easily hid-

den—we could sneak one in on the bus and no one would look up from their newspaper—is open to conjecture. The truth is more likely this: women fake so often that most men have no idea what the real thing is anymore.

Usually, we'll time it just as he's about to climax and, as one sex therapist put it, "Who can be bothered looking for giveaway signs when you're in the throes of experiencing your own pleasure?" Besides, outwardly visible signs of female orgasm aren't that obvious. Sure, our breathing gets heavier and quicker, and sometimes our whole body jerks with each spasm, but not always. Some men say they can feel our vaginas "quivering" with their tongue if we orgasm during oral sex, but that doesn't help much during intercourse.

Probably the most telltale sign is how sensitive our genitals are afterward. If you can touch her clitoris quite firmly immediately after she's gasped out the last "Oh yes," chances are she's telling lies. A few experts claim a dark red flush appears across the chest and shoulders for a split second, just after either sex orgasms, but again, who's together enough to notice?

We'd rather act than tell the truth because we don't want to dent that fragile male ego

Being the caring, nurturing souls that we are, women are loath to admit he's anything but perfect in bed. If he's trying his hardest to last and you're nowhere near coming, you'll fake it to put him out of his misery. Ditto when he's been down there licking for an hour but you just know there's no way you're going over the edge.

To get sex over with

If you're tired and longing for sleep, faking an orgasm gives him the signal it's okay to let go. The tragic part is a lot of women don't mind if they don't have one every time. Just because we don't climax doesn't mean we haven't enjoyed it. Sadly, men often react to being told this with disbelief. Because they orgasm most of the time, they think we're saying it just to be nice.

To save face

Some women feel like a failure if they don't orgasm at the touch of a breast (like our celluloid counterparts). That's the reason lying about orgasms isn't confined to the bedroom. If all our friends are owning up to multiple orgasms, why should we admit to none at all?

Why men fake
To explain a limp penis

His reasons aren't that different than ours. If he's tired, had a few too many, worried about work, or just not interested in sex right now, he'll pretend he's had an orgasm to explain why he's lost his erection. "If you feel it going down, you quickly let out a few grunts and moans, pump a bit harder, then pull out," said one guy.

How does he explain the lack of evidence? "If you've been giving her heaps of oral sex and she's already wet, she doesn't notice there isn't any sperm," he claims.

I'm a tad skeptical because semen has a pretty distinctive smell, but, according to the experts, ejaculate isn't a true indication that he's orgasmed, anyway. Kinsey and Miriam Stoppard both maintain orgasm and ejaculation are two separate processes and one can occur without the other. In other words, he can ejaculate without having an orgasm or orgasm without ejaculating.[4]

He's worried he'll hurt you

Men say women take it very personally when a man doesn't come, much more than he does if you don't. Because we think men's orgasms are automatic and inevitable, he's supposed to have one every single time or something's really wrong. We're not attractive enough, didn't turn him on enough, he's in love with the girl in his office . . .

What if I suspect my partner's just faked it?

If you suspect she's faked it and accuse her outright, she'll deny it and clam up. Instead say something like, "Darling, I love making love to you and want to give you as much pleasure as possible. What are the things I do that turn you on the most?" She'll be more comfortable to begin with focusing on what you do right rather than what you do wrong. When she's opened up, ask her to guide your hand (or tongue) in the future to show you the techniques that work for her. Say you read somewhere that lots of women like their clitoris stimulated during intercourse. The idea turns you on and you'd love to try it—what does she think?

If you suspect he's faked it, make light of it. If you think he did it because he was stressed or tired, when you come back from the bathroom say, "That's weird, there didn't seem to be much sperm this time. Maybe men are a bit like women and sex isn't so great when you're really tired." He probably won't confess, but it gives him the green light to say no to sex in the future.

If he never seems to have a genuine orgasm, he might be what's called a *retarded ejaculator*, an unfortunate term that simply means he can stay rock hard all night but can't ejaculate or orgasm. The cause is usually psychological—maybe he got a girlfriend pregnant in the past and is terrified it'll happen again. Alternatively, he may suffer from *retrograde ejaculation*. He feels an orgasm in his brain but the semen goes back down the urethra. Whatever. If he's *never* orgasmed with you, you've both probably acknowledged the problem by now. Suggest he book an appointment for a medical checkup with a doctor to see if there are any physical causes. They'll refer him to a therapist if psychological factors are at play.

Is it ever okay to pretend?

Some sex therapists (interestingly, all female) say if you have real orgasms with your partner 90 percent of the time, it's *not recommended* but acceptable if you fake 10 percent. It's a bit like telling your girlfriend she looks great in that new dress when it really does nothing for her. If he's doing everything right but you can't orgasm for your own reasons, sometimes it seems kinder to pretend.

Sex therapist Dr. Janet Hall claims there is an argument for encouraging women to fake it. She calls it "fake it till you make it." It's based on the assumption that if you act out the thing you want to happen, sometimes it will. Psychologists use the same technique on depressed patients: the act of smiling triggers hormones that make us feel happier so a forced smile eventually turns into a real one. If you want to orgasm, quicken your breathing, make noise, move your hips—do whatever you do when you really do have one. By reenacting the lead-up to orgasm, you may be able to push yourself over the threshold to the point where orgasm becomes involuntary.

The overwhelming majority of sex therapists give faking the thumbs-down—for a very good reason. If you *never* have an orgasm with your partner, it's pretty pointless pretending to. How are they ever going to learn to give you one if they think they're doing it already? The worst time to fake an orgasm is in the beginning of a relationship, which is, of course, when most women (and some men) do it. Keep *on* doing it and you've set up a pattern of behavior that's based on deception and dissatisfaction. He'll keep on using the same ineffectual techniques because he thinks he's turning you on; you'll remain frustrated and irritable every time you make love. Having the courage to open up and say "Actually, that does nothing for me" is difficult, but you really must.

❗ Approximately 40 percent of men admit women have faked orgasm with them; 40 percent aren't sure; 20 percent swear it's never happened. Ninety-two percent of women admit to faking orgasm at least once in their life.[5]

Communication is the key to good sex—and that's a fact. If either of you play ostrich—stick your head in the sand and refuse to talk about your needs—you're in trouble. Listen up, guys! Eighty-five percent of men are "stonewallers": people who refuse to talk through problems and fume in stony silence. Not communicating is a great way to ruin a relationship—not to mention your sex life. Open up. Faking orgasm isn't necessary if admitting to not having one isn't a problem.[6]

THE LONG AND SHORT OF IT

Some orgasms are so intense, your legs aren't the only thing that turn to jelly. "Marry me," you beg the guy who bores you silly outside the bedroom. The very next night, with exactly the same person, you come and it feels more like a sneeze.

Orgasms, like most things in life, vary depending on your mood, your partner, how turned-on you are, how tired you are, and, of course, on how you're having them. You might experience three massive contractions when he gives you oral sex, a dozen little ones when you masturbate. His orgasm intensity fluctuates, too. One night, he'll ejaculate enough semen to inseminate a small town, writhing about for what seems like hours; the next, there's a small sigh and not enough sperm to even warrant washing the sheets. Here's a brief guide to all the different orgasms both of you can experience.

> "Orgasms through oral sex feel more intense. If she's using her tongue and is a good fellatrix, she can do more than she can with her vagina. But the very best thing about them is you're completely in her control. In intercourse, you can vary the thrust speed and depth to control your own orgasm; with oral sex, she gives you one when she feels like it."
>
> Ian, 33, small business owner

The male orgasm

As he orgasms, engorged reproductive glands empty their contents into his urethra, expanding it to produce an erotically intense sensation. He ejaculates through a series of four or five contractions, usually one every 0.8 seconds. The male orgasm is straightforward biologically and it certainly sounds like there's not much room for variation. But there is. If he hasn't had sex for a while, he'll produce more semen than normal, making his orgasm

> **!** Only 30 percent of women can climax through intercourse without additional clitoral stimulation. It's thought these women may have a larger clitoris than usual so it's more easily "rubbed" by a thrusting penis.[7]

more prolonged. He'll "feel" the orgasm in his brain more intensely if his mind's not on other things, and if a lover brings him almost to the peak, over and over, before letting him ejaculate, all his senses will be heightened and the orgasm may feel fiercer. Alternatively, if he's having a quickie, it's a shorter but sharper feeling.

Vaginal orgasms

Because the inner walls of the vagina have nerve endings (not to mention highly sensitive points like the G- and A-spots), one third of women say they can climax this way. In contrast to clitoral orgasms, vaginal orgasms produce a more widespread, "warm wave" sensation. He can give you one through manual masturbation, fingers deep inside you, or through intercourse.

Clitoral orgasms

There's an assumption that vaginal orgasms are inferior to clitoral ones. They're not, just different. But the attitude stems from the fact that clitoral stimulation tends to produce more intense climaxes. Most women build to a high peak of pleasure that triggers a series of intense spasms and vaginal contractions. Unlike men, the degree, number, and time between the spasms varies dramatically from woman to woman.

Oral sex orgasms

Both sexes say orgasms achieved through oral sex feel different. Mouths and tongues are soft, gentle, and handily agile at stimulating a small area (like your clitoris or his frenulum). As a result, oral sex orgasms can feel stronger and more focused.

Masturbation orgasms

Some people maintain no one can give you a better orgasm than you can give yourself; others say masturbatory orgasms are short and perfunctory. Usually we climax more quickly, probably because our attention is focused on our own needs. Regardless, most people stop at one and few try to achieve . . .

Multiple orgasms

This is a term everyone uses differently. For some people, multiple orgasms simply means having more than one in a single sex session. Other people (more accurately) mean riding the wave of an initial orgasm until they've had two or three immediately in succession. Like simultaneous orgasms, a lot of couples are in desperate pursuit of multiples, thinking they've failed as lovers if they don't happen. Sensible couples break open the champagne if they do result, but don't worry too much if they don't.

In the 1940s and 1950s, Kinsey found only 8–9 percent of women were multiorgasmic. More recent research suggests 60 percent of us are at least capable of achieving multiple orgasms.[8] Women are slower to climb to an orgasm peak, so remain at the highly aroused "plateau" phase for longer than men do. If he continues gentle stimulation throughout our initial orgasm, it stops us moving to the "resolution" phase (when our body goes back to normal) and we're able to climb back up and have further orgasms. While our sleep hormones are released about half an hour after our first orgasm, men's kick into the bloodstream almost immediately after ejaculation. He peaks quickly and usually needs rest to build up semen (and energy) for further orgasms. Though new research suggests he can have multiple orgasms, it's unlikely he'll ejaculate each time. Sexpert Miriam Stoppard cites a study that documented multiorgasmic men who had between two and nine orgasms per session.[9] The trick seems to be to separate the process of ejaculation and orgasm. His body might not be able to physically ejaculate several times in succession, but his brain seems capable of registering the feeling of orgasm over and over. One technique to try: he (or you) press hard on his perineum (the area between his testes and anus) just before orgasm. This can sometimes stop ejaculation while he orgasms "mentally" and keeps him hard so he can go on to have another.

Simultaneous orgasm

This simply means both of you have an orgasm at exactly the same time. People on soap operas have simultaneous orgasms more often than they eat breakfast but it's a little different in the real world. The chance of both of you reaching a peak at exactly the same *second* is low but it is not unachievable. In other words, it's romantic to aim for simultaneous orgasms but unrealistic to expect them frequently. Because women take longer than men to build to the preorgasmic phase, you can up the chances of coming together by stimulating her until she's almost there before even starting whatever's necessary to make him come.

THE G-SPOT: MYTH OR MARVEL?

The G-spot (Grafenberg spot) was a bit like God. We wanted to believe in it even though we weren't really sure if it existed, and were scared to say "What a load of crap" in case we were the only person at the dinner party who wasn't having G-spot orgasms every five minutes. Men, particularly, seemed reluctant to admit they'd never found it on a woman.

"Have you ever found the G-spot?" I asked one man during an interview.

"Oh yes," he said confidently.

"Where is it?" I asked him.

"Oh, it varies," he said. "On some women it's just underneath the clitoris, on others it's underneath their breasts."

Somehow, I don't think this is quite what Grafenberg had in mind.

Ernst Grafenberg started all the fuss in Germany in 1944. He published a paper claiming there was an area in the upper wall of the vagina so erotically charged a woman was guaranteed to orgasm if it was stimulated. Fellow researchers pooh-poohed the idea so Grafenberg closed his mouth and kept it shut. About four decades later, a team of American psychologists also argued that women could have multiple orgasms, without clitoral stimulation, if the same area was stimulated. Again, the idea met with little support.

Since then, modern science has proved that our vaginal walls are pleasurably sensitive and there seems little doubt that there is definitely a "hidden area" that produces intense excitement when aroused in *some* women. But not all females appear to have one. The male G-spot (he had to get in on the act, didn't he!) is less controversial: it was identified almost immediately as the prostate gland. As for women, post mortems on females have failed to find a G-spot, leading some experts to believe in the only-the-lucky theory or that it is only visible when stimulated. Some still claim the G-spot is simply the whole of the front vaginal wall.

So, the debate still rages. Most sex therapists are convinced it does exist, a few fix you with a "not that old myth" withering stare if you even mention it. If you've found it, or what seems like it, you're the one jumping up and down whenever the conversation moves toward sex, waving the G-spot flag like crazy. If you've tried and failed, you're the one saying wearily, "Nice for some." To be honest, I didn't think I was a proud owner until quite recently. I don't know whether my lover found my G-spot, but he certainly hit on something in the general vicinity which made me want to shout *"Eureka!"*

How to find hers

The G-spot is a small cluster of nerve endings and glands near the woman's urethra or urinary tract. Because it only swells and stands out from the vaginal wall when aroused, the G-spot usually can't be felt unless it's stimulated.

The easiest way to find it yourself is to squat—maybe even sit on the toilet. Now, insert a finger into your well-lubricated vagina, curving it so you're hitting the front wall (imagine you're aiming toward your belly). Feel around a little, hopefully causing the G-spot to swell so you can pinpoint it, until you find a raised area that feels textured. Most experts say it's around the size of a large pea.

Some women find their first stimulation of the G-spot distinctly uncomfortable. It can produce similar feelings to wanting to pee. Empty your bladder first or sit on the toilet when you first try. If you relax into the sensation, the feeling will pass.

Hold your finger still to begin with, then experiment. Don't press hard and constantly—a gentle, stroking motion is better. Try stroking left to right and back again or in circles; in other words, so your fingers are *passing over* the G-spot without concentrating on it directly. G-spot orgasms feel different from clitoral orgasms.

If you have one, you may find you ejaculate a small amount of clear fluid (which isn't urine, by the way).

It's best if you lie on a bed, with pillows underneath your buttocks, for your partner to find it. It makes the area more easily accessible for him to follow the instructions above. Once found, he can combine G-spot stimulation with oral sex or while he's masturbating you. The best intercourse positions to hit the spot are woman-on-top or him behind (doggie-style).

How to find his

Just because you haven't found yours, doesn't mean you shouldn't try to find his (it might even give you some clues).

> "I was with an extremely liberated young lady once who inserted a vibrator into my anus. I felt intimidated at first, but when I let go, it was like wow! It was definitely the most fierce, overwhelming, total body experience I've had. I remember feeling an unusual 'full' feeling and thinking, 'This is what it must be like for women.'"
>
> Anton, 25, broker

Like the female G-spot, the male's is situated near the urethra. Unlike ours, his has a medical name—the prostate gland—and it has an organic function. There's another point of difference: while we can find our own, it's rather difficult for him to stimulate his because it's up his rectum. He can try (by lying on his back, knees bent and feet flat on the floor or knees drawn up to his chest, inserting his thumb and pressing against the front wall), but it's simpler if you find it for him.

Apply some personal lubricant to your finger (nails trimmed and clean) and get him to lie on his back. Gently insert the finger into his anus, then feel up the front rectal wall until you find something that feels like a walnut. Hold your finger still until he's relaxed, then start massaging firmly in a downward direction. He can draw his knees up to his chest once you've found it.

It can take a little while for him to orgasm (so make sure you're both comfortable) but it's worth the effort. If it works, you'll be in the unique position of having given him an orgasm without even touching his penis! Male fans claim not only are G-spot orgasms more intense, they ejaculate in a continuous stream rather than in spurts.

Once you're an expert, try massaging his G-spot while you're giving him oral sex or stimulate it during him-on-top intercourse positions.

One note about hygiene: always wash your hands after inserting fingers into rectums. If you touch your own genitals you can inadvertently transfer bacteria into your vagina.

THE *A(HHHH)*-SPOT

Just when the search party finally returned from the G-spot expedition, scientists came up with another supposed instant orgasm button. This one's called the A-spot. A hot spot accidentally discovered in early 1996, it's officially called the "anterior fornex erogenous" and is located on the front wall of the vagina, a third of the way down from the cervix.[11]

Stumbled upon during an experiment to find a cure for vaginal dryness, scientists were amazed to find an astonishing 95 percent of women became massively turned-on when they stimulated this particular area. Many had their first orgasm or found it led to more frequent and intense climaxes. I'm obviously one of the 5 percent. Despite faithfully following the instructions, nothing much happened to me. But that's not to say *you're* not going to think it's the best invention since tampons.

According to the research team, stimulating the A-spot not only made women wet within 10 minutes, it led to multiple orgasms. Because their vaginas were more lubricated, the women said they felt more excited, both mentally and physically. Usually, our lubrication slows down or stops after one orgasm. Theirs continued—so they did, too.

To find your A-spot, wet two fingers and slide them inside your

"When I first went out with Scott, he was always fiddling around inside me and I thought, 'What's he doing?' The third time we made love, I found out: he was looking for my G-spot. And he found it. I can't orgasm from that alone but if he has one hand stimulating that and the other on my clitoris, I'm putty."

Marie, 20, secretary

vagina, stimulating it until you (hopefully) hit a small mass of spongy material a third of the way up the front wall (curve your fingers and aim toward your stomach). This is the G-spot.

Continue upward to find your cervix. It feels like the very round end of a nose. Move back until you're about halfway between your G-spot and your cervix. That's the A-spot. It's a smooth area that's extremely sensitive to touch. Now slide a finger up and down over the A-spot or try moving in a clockwise then counterclockwise direction.

If you want to strike it lucky during intercourse, opt for positions where the penis hits the front wall of the vagina: him behind (doggie-style) or you sitting on the edge of the bed and him kneeling before you.

DEEPER, LONGER, BETTER, MORE . . .

Up the number and intensity of your orgasms by trying any (and all) of the following.

- **Don't race to get to the finish line.** The longer you've spent on foreplay, the more enhanced it will be for both of you.

- **Slow his down, speed yours up.** You envy the fact that he can orgasm with one hand behind his back (literally); he's jealous of your ability to hover in the oh-Jesus-I'm-just-about-there stage for ages. Anything that delays his orgasm will increase his enjoyment; anything that makes her more easily orgasmic will increase her pleasure potential.

> **❗** *Partner sex often follows a 3-2-1 pattern: three minutes of foreplay, two minutes of intercourse, and one orgasm—his.*

- **Teach him control.** As you're stimulating him, get him to tell you how he's feeling by rating it on a scale of 1 to 10 (10 being the point of no return). Drive him to distraction by revving him up to a seven or eight, then slowing it down again, several times over, before letting him go all the way.

- **Alternate oral sex with intercourse.** If he's too close to coming, change activities. Get him to give you oral sex until he feels more in control.

- **Touch his penis frequently.** The more often your hand, tongue, or vagina touches it, the less sensitive he'll be and the longer he'll last.
- **Don't be a clock-watcher.** Stop wondering whether his tongue's gone numb, wipe out the "If I don't come soon, he's going to miss the game" thoughts. The best lover in the world is the man who says, "Take your time honey—I love doing it to you as much as you like receiving it" (and means it). You can't fight biology; both of you should accept that it's more complicated for you to have an orgasm than him.
- **Give her a head start.** Give her an orgasm through oral sex or masturbation *before* intercourse. Give him one orally, so his second intercourse orgasm lasts longer.
- **Don't try too hard, and don't freak if you don't have one.** Remember when you were a kid and tried to touch a rainbow? Orgasms can be just as elusive. Reach just a little higher, you think, and you'll have one but the next minute it's slipped through your (or his) fingers. Lots of women move steadily toward the point of having an orgasm then, out of nowhere, something intrudes. *I forgot Jane's birthday last week*, your brain inappropriately throws up, or you hear your roommate's key in the door or remember you have to confront your boss in the morning. Your orgasm potential's disappeared, not forever, but certainly for that session. The same thing can happen if he changes technique or rhythm at the wrong time; everything that has built up fades away. Trying harder will only makes things worse. Instead, accept that you will have one next time you make love (making sure it's sooner rather than later) and you will. Stress out about it, start tormenting yourself with thoughts like "That's it. This is going to happen every time and I'll never have one" and you'll set up more psychological roadblocks than the average detour.
- **Masturbate with him rather than alone.** If you don't have an orgasm during intercourse, give yourself one afterward. He can watch or place his hand over yours.
- **Don't treat her clitoris like it's an elevator button.** Some men think the more they press it, the quicker you'll zoom to

the top. Most women climax if you work around the base of the clitoris rather than touch it directly.

- **Prime yourself for sex by turning yourself on beforehand.** When he's talking to friends, think about what that tongue will do to you later, how much better his fingers would feel inside you rather than wrapped around a beer glass.
- **Stop worrying about what you look like.** If your partner isn't someone you can let go with, without fear of criticism, they're not the right choice. In or out of the bedroom.
- **Show each other how to do it.** Not like an army commander where you're shouting "Left" and "Right" but "Mmm, that feels fantastic when you do it really slow," or "God, that's great. Do it harder."
- **Masturbate more.** Researchers claim it increases your sexual appetite because the more sex we have, the more our bodies expect.
- **Make noise.** It sounds and feels sexy.
- **Get wet.** It doesn't mean you're not turned-on if you're not lubricating like crazy; you might just be at a different stage of the menstrual cycle, stressed, or tired. Accept that sometimes you'll need to add artificial lubricant.
- **Both do Kegel exercises.** Women do them to tighten their vagina and give them more control over orgasm; men can use the same genital workout to orgasm more frequently. (See page 86 for details—the same technique works for both.) The experts maintain male masters of Kegels can become multiorgasmic. He can try contracting his PC muscle hard, for five seconds, as he's hovering on the brink of orgasm. Reportedly, this delays ejaculation but he'll "feel" an orgasm in his brain. Potentially, he could climax several times before having an ejaculatory orgasm.
- **Give him a squeeze.** Squeezing the base of the penis firmly for a few seconds can delay ejaculation.
- **Fantasize guilt-free.** Many women and men use fantasy to launch themselves into orgasmic orbit; some can't achieve one without it. Quit the guilt trip. Your partner can't read your mind, remember?

HOW TO MAKE YOUR ORGASM LAST 1,790 TIMES LONGER

Imagine an orgasm that lasts a full thirty *minutes* instead of seconds, with bonus, occasional deep contractions occurring up to twenty-four hours afterward. This is the extraordinary promise of two American sexologists who've pioneered and perfected the Extended Sexual Orgasms (ESO) technique. Psychiatrist Alan Brauer and psychotherapist Donna Brauer claim if you faithfully follow the four steps of their sexuality program, *every* woman is potentially capable of experiencing a continuous orgasm of ever-increasing arousal lasting thirty minutes to an hour or more.

Of course, there is a catch. The "training" that ESO requires will make your gym regime pale by comparison *plus* your partner has to be motivated, sexually educated, and capable of following explicit, often complicated instructions. On top of that, not all of us *want* to experience an impromptu orgasm while admiring the roses with our eighty-seven-year-old neighbor, twenty-four hours after doing it, but . . . for those who want to give it a whirl, here's how to.

The ESO technique

You prepare for a female ESO orgasm by working through stages 1 through 3 on your own and involving your partner in stage 4. It's not something you can pick up and try tonight; allow at least one month. (I've only detailed the female orgasm here. If he also likes the idea, ask your local bookstore if they stock the ESO book or flip through a Tantric sex guide which has similar techniques.)

1. Change your attitude about sex

According to the Brauers, everyone resists pleasure. Some of us are plagued by a deep-rooted fear of sex (the legacy of overstrict parents or a religious upbringing perhaps), others have more superficial sex worries (like suddenly wondering if we've fed the cat or if our thighs look fat). Either way, intrusive thoughts during the act need to be challenged with "cognitive restructuring." Every time you think a negative thought, suggest the Brauers, replace it with "I'm calm" or "Relax. I'm having a good time."

2. Develop your PC muscle

See the Kegel exercise guide on page 86 to find out how to exercise your vaginal muscles. The Brauers also suggest you do "slow clenches" (squeeze and clench to the count of three before releasing), "flutters" (squeeze and clench as quickly as possible) and "push-outs" (bearing down as if trying to go to the bathroom using your stomach, anal, and PC muscles). Do this for two weeks before starting stage 3.

3. Masturbate regularly
Concentrate on what strokes suit you, the speed, pressure, and rhythm. When you're convinced your attitude toward sex is positive, your PC muscle is toned, and you know your body's responses intimately through masturbation, progress to stage 4.

4. Train your partner
This is the fourth and final stage of the program, and the most complicated. It is divided into three steps:

Step one. You lie down, he sits or kneels cross-legged beside or in between your legs. He applies a personal lubricant to the whole of your vaginal and perineum area (the section between your vagina and anus).

He "teases" you by lightly brushing and stroking all the genital area *except* the clitoris and inside the vagina.

Stimulation moves to the clitoris. He strokes, slow and steady, circling the clitoris with his finger once per second, while you tell him what feels good, what doesn't.

Step two. He continues clitoral stimulation while you use your PC training to flutter, slow clench, and push-out as he's arousing you. Concentrate on your breathing. Don't hold your breath, and aim to breathe at least six times a minute, breathing deeply from your stomach rather than shallow breathing from your chest.

If you're doing everything right, an orgasm isn't too far away. As you feel the onset of a climax, he should watch for regular two-second contractions in your genital area, which means you're about to orgasm. Once the contractions start, he switches from stimulating your clitoris to the inner vaginal walls. Using his fingers, he can either push them in and out or sweep them in circles and in and out of the entrance. If he can locate your G-spot, stroking with his fore or middle finger is another option. Again, it's imperative he maintains a regular, slow rhythm.

Step three. After your orgasm subsides *but before the contractions stop entirely*, he'll feel the vagina start to draw back or "pull away." This is the "coming down" period, usually the point where most couples stop. But in ESO, your first orgasm is only the beginning and the aim is to continue the contractions. He lightens his strokes inside until you give a signal you're ready for more before again upping the frequency and pressure. At the first sign of a pause in the vaginal contractions, he moves quickly back to the clitoris and continues stroking as before. This should trigger further contractions, at which point he moves back to stimulating the inner walls of the vagina.

Your partner continues switching back and forth from vaginal to clitoral stimulation until your contractions occur every one to five seconds. He then continues for about fifteen minutes until the "coming down" periods (where the vagina "pulls away") occur less and less frequently and the contractions start to become continuous. When the vagina pushes out in a continual wavelike motion, you're in the final phase.

Now he needs to get into a position where he can use both hands (and keep his balance) to stimulate the clitoris and the vagina *simultaneously*. The result, claim the Brauers: wave after wave of orgasms, the like of which you've never felt before!

IF YOU'VE NEVER HAD AN ORGASM

Personally, I've never met (or even heard a whiff of a rumor about) a man who's *never* had an orgasm. But I can name at least six women off the top of my head who did (or, miserably, still do) fit the bill. For that reason, this section is devoted to females. While an extremely small percentage of men do suffer from *anorgasmia*, the inability to have an orgasm, the causes are

> "I've never ever heard of a guy who's never come. If a guy told me that, I'd be like 'What?' and pack him off to the nearest doctor. I don't think I'd believe him; it sounds too weird."
>
> Peter, 42, vet

usually physical (see "Faking it," page 96) or deeply psychological (and therefore best dealt with by a professional therapist).

A tiny percentage of women do "miss" orgasms. Their vaginal muscles contract but they don't register any sensation in their brain. It's rare, and the cause is usually psychological and best solved by a professional therapist. For most anorgasmic women, however, it's more likely caused by a lethal combination of a strict (particularly religious) upbringing and a lack of understanding about their own bodies. For that reason, it's a good idea to read about masturbation in Chapter 1 first. This will give you a basic idea of your sexual response system and guide you, step-by-step, through masturbation, the surest route to orgasm. Armed with the facts, you can then work through the following action plan—and be well on your way to working out what all the fuss is about!

1. Change your attitude by educating yourself

The most common obstacle to having an orgasm is your attitude to sex. If you've been brought up to believe it's "bad" or "dirty" or even "unladylike," you probably feel uncomfortable touching your genitals or letting your partner touch them. The "good girls don't" inhibition factor is covered in the masturbation chapter (see page 10). If this doesn't help, book a few sessions with a female sex therapist (call the American Psychological Association at 202-336-5500 for referrals). The therapist will help you work through your feelings.

> ❗ *Only 15 percent of men say they're certain their partners always have orgasms during lovemaking.*[12]

2. Accept that you have to "learn" how to orgasm

Female orgasms aren't automatic. In other words, you're not going to accidentally have one while doing the ironing. It's also extremely unlikely that you'll have your first orgasm with a partner. Practically *all* women have their first *on their own*. So if you're waiting for some magical lover to transport you to heaven, stock up the cupboards—you're in for an awfully long wait. Instead, invest in a few good sex books. This book will give you lots of practical information, but you might also want to scour the shelves for books that focus specifically on the emotional barriers to orgasm. Keep reading and researching until you feel good about sex, confident that you understand how your body works, and know the basic techniques most women use to orgasm.

3. Accept responsibility for your own pleasure

Do you think it's his responsibility to "give" you an orgasm? No one can "give" you an orgasm; you have to "take" one yourself, by guiding and telling him how to do it. It's not like a five-course meal where he slaves in the kitchen and you get to do nothing but lie around until you're ready to savor the results. Orgasms happen when both of you know what you want and how to get it.

4. Teach yourself how to masturbate

Chapter 1 describes how to masturbate for the first time and outlines other techniques to try. You'll learn more about your body and its response system if you use your fingers but using a vibrator is also a good idea. Any good department store sells personal massagers, ostensibly designed to massage shoulders but more often bought to massage clitorises. The saleswoman won't know what you're buying it for, so just let her babble on in the background while you check to make sure it's got some sort of flat, small, round attachment. You won't put it inside but hold it against the *mons* (the fleshy bit covered by pubic hair).

Once you've bought it, refer to Chapter 1 for instructions on how to masturbate using a vibrator. If you don't orgasm with this technique, see a gynecologist to check for any physical problems (physical impairments to orgasm are rare and treatable so practically all women are capable of them). Otherwise, let it rip and have as many orgasms as you can handle before collapsing in a happy heap.

Sorry, but the vibrator is now banished to the back of the closet until you can teach yourself to climax using your hands. Unless you want to always use a vibrator with your partner, you

> ❗ *Experts estimate that between 10 and 15 percent of women never reach orgasm during sex or masturbation. The same number can only climax through masturbation.*[13]

need to know how to do it manually. Again, turn to Chapter 1 for details on techniques.

5. Teach him how to do it

Once you've masturbated yourself to orgasm, it's time to tell *him* how to do it. Chapter 2, on foreplay, is peppered with suggestions about how to talk to him about sex, as are all the chapters in the book.

6. Change your mind-set about your body

Many women don't orgasm because they think their partners can't possibly find them attractive. Let's get one thing straight right now: an overwhelming majority of men are turned on by a naked woman's body, no matter what shape it's in. However, if *you* aren't happy with yours, do something about it. Join a gym, get a makeover, eat healthily, then splurge on some new clothes. But accept what nature has handed out: ignore the faults, play up the good parts, and learn to love every inch.

7. Stop trying so hard

A watched pot never boils. Your mind should be focused on how pleasurable the sensations are, not on "Please God, let me have one." The more you worry about it, the more your body will tense and make orgasm impossible. Try a bit of reverse psychology.

In the quest for orgasm, 75 percent of women rate foreplay as more important than intercourse. About half the men surveyed by sexpert Susan Crain Bakos say they don't get as much foreplay as they'd like to make their orgasms more intense.[14]

When you masturbate or make love, tell yourself you're *not allowed* to have an orgasm, that this session is strictly for research purposes. You'll relax more and may well end up scoring a goal.

8. Make time to pleasure yourself

My friend Sarah was trying to teach herself to orgasm through masturbation but to no avail. When I asked her when she masturbated, she answered, "When

Ben [her two-year-old] is finally asleep." Sarah's body didn't need an orgasm, it needed sleep!

For her birthday, a few of us (including her husband) all chipped in and sent her away for the weekend, solo, to a luxury resort. Tucked in her luggage was a vibrator. A blissful forty-eight hours of peace and she'd not only had one orgasm, she clocked up a dozen.

9. Rethink your relationship

"You're fat," "No wonder you can't have an orgasm, you're no good at anything," "You're not a real woman," "You're frigid"— if your partner says or insinuates negative things about you, your body, or your inability to climax, getting rid of *him* is the simple solution to your problem.

IF YOU USED TO REGULARLY ORGASM BUT DON'T NOW

- **Have you built a mountain out of a molehill?** Most men, at some stage in their life, hit an occasion when they can't get an erection. Those that shrug and think, *So what? I was tired*, usually have no problems next time around. Those who think the end of the world has arrived find it's the beginning of a period of impotence. Women are the same. If you don't orgasm when you expect to, consciously dismiss it as a fluke. Thinking you won't have an orgasm is a self-fulfilling prophecy.

- **Are you happy with your partner?** Is it all men or just this man? If you've recently found out he was unfaithful, your body is protesting as much as your heart is. If you generally aren't sure of him or don't trust him, you won't relax enough to climax. Mr. Nice Guy can also be an orgasm dampener. Are you frightened he'll think you're a slut if you let go of your inhibitions?

- **Are you particularly stressed or tired right now?** Your body can't orgasm because it's too busy struggling with other issues—like keeping your heart pumping or your brain from exploding. Skip the orgasm mission; take a vacation instead.

5

Sexual Etiquette

Searching for Mr. or Ms. Compatible without making a complete fool of yourself

●●●

The old sexual etiquette book's a mess—things crossed out and things added in all over the place—and quite frankly, I think it's the job of whoever invented the Pill to do the rewrite. Pre-Pill everyone knew exactly what was expected of them: no sex before marriage (and not too much after it either). Then along came that tiny, innocent-looking tablet and quicker than you could say "flower power," those nice, orderly sexual mores were scattered to the wind.

No longer watching for a bun in the oven, women got out of the kitchen and raised temperatures elsewhere. Everyone flopped around on lumpy beanbags and gazed through dope-dulled eyes at globs of wax floating about in Lava lamps, trying to remember who they *hadn't* slept with so they could experience the free love phenomenon yet again. The advent of AIDS sent most scurrying back to the relative safety of monogamous relationships, but the damage was done. The rules of old no longer existed and no one's had the foggiest as to what's normal or expected since.

Not that it's stopped us from doing it away. Most Americans start having sex before they hit sixteen (the youngest of all nationalities polled in a worldwide survey!). The majority of people in the Western world are sexual veterans by age twenty-one.[1] In fact, we're encouraged to experiment with several or lots of different partners to avoid a *new* no-no—settling down before we're "ready." If you do defy your friends and get hitched, husbands and wives are urged to go out separately and see friends solo. "Space" is the new buzzword. So we go out alone, end up with someone else, get caught, then divorced and it's back to square one, the singles bar—bruised, battered, but determined not to miss out on what everyone else seems to be having.

It's astonishing any of us bother dating at all given the minefield of potential disasters that go along with it. Because there really is *no one right answer* to today's between-the-sheets dilemmas, most of us seem to invent our own rules as we go along. But there *are* some broad guidelines emerging. Here, some hopefully helpful solutions to a selection of the most common questions asked by men and women in, or contemplating, a new relationship.

❗ *Eighty-four percent of women are not satisfied emotionally with their relationships. Twenty-six percent of single, never-married women (20–30) aren't interested in getting married. Forty-six percent of divorced women do not want to marry again.*[2]

DATING DILEMMAS
How do I tell if she's interested but just playing hard to get?

Even if she is test-running the "treat-'em-mean-keep-'em-keen" theory, she's probably giving out *some* signals. Does she look you straight in the eye when she talks to you? Does she always seem to be near you even though she pretends she'd rather not be? Do you catch her looking at you when she doesn't think you're looking at her? If you're not even close enough to put any of these theories to the test, there's no alternative but to pick up the phone and ask her out. If she's busy the night you suggest, she'll suggest another if she wants to see you. She didn't? She's not playing hard to get, she is hard to get (that is, give up now).

Is it okay if I call to ask him out? Don't men always like to be the one who conquers?

Some of the most confident women I know still won't pick up the phone to ask a man out on a date, which isn't very fair when true equality between the sexes means sharing the male pressures as well as pleasures. The first move—which means facing a possible slap-in-the-face rejection—is still usually left up to him (even though most men I know said they'd be stoked if a woman called to ask them out). So strike one for sisterhood and pick up that phone if you like someone. If he instantly thinks you must be (a) desperate to do him, (b) hard up, or (c) one of those "ball-breaking career women," it's better to find out he's a jerk *before* you waste time waxing your bikini line.

Who pays on the first date?

Whoever asked who out. If that's him, he'll usually expect to cough up the cash, but that doesn't mean you shouldn't offer. Forget the notion that letting him pay for your meal means you owe him something (sex, for instance). If during the date you start to think he *is* assuming that, feign sickness and leave. Otherwise, graciously accept his offer to pay even if you're squirming because you earn *twice* as much as he does. He's not being a chauvinist or playing power games, just doing what he thinks he should. Split the bills from then on or take turns paying. Most couples split expenses proportionate to their respective salaries. The poorer partner can even the score by doing things that require less cash (cooking dinner at home, supplying the wine, etc.).

What if I really don't like her after the first date. Do I have to take her phone number?

No, though lots of guys do because it's far easier to say "I'll call you" then disappear into the night. (Look up "bastard" in the dictionary and you'll find their picture.) If you haven't enjoyed yourself, take a deep breath and say something like, "Thanks. It's always nice meeting new people. Perhaps we'll run into each other again." She won't wait by the phone, and you won't feel guilty for making false promises.

What if he said he'd call then doesn't?

Give him a little time to gather courage (he'll often take longer to call if he's really keen) but as a general rule, the old theory that if he hasn't called within three days he isn't going to is pretty accurate. If you went out on Saturday and he hasn't called by Wednesday, he's not calling. Either accept it or call him. If you slept together and he doesn't call the next day, it's also unlikely he's going to. He hasn't had an accident, his mother's not dying in the hospital, and there's nothing wrong with your phone.

I'm too scared to make the first move in case I'm accused of date rape. How do I get her to?

Be honest. Say, "This whole date rape issue has really upset me. I'd hate to think a girl thought I was putting the moves on her when she didn't want me to. So, I'll leave it up to you to call the shots."

Any girl who doesn't think you're a sweetheart after a speech like that isn't worth dating. She probably won't unzip your jeans within the next sixty seconds, but she may give you an unmistakably passionate kiss that hints she wants more. If you think she does, ask, "Can I take things further?"

> **❗ Number of men who admit they've tried to get a girl drunk or high to get her into bed: 30 percent. Men who'll go "as far as she'll let me" on a first date: 28 percent.[3]**

How do I initiate sex with a new guy without coming on like I'm desperate?

Most men will love it if you *do* seem desperate for sex. But I identify with your dilemma. The old "I'll just slip into something more comfortable" routine goes down well in a James Bond movie, but the only time I've ever said it in real life, I meant it—and came out in sweatpants and slippers.

If you're stuck at the quick-peck-on-the-cheek stage, he's either gay, wants the two of you just to be friends, or he doesn't think he has the green light to progress any further. Are you sure you're sending the right signals? Women who are ready for sex go further than holding eye contact—they move closer, touch the guy a lot, linger over that good-night kiss.

One way of getting the message across loud and clear but in a subtle way is to ask him over to dinner (complete with candles, romantic music, and a sexy outfit). Give him a hug in the kitchen then a sexy kiss; afterward, sit next to him on the couch and put your legs on his lap. Later, initiate some passionate kissing—most men won't need more than that to take things from there.

If he still sits there with his hands shoved between his knees, behave like the liberated woman you are: tell him outright you want to make love to him. If he reacts as if your invitation is promiscuous or unladylike, he'd be a bore in bed anyhow.

When is it okay to sleep with him so he won't think I'm easy?

Plenty of people regret sleeping with someone too soon, not too many people regret waiting it out. There's no magic formula but there is a sexual double-standard. Some guys will think you're "easy" if you sleep with them after dating every weekend for six weeks, others won't judge you if you sleep with them the first night. The "norm," if indeed there is one, is probably after at least three or four dates. (But what constitutes a date? Is a Friday through to Sunday stint one or three?)

When you sleep with each other depends very much on what you want from the relationship, how well you're getting along, your sexual pattern, morals, upbringing—a whole host of issues. Don't make the decision if you've been drinking heavily and don't do it until both of you feel comfortable with each other.

Whose responsibility is it to provide the condom? Will he think I'm a slut if I do?

Both of you should always carry condoms. It's a shared responsibility. If you're single, it doesn't mean you sleep around; it means you're sensible and (like a good Girl Scout) prepared for anything. If you're married with six kids, on the Pill, and produce the condom, it's a little fishy but even then (especially then), prudent. If he gives you a withering "What sort of girl are you?" look when you grab one, put it back in your handbag, put your clothes *on*, and leave.

I start out with every intention of using a condom but it all flies out the window if I've had a few drinks and get carried away. When is the right time to bring the subject up and the condoms out?

We've all woken up the morning after and felt sick from more than just the hangover. "Did I or didn't I?" your groggy brain tries to deduce, then you find it, there in your bag, still in the wrapper.

Many people righteously carry enough condoms to solve the world's population problem; not so many actually use them. Unfortunately, a condom won't protect you against HIV (the virus that can lead to full-blown AIDS) unless it's actually on his penis. You'll be more inclined to practice what you preach if they're within reach, so keep some near the bed as well as in your purse.

When's the best time to talk about safe sex? Somewhere between the first drink and taking your clothes off. Make it a personal rule to discuss—and produce—condoms while you're still fully clothed. You'll be far less likely to get so turned-on that you conveniently forget.

Don't say, "You might have AIDS, I think we should use a condom," but "God, I'm so turned-on. I think we'd better get a condom out now because once we start, there's no way we'll want to stop." In other words, don't *suggest* using a condom, take it for granted that you will. If he tries to talk you out of it or refuses to wear one, give sex—and him—wide berth.

> **❗** *An unfaithful boyfriend can do more than break your heart—he could give you cancer. If he's playing around and not using condoms, he ups your chance of contracting a strain of HPV (human papilloma virus), which is strongly linked to cervical cancer.*

When is it acceptable not to wear condoms?

Many couples decide to get tested for AIDS when they've been going out a while, don't want to have sex with anyone else but their partner, and don't want to continue using condoms. Before being tested, make sure you haven't had unprotected sex (sex without a condom) for at least three months; the result will be inconclusive otherwise. Keep using condoms until the test results come back. If you both test negative and are committed to being monogamous, you've reduced your risks substantially.

Note I said *reduced* your risks. Unfortunately, there's no way of telling whether your partner will be faithful or if he or she will use condoms if they do have sex with someone else. (Make sure you organize alternative contraception if you don't want to get pregnant.)

I want to ask my new lover how many lovers they've had so I can determine how risky they are as a sexual partner. How do I approach it?

Are you serious? It's not worth wasting your breath. For a start, how do you know he or she is telling the truth? How do they know all their previous partners were telling the truth? Even if they have only slept with their childhood sweetheart, it doesn't mean they're not carrying HIV. You can become infected from just one encounter of unprotected sex and the risk doesn't necessarily increase with the number of partners you've had. The guy who's slept with 1000 women but used a condom every single time is safer than the man who's had unprotected sex six times. Skip the pointless chitchat; put on a condom instead.

> ❗ *Average number of sexual partners for most American men: 13.1. Average number for American women: 5.8. Global average: 9.5. The American average tops the poll at 14.3.*[4]

I have genital herpes. How do I tell my new man?

Start by reading the "Fessing up: How to tell a lover you have an STI" section. It's not that difficult. Honest.

TEN WAYS TO GUARANTEE A SECOND DATE

1. Forgive each other for being clumsy. So he knocked wine all over your new suit or your potato shot straight off the plate and flew across the restaurant. So what? You're looking for a partner not trying to impress a new boss.

2. Fill the silences. You're both fiddling with napkins and frantically searching for something, *anything*, to say. Those silences can be unnerving but (I hate to say it) women are usually better at filling them up. Put him out of his misery by making small talk; the more relaxed you are, the more comfortable he'll be. Now's not the time to launch into a history of your gynecological problems or how that bitch in the office is making your life miserable. Also steer clear of a long list of criticisms of your last boyfriend. Other than that, you don't really have to censor your conversation too much. There's not much point in pretending to be someone you're not—they're going to see the real you at some point!

3. Have a sense of humor. If he stumbles over his words, she trips, make a joke of it. Laugh your way through those difficult, awkward situations. If she's talking to you with a piece of spinach lodged charmingly between her front teeth, tell her. And don't be scared to say, "God, don't you wish we could fast forward to our second date? I'm a bit nervous."

4. Tell them they look nice: "What a great jacket," or "Wow, you look fantastic." You've both spent *hours* examining your reflection; make each other feel it was worth it.

5. Be honest. Say, "I was really pleased you called," or "I'm so glad you accepted my invitation." There's nothing wrong with admitting you like someone.

6. Help choose the venue so you can share the blame if it's awful. The service is laughable, the food inedible—does it really matter? Tell a funny story about the time you chose a restaurant that everyone hated. It's not the customer's fault if the venue doesn't live up to expectations.

7. Don't judge them too much on what they say. You're both nervous and likely to say something silly, or maybe give

impressions that aren't accurate. Don't criticize each other the first time around. Ease up a little.

8. Enjoy yourself. If you're starving, order an appetizer, main course, and dessert, even if your partner orders a salad. If you hate red wine, say so. Be yourself. It's a date, not a job interview.

9. Ask them out at the end of the night if you've enjoyed yourself. There's a weird date protocol out there that decrees you're meant to say, "I'll call you" instead of "Can I see you tomorrow?" even if you're both desperate to. If you really got along well, there's nothing to stop either of you from making arrangements there and then. Besides, it saves that post-first-date, pre-second-date panic that everyone struggles with if they've had a fantastic time. She thinks, "He's far too attractive/intelligent/cool to want to see me again." He thinks, "She's figured out I'm not rich or sophisticated—especially since I dribbled spaghetti down my chin/left a meager tip/spilled the wine." Deal with it by making the date on the spot.

10. Don't finish the evening with sex. Sometimes it seems to be and is the natural thing to do. If this applies to you, you'll know it. Most of the time, though, it's a mistake. If you're desperately attracted to each other and getting along well, what's the rush?

CASUAL SEX

We don't always have sex with people we love. Sometimes we'll quite happily do it with someone we don't even want to spend a whole day with. Why? Because we can lust after someone without necessarily wanting to get involved. While one- (or two- or three-) night stands aren't terribly satisfying long-term, sometimes, for a number of reasons, sex without romantic involvement is all you want. If you're in that head space right now, these are a few of the etiquette trouble spots you may have to negotiate.

If I'm only interested in having sex, should I say something *before* sleeping with them?

Yes. It's wholly unfair, disrespectful, and unforgivable to whisper sweet nothings that really are nothings. As you're having dinner or drinks say, "Look, I thought you should know I've just come out of a long-term relationship/I'm really busy at work right now, and I'm not interested in a serious relationship. I think you're gorgeous and I'd love to have fun with you but if you're looking for more, I'm the wrong person." If you end up in bed together after that, fine. You both knew the score.

Whose place should we go back to?

If you're a guy, it probably doesn't matter. If you're a girl, it matters a whole lot. Don't even think about letting some guy you've just met at a bar or a nightclub take you home to his place, even if you *do* fully intend to have sex. He might seem harmless but you can't judge by appearances or by chatting to him for a few hours if someone's violent or psychologically unstable. (If you're tempted, just remember that serial killer Ted Bundy was described by all who knew him socially as "a nice guy.") If you take him back to your place, make sure your roommate is home and alerted. Also remember he now knows where you live. If you check into a hotel or do go back to his place, call a friend first and leave the address and phone number. Ask them to call you in half an hour to make sure everything is okay.

! *Will your relationship survive? A crucial giveaway is how positively you both recall your early times together. In one study, researchers had a 100 percent success rate predicting who would split three years later, based solely on negative reminisces.[5]*

What if I don't want them to stay the night? How do I leave without offending them? Somehow, I always end up cooking breakfast for people just to be polite.

Regardless of whether you're talking about a one-night stand or the future father or mother of your babies, it's rude to jump up and into your clothes before the sheets have even settled. If you're at their place, a good way to work up to leaving is to suggest a nightcap (a drink or a cup of coffee). Then, get up and get dressed while they're making it and move into the living room. Even if you drink it in bed, it's still a pretty easy way to break the mood. When you've finished, just yawn and casually say, "I should be going." If they ask you to stay, say "I'd love to, but I have a huge day tomorrow and really need some sleep." If you *do* want to see them again, you can follow it through with, "But on Friday night, I'd love to stay over." If someone's settling into *your* bed, try the nightcap trick again (dressed, in the living room). They really have no choice but to put their clothes on and join you. If they still don't get the hint say, "My roommate and I have an arrangement that no one sleeps over," or "I'm really sorry. I can never sleep with someone in my bed and I have to be up really early. Can I call you a cab?"

What if I'd like to see him/her again for sex but don't really want a relationship?

If you were honest *before* you got into bed, all you need to do is call. If you weren't, you'll need to say something like, "That was fantastic and I'd love to do it again but I think I should tell you I'm not interested in anything serious. Are you happy just with a casual relationship?"

My best male friend and I are both single and have high libidos yet neither of us wants to sleep around. I think the ideal solution is to sleep with each other as friends until one or both of us gets involved. What do you think?

It can be the very best or the worst idea you've ever come up with. I know one couple who carried it off successfully but I suspect they were the exception to the rule. They were both able to separate sex from love and neither had ulterior motives. I know of another couple who now don't speak because of it. It's incredibly difficult to sleep with someone regularly and not become emotionally attached. After all, you already like the person as a friend, so if you also have great sex it suddenly seems *logical* to become a couple. Sometimes people do. Other times, one wants to, the other doesn't and "my friend Mary" becomes "that heartless bitch." Is it worth risking the friendship?

If I always use condoms, do my partners need to know if I have more than one lover?

Yes, it's called being honest. But once you've made it clear that the relationship is not monogamous, there's no need to dwell on it. They don't need to know when you've slept with someone else or who the person was. So long as they're aware it's not an exclusive relationship, it's really none of their business.

It's over, but I'd like to be friends. Does that ever work?

Yes. Many ex-lovers are now very special friends, but there are a few factors common to all these friendships. It usually doesn't work if one of you is still in love with the other, if the trust between you was broken (by an affair, for instance), or if the breakup was particularly nasty. It works best if the split was mutual, you live close by or share lots of mutual friends (so it's easy to see each other), you've got common interests and *no longer want to be a couple*. That's the magic ingredient: if one of you is secretly hoping the friendship will lead to you getting back together, it can only end in more tears.

I'm pregnant, but have only been going out with my boyfriend for a few months. While the relationship is nice, it's not serious, and I fully intend to have an abortion. Do I have to tell him?

I would. Not only is it the decent thing to do, he has a right to know for fertility reasons. If he has trouble fathering a child later on, it may help to know he was fertile at some point. Besides, a pregnancy—even an unwanted one—involves two people. Both of you had sex, both knew the risks. He doesn't have the right to tell you what to do about the pregnancy but he does have the right to know he's fathered a child. You're concerned he'll force you into keeping the baby? Play your cards close to the vest. Tell him you're pregnant and thinking about having an abortion, calmly explaining the reasons why you don't want to keep the baby. If he starts threatening you, tell him you'll think about what he's had to say, then leave. Make your appointment with a clinic or your doctor as soon as possible and don't tell him where or when. Legally, he can't stop you, but it could be messy if he turns up.

Why do I only find "bad boys" sexually attractive? I've been out with nice ones but they leave me cold.

Women who like bad boys fall into two categories. There are girls who wouldn't dream of settling down with one but thoroughly enjoy the sex. Then there are women who only go out with bad boys and spend most of the time miserable because they desperately want these men to love them. Several "popular" psychological theories attempt to explain both cases.

If you fall into the first category, I bet you describe your family and childhood as "eccentric." Think about it. What do bad guys give you that good guys don't? Excitement. Drama. (They can only cause you heartache if you let them.) Now think back to your childhood. Would you describe it as quiet, peaceful, serene? *Are you kidding?* I can hear you say. You're attracted to the drama of bad-boy relationships because you're re-creating what is familiar. If home was frenetic—your parents had strong personalities and argued constantly, one (or both) had an affair, or you had a brother or sister whose antics turned the house into something resembling the set of a soap opera—then you were brought up to believe that constant tension is normal. It's not, and if you're only treating bad boys as a boy toy, you've already figured that out.

If you're in the second category, the tension at home was probably more sinister than exciting. Maybe your parents fought viciously, ignored you, or perhaps there was violence or even abuse. Our parents' relationship is often what we base our relationships on: subconsciously, we try to re-create them. If you have a history of always hooking up to guys who are bad for you, make an appointment to see a good therapist, even if you don't identify with *any* of the theories listed here.

SEX FOR SEX'S SAKE: THE RULES

If you've just come out of a long-term relationship (and can't bear to dive into another), haven't got time for a love affair because your career is all-consuming, or have simply met someone who makes you boil below the belt but leaves you cold above, a lust affair could be *just* what the sex therapist ordered.

Men have been having sex affairs since God said, "Let there be light" (even if their partners didn't realize). Now, lots of confident girls with raging libidos and a guilt-free attitude are also able to separate sex from love. They're not searching for Mr. Right or even a commitment for a date on Saturday night: all they want is good sex and a good time.

> **Women with the highest education report having the greatest number of sex partners—twice as many as any other group of women—as well as the most sexual experience before marriage.**[6]

If that's you, go for it! But be careful, not just with your sexual health and personal safety but with your emotional health as well. Just because there's no commitment to be monogamous doesn't mean either of you has the right to treat the other badly. If you're going to indulge, here are the rules:

- **Refuse to feel guilty.** If you suffer even the faintest twinge of guilt, sex-only affairs aren't for you. If you find you're waking up feeling depressed or bad about yourself, don't do it again. People in casual relationships are exploiting each other—which is fine as long as that's what they both want. Just remember there's a huge difference between having sex and making love. He's not going to send flowers, she's not going to call to say good night. So there's no reason to pretend you "don't usually do this sort of thing," even if you don't. If he thinks you're a bit easy, who cares?
- **Use condoms every single time.** If I have to explain why, you're not a candidate.
- **Use backup contraception.** Again, for obvious reasons.
- **Do it for the right reasons.** Casual sex may make you feel sexy, attractive, and desirable, but it won't make you feel special or loved. If you're having sex just to get the hug at the end, stop kidding yourself. Lust affairs are conducted for sheer pleasure. Don't sleep with someone simply to reaffirm your attractiveness.

- **Let go of any inhibitions.** A lot of women find they're much less inhibited with a guy they don't care about. After all, does it matter if he thinks you're fat or kinky? If you've always wanted to have someone tie you up and lick whipped cream off your body, this is your man.
- **Don't broadcast your affairs.** Some women will brand you just as readily as some men will. It's your business, not theirs.
- **Stay in control by being honest with each other.** Establish up front that you want uncomplicated sex and not a relationship. If you feel yourself falling for this person, let him or her know. They might feel the same. If they don't, stop seeing them and find someone else. Great sex isn't worth a broken heart.
- **Be nice to each other.** He's got a body that makes you wet just looking at it? Tell him. She's so erotic, you're convinced she'll be in your fantasies forever? Ditto. Compliments don't equal commitment.
- **Pick your partners carefully.** If you feel like sex and don't meet someone who measures up, go home and masturbate instead. Choose partners who you like and who make you feel good about yourself. Other people's husbands, wives, girlfriends, and boyfriends are off-limits; and don't sleep with friends of friends unless you can cope with the rumor mill.
- **If you're female, don't put yourself in risky situations.** Be super-safety conscious and trust your gut reactions. If you feel it's wrong and the guy's a bit sketchy, don't do it. It's safer to take him back to your place (with a roommate home and in the next room) than it is to go back to his. If you've seen him a few times and trust him enough to go to his place, leave his address and phone number with someone *you* trust.

THE "I AM WHO I GO OUT WITH" TRAP

Because women are naturally caring and nurturing, there's a tendency for some to get "lost" in relationships. Instead of going out, they *merge* with their boyfriends, losing their individuality in the process. This is not healthy.

It's easy to tell if you fit into the "women who love too much" category. Did you become a sports nut even though you *hate* football, just because your last boyfriend was one? Did you ditch the suits for loose dresses and grow your hair out when you went out with the crunchy type? Are you prepared to do just about anything to make him happy, even if it means forcing down steak and a potato when you'd really rather have pasta and a salad? Given time, you'll spend so much of your life pleasing your boyfriends, you'll completely forget what pleases *you*. You become what you think they want you to be—and that's dangerous.

The fact is, if you lie down like a doormat, people will walk over you. *You* think you're being supportive and easygoing, he thinks you're a pushover and treats you like one. Your self-esteem plummets when he loses respect, and you find yourself putting up with inexcusable behavior just because you're now too frightened and vulnerable to be alone. Don't let yourself get to this point. The more you retain your individuality—your friends, your career, a life *apart* from him—the more successful and satisfying your relationship will be. Men respect confident women. He can't treat you like dirt if you don't let him.

SECOND-TIME ROUND

Relationship breakups *hurt*. It doesn't matter who dumped who, whether you're heartbroken or relieved that it's over, the end of any serious relationship means a dream is shattered. You loved each other once, you probably thought it would last forever, now it's over. The most confident person is plagued by insecurities for at least a little while afterward—and if you aren't, you should be.

There's a certain amount of "cleaning up" that's necessary after a serious split. You may need to sift through any accusations thrown at you—some trivial (Is my nose really too big?), some serious (Do I have a problem with commitment? Am I a good mother/father?). You also need to reestablish yourself as "one" rather than part of a couple. This takes time. Rush through the recovery process—kid yourself you're over it and ready to start a new relationship too soon—and you'll carry the baggage from the old one all your life.

The first few months will be painful—maybe it'll take years for the sharp pain to recede to a dull ache—but eventually you *will* wake up one morning and forget to be miserable. It's usually around this time that the blinders fall off and the world suddenly seems full of gorgeous, yummy (*Gosh! Check that out!*) people. Your libido kicks back in with a vengeance and hovers dangerously high. You start masturbating like crazy and even the fat little man at the newsstand or the woman pushing the stroller in the supermarket seems possible dating material. Congratulations! Months ago, you never would have thought it possible but you're not only ready to date again, you're ready for sex, maybe even another relationship! Here's a few of the common dilemmas second-time-arounders have to deal with.

I split from my husband six months ago. My girlfriends have dragged me out to singles places a few times but everything's changed. I don't know the rules anymore, sex seems different—and I feel lost.

I remember walking past a particularly dreadful singles bar one night, arm-in-arm with my husband, thinking, "Thank God I don't have to do *that* again." A few years later, we split and (*groan!*) there I was, back on the dating scene. The first few times I went out, I felt truly awful. I'd forgotten how to do all that silly get-to-know-you talk and everyone seemed younger, prettier, and more together than I was. It felt different because I was different. Premarriage, I was the quintessential nightclub queen: capable of chatting up men, downing a gin and tonic, smoking a cigarette, and keeping an eye on my friend's handbag, all while I was on the dance floor. Post breakup, I felt about as groovy as the shiny disco balls that had magically disappeared from the ceiling of every nightclub.

Things appear to change fast in dating land but, believe me, it's mostly surface stuff. Your girlfriends could write you a long list of the "new rules for the 90s" but if you looked closely you'd see they're just rewritten versions of the rules you already know. The only thing that has changed is the danger factor. If last time round you feared getting herpes, this time you're dealing with AIDS. The only real new rule is this: you *must* use condoms.

You feel misplaced not because the scene has changed, but because you have. It's like tackling that previously mastered tricky soufflé again when you haven't made it for years. You're apprehensive because you're out of practice. Being single is great fun when you're feeling fabulous, not so great when you're vulnerable—and everyone is after a breakup. The prospect of finding a partner amongst all those strangers seems about as likely as finding a match to half the dinner service you're now left with. Do yourself a favor and avoid the pickup places for a while. Avoid them permanently if you like. Stick to parties and dinner parties with friends or nights out at restaurants until you feel a little more in control.

How soon is too soon to take a new lover?

It's probably not a good idea to bring the girl you picked up at a nightclub to a friend's dinner party the week after you split from your wife, but it's really up to *you* to decide when you're ready. Just be aware of your real motivations. Lots of people who quickly jump feet first into a new relationship are really just wanting a warm body in their now cold bed, trying to ease the pain or loneliness. If that helps you get through and your new partner is aware of it, fine, but you still have to confront the issues, and this is probably best done alone.

When you date again depends on how long you were in your previous relationship, how serious it was, and the nature of the breakup. It takes some people years to get over those awful feelings of hurt, vulnerability, pain, or anger. Others find they did their grieving while still in the relationship—it ended emotionally years before they physically moved out—and are ready to date within weeks.

If the split was sudden, bitter, and painful, you'll probably want to shut the door and hide away for a while. If you've got kids, you'll need to devote time to helping them get over the split. In other words, there's no acceptable time frame that applies to everyone.

Also recognize that there's a difference between taking a lover and getting involved again. Every person you go out with doesn't have to be a prospective long-term replacement. If you meet someone who's fun, who you can rediscover sex with but not much else, great! Don't feel guilty, just enjoy.

Another word of advice: you've probably been leaning heavily on your friends and family during the split-up, letting them know how you feel at every waking moment. If you're ready to have sex again, you're ready to wean yourself and stand on your own two feet. By all means, have a laugh with a pal or a girlfriend over what you've been up to but don't feel obliged to confide all the intimate details. You don't need their permission. You're an adult.

I can't imagine stripping naked in front of a total stranger. I'd be far too embarrassed. My body was great the last time I was dating, but now I'm older and I've had a child.

I don't think too many people *would* feel comfortable stripping naked in front of a total stranger! But the man you *want* to take your clothes off for won't be. Forget any preconceived notions you have about having to climb into bed on date three. Have sex when you feel ready—when you know, trust, and feel comfortable enough to sleep with him without being judged. Unless you're planning on dating a sixteen-year-old supermodel, your new lover's body isn't going to be perfect, either. While you're frantically sucking in your stomach or worrying about how big your butt is, he's nervous the light's hitting that not-so-well-concealed bald spot and that the arms you're grabbing on to aren't as muscular as your ex's were.

Accepting that our bodies age is just another icky fact of life. Eat well, exercise often, dress to conceal your faults, and make the most of what you've got, then relax about the rest. Besides, would you swap that gorgeous child of yours for your previously flat tummy? Not in a million years!

My old partner knew my body inside out. I don't know if I can be bothered teaching someone all over again.

Oh, I agree. How boring (yawn)! What an absolute pain in the rear to have some gorgeous new lover rediscover all your known sensitive spots (and some you never knew you had). How tedious to have to guide his or her deliciously sexy tongue to all the right places. How positively awful to have to spend all day in bed, fueled by champagne and oysters, taking this new angel on a guided tour of your body. I'm with you—it must be dreadful to have to say "Oh yes, that's it, right there" . . . get my point?

I was ho-hum about sex with my husband, now I can't get enough of it with my new lover. The ironic thing is, technically, my husband was probably better in bed. I feel guilty, like maybe if I'd tried harder with him, we wouldn't have split.

I bet you *did* try hard with your husband, at least at some point. But there's something decidedly unsexy about being married. We "live in sin" as lovers, but once that band of gold's slipped on our fingers, we become "husband and wife"—respectable people granted official permission by society to have sex. No wonder lots of people don't want to! Spending all Sunday in bed making love somehow seems frivolous when you're married (and really should be working on that renovation). Add to that problems in the relationship, which you obviously had or you wouldn't have split, and you can start to see why sex maybe wasn't that wonderful.

You can't have great sex with a long-term partner unless your relationship's also great. You broke up for a reason. Whatever that reason was, it had to affect your sex life somehow. Sex with your new lover is wonderful because he's not your husband and you're not struggling with relationship problems. Plus he's new (anything new always seems more exciting) and, I bet, more passionate. Lust and enthusiasm can beat the hell out of technical skills (though it's always nice to get all three). Stop feeling guilty. Even if you did make some mistakes, it's over. Let go of the past and let yourself enjoy what sounds like an enviable sex life with your new man.

I've just started dating again and a guy twelve years younger than me has asked me out. I like him but fear he sees me as a desperate, older woman.

I'll let you in on a secret: the single, older woman—yesterday's "old maid"—magically transformed herself into the new sex goddess while you were playing house. There are lots of young men out there who've discovered that dating an attractive, well-preserved older woman can be a lot more fun than seeing someone who still works a shift at McDonald's. The guy who asked you out sees you as confident, experienced, and worldly. He's hoping like hell you'll sleep with him because he's heard (quite rightly) that older women take control in bed, are more sexually adventurous, less inhibited, and more likely to let him lie back and enjoy for a change. Go out with him. Turn all his fantasies into reality. Enjoy him as an ego-boosting, marvelous affair. He probably won't be sitting next to you in a rocking chair when you're sixty, but he could be Mr. Right for now.

What do I tell my kids when I meet someone? When should they meet him? Can he *ever* stay over?

It all depends on how old your children are, when you split, how well they're coping with it, their personalities, their relationship with the estranged spouse, the person you're dating, and how serious your relationship is. Phew! For some time after the breakup, your children will probably be more clingy than usual. They'll be feeling as insecure as you are and worried you'll "abandon" them as well. They've only seen you act romantically with Daddy or Mommy and seeing you hold hands or kiss someone else will be upsetting initially—especially if they're secretly hoping for a reunion (and they nearly always are).

Personally, I wouldn't tell them about, or introduce them to, people who you know aren't going to be long-term material. What's the point? Tell them you're going out to have fun with some friends and let them wreak havoc on the baby-sitter. Once you decide you've met someone special, introduce your new partner the same way you would any friend. Get him to pick you up from home initially, then maybe invite him for dinner with other friends. Don't be overtly affectionate if they seem upset. Give them time to get used to the person as a friend rather than a father substitute.

Accept reality. You can control kids only to a point. Tell them it's forbidden to wander into your room late at night and they'll still wrap that little hand around the doorknob and do it. ("Are you hurt, Mommy? Why are you groaning?") Making out in the kitchen where they can see you or letting your lover sleep over when they're still at the stage of crying themselves to sleep over the loss of a parent isn't right. Take it slow. You know your children; you'll know when they're ready to accept that you have a lover. Don't force a new person down their throat and insist they like him—or her—but don't let them dictate your life, either. Your kids are important, but your happiness is equally so.

What if my children disapprove of who I'm going out with?

They probably don't dislike the person you've chosen, just resent sharing you and, of course, would prefer you to be back with their *real* mom or dad. They're hurting and highly vulnerable after the split. One person has left them so they want all your attention and if you're giving it to someone else, they feel threatened all over again. Reassure them until you're blue in the face, load them up with so much affection, they *can't* feel left out. Make them feel involved when your new lover is around and insist he or she treats them with respect and kindness (even if they are being difficult little buggers). Explain that this person won't replace Mommy or Daddy but that you enjoy their company. It's especially easy for teenage kids to sit in moral judgment of what you're doing—remember

> **!** *Women spend their 20s wanting a caring, sharing man in bed—just when men are only interested in sex, say psychologists. The opposite happens in our 30s. Women become more sexually adventurous and insatiable, men turn sensitive. A good argument to match older women with younger men.[8]*

how superior *you* used to feel at fifteen? Let them know you love them desperately, but this person also makes you happy.

What if his or her kids don't like me?
You can't make children like you. They'll be especially hostile if you try too hard or (God forbid) try to become a replacement for the parent who's left. Be nice, be kind, spoil them a little. Talk to them even if they ignore you. Refuse to get angry if they treat you badly. Ask your partner if there's anything you do that upsets them, and for hints on how to win them over. She or he should also be making an effort to ease the situation on your behalf. If, in time, they're still hostile, there's nothing much you can do but live with it or move on.

Do I have to tell every new lover I've got kids? I find it turns guys off.
Not if it's just for sex, but otherwise why not? Are you going to lock them in the attic whenever he's around? Remove all evidence (just try, bet you can't do it) every time he visits? It's unrealistic and illogical. If your new lover's going to turn white and start shaking because you tell him straight off you've got a child, he's going to run *screaming* into the sunset when you do tell him later, feeling (understandably) duped. And it'll hurt you a lot more then. You come as part of a package—you and your kids. If your lover can't accept that, it's *his or her* problem. What are you going to do? Give them away to charity?

How do I tell if I've fallen for my new lover out of fear of being alone? I don't feel I can trust my feelings. What's this I've heard about "transition lovers"?
If you feel you can't trust your feelings, you can't. You're at the stage where you're ready to go out with someone but probably not at the point where you want to (or should) commit. You won't know if your feelings are real until you feel confident again, happy with your own company and capable of making it alone; in other words, when you're at the point where, while you might *want* a relationship, you don't *need* one. Handle the situation in the

meantime by letting your new partner know you're still working through things and while you think they're fantastic, you're a little unsure of your feelings. Don't let anyone pressure you into committing before you're ready.

Transition lovers is a term some psychologists use to describe the first relationship after a big split. Often, we hook up with people before we're really ready, and while we might *think* we're madly in love with them, subconsciously we're using them to get over insecurities and to fill the well of loneliness left by our last relationship. It's not until we feel more ourselves that we realize we don't love them after all. This doesn't

> **Come on guys! According to Shere Hite, 72 percent of women say they're the ones who are forced to bring up problems that need talking through. Sixty-three percent of men prefer to solve arguments by (you guessed it!) having sex.[9]**

mean *all* relationships that happen right after the split will end; some people do find a new partner quickly and stay with that person, happily, forever.

My new girlfriend has the ex-husband from hell. I'm sick of hearing about him and he's now causing problems with us.

Your girlfriend's marriage is finished. *Kaput.* There's obviously no chance of friendship so her ex should be out of her life completely if they're divorced and don't have kids. If they do, it's not an amicable split, so she should see him only when he picks the kids up or drops them off. Better still, she should arrange for him to pick them up from a sympathetic friend's place. In other words, if he's still causing her trouble a year or years down the track, she's letting him—probably because she feels guilty. If he's bitter, chances are she's the one who left. She figures if he treats her badly, it's her punishment for walking out. Tell her you're sick of talking about him and she needs to let go, to get him out of her life and get on with hers. If she can't, pack her off to a good counselor for some therapy or tell her you're not interested in continuing the relationship until she's sorted out the problem.

FIRST-TIME SEX AFTER A LONG-TERM LOVER

You've been out to every restaurant in town, they've been to your place, you've been to theirs, and now it's crunch time. Which is why you're in the bathroom, ostensibly brushing your teeth (for the last twenty minutes), while your about-to-be-lover waits in the bedroom, wondering if you have any gums left. *Don't be ridiculous*, you lecture yourself in the mirror, *You've had sex hundreds, probably thousands of times before. Yeah*, says another little voice, *but with the same person for the last ten years.*

First-time sex with a new lover, after years with an old one, *is* heart-thumping stuff. Part of you can't wait to give it a whirl (no prizes for guessing *which* part) but your brain would stay happily celibate for another 100 years to avoid any embarrassment. But come out of that bathroom you must (the window's usually far too small to escape from). Just keep the following points in mind.

- **Don't panic if you feel as nervous as a virgin.** In a sense, it is like losing your virginity all over again. Don't fall into the same trap you did back then and expect that it's going to be wonderful. You've fantasized about it, so have they, and reality hasn't got a hope in hell of matching expectations.

- **Admit you are nervous.** If the thought of this lover gazing at your flesh makes you faint, leave your underwear on and slip under the sheets. Say, "I haven't had sex with anyone but Martha/Martin for years. I feel like a teenager." It'll ease the tension for both of you. You're not the only one who's under pressure. Your new lover feels they have to at least measure up to the standard set by your ex—and that's pretty difficult when your old lover's a few hundred practice runs ahead of them.

- **Stick to the basics.** If you're really nervous, this is one situation where I advocate just getting through. Kiss, have some foreplay, do the deed. Get it over with, let most of your anxieties evaporate, *then* you can concentrate on getting to know each other properly (and don't be surprised if after all that fuss, you're actually ready for a repeat within the next half hour).

- **If it's awful, admit it and laugh.** Say, "That was *such* a disaster because we were so nervous. But now it's out of the way we can relax and really get to know each other sexually." It's not a big deal if she didn't lubricate or orgasm or if he couldn't get an erection, lost it, or came too quickly. It doesn't mean you're not compatible in bed. It doesn't mean you should have stuck it out with your ex. It just means you don't know each other's bodies, desires, or needs yet.

- **Accept that you may feel sad afterward.** For many people, especially women, sleeping with someone new marks the true ending of the previous relationship. It'll hit you like a lightning bolt: My God, it really is over. Even if you broke out the champagne when your ex left, don't be surprised if you have a post-coital grief attack. Cry, *sob* if you must, but don't shut your new lover out. If you're open and explain your emotions, this person should understand. Remember, an ending is often the glorious beginning of something even better.

6

Contraception and STIs

Avoiding pregnancy and the lumps, bumps, and
things that itch in the night

• •

Sex can give us the most pleasurable moments of our life—and
the most painful. Getting pregnant by the waiter in Greece who
did more than lay your table or discovering a T-shirt wasn't the
only thing your ex left behind are both very real consequences of
not treating sex with the respect it demands. Don't kid yourself:
having sex can be dangerous. Terminating an unwanted pregnancy
is not fun. Getting very, very sick from a sexually transmitted infection (STI) is not fun. Dying from AIDS isn't ever on the top of
our "Things I want to do this year" list. And if you're not careful,
all can happen to *you*, no matter how "nice" you are.

Have I put you off sex for life? If you're not prepared to take
the associated risks seriously, I truly hope I have. But the fact is,
most of the "nasties" of sex can be avoided. With all the contraceptive choices available today, you'd have to be a complete dud
not to find a method that suits both you and your partner. That
removes the pregnancy risk immediately. Condoms (used properly
and every single time) significantly reduce the risk of sexually transmitted infection. Add a good dollop of common sense and sex
education and your chances of catching one drop to almost zero.
At the risk of sounding like your mother, reading this chapter will
not only save you heartache, it could save your life.

HOW NOT TO GET PREGNANT

The ideal contraceptive is 100 percent effective, easy to use, and economical—with no known side effects. Unfortunately it hasn't been invented yet. But here's the good news: not only are traditional methods of contraception being constantly improved, there's some new kids on the contraceptive block that you may never have heard of. So while there's no such thing as a *perfect* contraceptive, for most women there's one that comes pretty damn close! This is a list of the latest and greatest contraception around, to help you find a hassle-free method for your personality, lifestyle, and relationship. Since most women take responsibility for contraception, I've devoted this section to them. I've listed the prices for contraception as a comparative guide only. They were correct at the time of publication but may increase over time.

The symptothermal method

It sounds complicated, and it is, but if you're the "herbal" type—drink green tea, own CDs of whales singing, and recycle *everything* (including what the cat threw up on the carpet)—this could be the method for you. It's totally natural and completely cost-free but, alas, only for the truly dedicated: "fussy," "messy," and "time-consuming" are adjectives that immediately spring to mind.

How it works

The symptothermal technique aims to pinpoint ovulation (the most likely time to get pregnant) by reading the body's signals. You use a combination of the calendar, mucus, and temperature methods to work out what days to avoid intercourse. By combining the three natural methods, you up the effectiveness rate considerably.

The calendar method: Ovulatory cycles are usually around twenty-eight days. It is assumed that ovulation takes place mid-cycle, that the released egg will die after twenty-four hours, and that sperm live for no longer than three to five days. Note I said *assumed*. One of the problems with this method is that everyone's body behaves differently. To be totally accurate, you should write down when you start and finish your periods for at least six months (eight to twelve if possible) to work out your own personal menstrual cycle. It's then a matter of counting up the number of days between each period and doing some rather complicated math. If you're truly devoted, invest in a book detailing the Billings method (the name of the people who formulated it). It's far too complex to summarize here—and not terribly reliable even if you do master it.

The temperature method: There's a minute increase in our body temperature following ovulation (in the range of 0.36 to 1.08 degrees Fahrenheit). The theory is that by taking your temperature daily with a thermometer (either in your mouth or vagina), you'll know when ovulation has occurred and shouldn't have sex for three days after your temperature has risen.

The mucus method: Around ovulation time, vaginal mucus (the clear or whitish discharge that comes out between periods) is clearer and thinner; after ovulation has occurred it becomes sticky and tacky and stretches like chewing gum. Recording changes in your mucus, again over a period of months, helps pinpoint when in your cycle you tend to ovulate. Some months, the mucus may change from clear to tacky on day 14 (day 1 is the first day of your period), others on day 18. If a pattern forms, you can get a rough idea of when ovulation usually occurs (and avoid sex around those days in the future). It's best to test mucus at night, just before you go to bed.

What's good about it
By combining three natural methods, you up the effectiveness rate considerably. It's natural and involves no chemicals or equipment.

The bad news
It requires a lot of effort and it's horrifyingly easy to miscalculate. The method relies rather optimistically on ovaries and sperm behaving in a predictable manner; infections, viruses, and other health problems can cause false readings for both temperature and mucus.

Best suited to
Long-term couples trying to space a family.

Protection against HIV and STIs
None.

The failure rate
The theoretical failure rate is 2 to 5 percent but the actual failure rate is more like 15 to 20 percent.

Do I need to see a doctor?
No, but you might like to buy a few books on the subject so you know exactly what you're doing.

How easy is it to use?
It's complicated.

Is it expensive?
The price of a thermometer.

How enthusiastic will he be about it?
If you're long-term and it doesn't matter if you have "an accident," very. Sex is totally natural, and he doesn't have to do a thing.

The withdrawal method
How it works
You probably used this method when you were a teenager. He removes his penis from your vagina before ejaculation (coming), so there's no sperm inside you and little chance of you getting pregnant. Preejaculatory fluid (the stuff that comes out before he orgasms) does contain some sperm, but it's unlikely to cause pregnancy. This method requires strong self-control on his part and many couples find it emotionally and physically unsatisfying, for obvious reasons.

What's good about it
If he's experienced, it can be quite a successful method of contraception. It's natural, has no side effects, and costs nothing.

The bad news
You need to trust your partner implicitly to withdraw at the right time.

Best suited to
Couples in long-term relationships who could cope with an unexpected pregnancy.

Protection against HIV and STIs
None.

The failure rate
It depends on whether he withdraws every single time. Family planners put the failure figure at once every four years with experienced couples.

Do I need to see a doctor?
No.

How easy is it to use?
There's no effort required on your part.

Is it expensive?
It's free.

How enthusiastic will he be?
He may feel "robbed" of the grand *finale* of orgasming inside you. Good self-discipline on his part is a must.

The condom
Condoms, as well as diaphragms and cervical caps, prevent pregnancy by providing a physical barrier between the sperm and egg. Each is an ideal alternative if you don't want to, or can't, take the Pill and are prepared to do a little preplanning.

❗ **Number of condoms sold by a popular bicoastal condom shop per month: upwards of 30,000. Number of different varieties stocked: 300.[1]**

For maximum effectiveness when using a condom, use a spermicide as well—possibly one containing the purported AIDS-fighter, Nonoxynol-9. (In the laboratory, Nonoxynol-9 had some effect against the HIV virus but no one knows if it's equally effective in the human body.[2] Still, there's no harm in hedging your bets!) You can buy spermicides from any pharmacy.

How it works
The condom was virtually ignored when the Pill appeared on the scene; now it's back in vogue because of AIDS. A very thin but

strong latex (rubber) sheath, it's designed to fit over his erect penis and catch the sperm in a pocket at the tip. The main complaint? Intercourse doesn't feel as pleasurable. For this reason, scientists are currently researching a plastic condom that conducts heat more efficiently and feels much more like the "real thing." A condom with a looser end (which apparently feels better for him) is also in the trial stages.

What's good about it

It's a great germ stopper. Not only does it stop sperm, it helps prevent you catching viruses like HIV (which can lead to AIDS) as well as blocking bacteria that carry other nasties like gonorrhea.

The bad news

Condoms only protect you against pregnancy and diseases if they're used properly, each and every time you have sex, and if they don't break. Breakages and tears are usually your fault not "the bloody manufacturer." If you haven't put the condom on properly and squeezed the air out of the end tip, an air pocket can form that heats up (as you two do) and expands during intercourse, causing the condom to burst. Use plenty of water-based lubricants like K-Y to prevent splitting but avoid oil-based lubricants like baby oil and Vaseline, which can weaken the latex.

Best suited to

Couples prepared to wear a condom every single time they have intercourse and put up with a decrease of sensation; anyone who's single and planning on having more than one sexual partner.

"It was the first guy I'd ever slept with purely for sex. We used a condom but he obviously didn't put it on properly because it kept sliding off. We put on a new one but when he withdrew, found it had a huge tear in it. I was scared stupid. It wouldn't have been so bad with a boyfriend but a guy I didn't know and sure as hell didn't want a baby with? I got the Morning After Pill and a checkup for STIs that week, then waited three months for an AIDS test. Now I provide the condom, I put it on and make sure we use lubricant."

Jenny, 26, secretary

Protection against HIV and STIs

Condoms will protect you against HIV if you use them each and every time you have sex and they don't break. As HIV can be present in preejaculatory fluid, you must put the condom on before any kind of penetration and before it even touches your genitals.

> "Condoms. I hate them. I can't stand them. I use them for safety but can't wait to get to the point where we're serious, can get tested and dispense with the damn things."
>
> Phillip, 27, promotions manager

The failure rate

Somewhere between 1 percent and 60 percent because it all depends on how often they're used and how; 30 percent is probably a realistic figure.

Do I need to see a doctor?

No.

How easy is it to use?

Some couples complain that condoms interrupt the "flow" because they have to stop sex to put them on. But it can become part of foreplay if *you* put it on for him (go on, at least try to do it with your mouth); besides, a seasoned condom user needs only a few seconds to prepare.

Is it expensive?

Around $5 to $10 for a pack of twelve, one-use only, depending on the brand and whether it's prelubricated or has spermicide. A tube of spermicide costs between $8 and $17.

How enthusiastic will he be?

Probably not very. You've heard the jokes (it feels like having sex with a raincoat on).

HOW TO USE A CONDOM

1. Be careful when you're unwrapping it. Don't rip the packet open with abandon (and don't even think about doing it with your teeth). Rings and fingernails can snag and while condoms are tough, they're not *that* tough.
2. Wait until he's erect. Put the condom on *before* the penis touches the vagina but only when he's hard.
3. Leave the condom unrolled and squeeze the tip to get rid of any air. Hold it against the tip of the penis, then . . .
4. Gently unroll the condom, all the way down to the base of the penis. Smooth out any air bubbles once it's on. Apply some extra *water-based* lubricant on the outside of the condom even if it's been prelubricated.
5. Have fun—guilt-free!
6. Withdraw the penis *immediately* after ejaculation while it's still erect. One of you should hold the condom firm at the base of the penis while he withdraws, to stop it slipping off or any sperm leaking out.
7. Point the penis downward and slip the condom off carefully.
8. Remember you can only use a condom once. If you want to have sex again, get him to wash his penis and use a new one.
9. Tie a knot in the used condom, wrap it in paper, and put it in the trash. Don't flush it down the toilet—it's not biodegradable. Do you enjoy catching your toes on used condoms while walking on your local beach?
10. Score full marks for putting it on with your mouth. If you can cope with the taste, unwrap it and place it (unrolled) on the top of your tongue, the open end facing upward. The first time, cheat and use your fingers to position it over the penis head, then use your tongue and mouth to unroll it.

The female condom (femcondom)
How it works
It appeared amidst a fanfare of publicity but there is currently only one brand on the market. A soft, loose-fitting plastic pouch with a soft ring at each end, the ring at the closed end is inserted into the vagina, holding the condom in place. The other ring is exter-

nal and partly covers the labia. Like the male condom, it works by acting as a physical barrier, stopping sperm entering the vagina.

What's good about it
It does have advantages. Because the condom covers the labia as well as the vagina, it helps protect against herpes and other STIs, reputedly including HIV. It's readily available in drugstores and supermarkets.

The bad news
The general consensus of women who've tried it? Distinctly negative ("It feels like having sex in a plastic bag"). It can also be noisy, may irritate the vagina or penis, and can be difficult to insert. The outer ring may slip inside the vagina during intercourse.

Best suited to
Women who are allergic to latex or spermicide and want protection against STIs.

Effect on future fertility
None.

Protection against HIV and STIs
Because it covers the labia, it does offer some protection against STIs and reputedly HIV.

The failure rate
The typical failure rate during the first year of use is 25 percent.

Do I need to see a doctor?
No.

How easy is it to use?
If you've got short fingers or are squeamish about touching your genitals, it's not for you (unless you let him insert it for you).

Is it expensive?
Around $2.50 per condom.

How enthusiastic will he be?
Not very. He may even prefer pulling on his own protection.

The diaphragm
How it works
The diaphragm is a shallow dome of thin rubber with a firm, flexible rim. It looks like a tiny alien spaceship and can seem just as mysterious, according to frustrated users. You put it inside your vagina so it covers the cervix and tucks in behind the pelvic bone, held in position by the pelvic muscles. There are three types available in America: flat-spring, coil-spring, and arcing-spring, with fit and ease of insertion the main differences. The diaphragm isn't a popular method of contraception—in our "instant" era, no one wants to prepare for sex. You need to be fitted for one by a nurse practitioner, your doctor or gynecologist and change sizes after a baby, pelvic surgery, or significant weight loss (10 pounds or more). You'll be shown how to insert it then left for a little while to "practice"—and practice you will, because for some women insertion is difficult. Lots feel squeamish, others can't quite get the hang of it. But once you do, it's a ten-second job. It's a good idea to buy two diaphragms and leave one in continuously so you're always prepared. (The best place to carry a diaphragm is in your vagina, not your handbag!) Swap over every day or, if you only have one, take it out (but not before six hours after intercourse!) and wash and dry it before reinsertion. If it starts to smell, wash in one part vinegar, four parts water.

> **!** *An Australian survey found that 66 percent of women let trust interfere with their decision on whether to use a condom. In other words, factors like "But I love him" and "He's a nice guy" stopped them from using protection. Romantic but hideously dangerous.[3]*

How it works
The diaphragm needs to be left in for six hours after intercourse to ensure all the sperm are dead. Up until a few years ago, most women were advised to apply spermicide around the rim of the diaphragm to kill any renegade sperm but all that did was cause it to slide around. If you still feel safer using spermicide, avoid the

rim. There's no need to reapply it each time you have sex, just when you first insert it.

What's good about it
The diaphragm is fairly free of side effects, it's cheap, and relatively reliable in capable hands. When fitted properly and inserted correctly it usually can't be felt by either partner—and if you leave it in permanently, there's no preplanning required.

> "My girlfriend had a diaphragm fitted and we had no end of problems. I could feel it inside and while it didn't hurt, it was irritating. She got constant urinary infections and used to disappear for ages inserting it. It was a major disaster."
> David, 25, psychologist

The bad news
Lots of women find insertion difficult; others find the whole thing messy. Some women with persistent urinary tract infections claim it makes them worse; others believe diaphragms are plain uncomfortable, though this is usually the result of being fitted with the wrong size or inserting it incorrectly. A very small amount of women are allergic to latex and/or the spermicide.

> ❶ Oral contraceptives have been around for 2000 years. The ancient Romans used the sap of now extinct plants to "not only prevent conception but destroy an existing one."[4]

Best suited to
Women with strong pelvic floor muscles to hold the diaphragm in place and who are comfortable with their bodies.

Protection against HIV and STIs
No protection against HIV but it does help protect you against chlamydia and gonorrhea.

The failure rate
Theoretically, the failure rate is 4 percent but in practice it's much higher because, like the condom, people don't use it properly every single time they have sex.

HOW TO INSERT A DIAPHRAGM

1. First, rescue it from him—he'll think it's a scream and whiz it around the room like a Frisbee. You'll be less enthusiastic when it twangs out of *your* hands while you're struggling to insert it and it flies across the bathroom (again). But persevere you must. Master the insertion part and the rest is simple.

2. Stand with one foot on a chair, sit on the toilet, squat, or lie down with your knees bent for insertion. Experiment with each position until you find the one easiest for you.

3. Feel with your fingers where the diaphragm is to sit—locate your cervix and pubic bone, as shown by the doctor who fitted you.

4. Squeeze the edges of the diaphragm into a long, narrow shape between your thumb and first finger.

5. Hold the vaginal lips apart with one hand and use the other to insert the diaphragm into the vagina. Press down along the back wall of the vagina (the side nearest your rear end) until the far rim passes the cervix. Then, tuck the front rim up behind the pubic bone.

6. Check it's in place properly by feeling your cervix through the latex. It should be completely covered.

Do I need to see a doctor?
Yes. You need to be professionally "sized" initially.

How easy is it to use?
It's complicated at first, but once you're in a routine, changing diaphragms becomes part of your daily toiletry routine.

Is it expensive?
They range from around $13 to $25. Diaphragms usually last about two years unless you're wearing the same one continuously, which will cause it to deteriorate more quickly.

How enthusiastic will he be?
Some men claim they can feel the diaphragm with the head of their penis; most don't notice.

The cervical cap

How it works
The cap works like a diaphragm but it's smaller. A firm, cup-shaped or dome-shaped device, it sits snugly over the cervix and is held in place by suction. Some women find it more difficult to insert than the diaphragm—you need to have a reasonably long cervix and to be able to reach it easily. Caps are generally only available through family planning clinics and selected doctors.

What's good about it
Because it's smaller than a diaphragm, some women find it more comfortable.

The bad news
It's design is also a disadvantage because it can be knocked off during intercourse. The cap isn't advised for women plagued with urinary tract infections.

Best suited to
Women with weak pelvic floor muscles who can't, but would like to, use the diaphragm.

Protection against HIV and STIs
Same as the diaphragm—no protection against HIV but it protects you against chlamydia and gonorrhea.

The failure rate
One study put the figure at around 18 percent.[5]

Do I need to see a doctor?
Yes, for the initial fitting.

How easy is it to use?
Some women find it harder to insert and remove than the diaphragm.

Is it expensive?
Around $25.

How enthusiastic will he be?
Very. He's unlikely to feel it.

The intrauterine device (IUD)
How it works
The IUD has suffered some pretty bad press over the years—mainly due to a faulty IUD, the Dalkon Shield, which raised questions about the safety of *all* IUDs. The Dalkon Shield is no longer available and the World Health Organization, the American Medical Association, and the American College of Obstetricians and Gynecologists stand by their claim that all the *other* IUDs remain one of the safest, most effective reversible methods of birth control for women around. It's a fantastic method for the right person because once it's in, you can leave it there for up to ten years. Immediately effective on insertion, remove the IUD and its contraceptive effect is also immediately reversed.

> "The Pill made me sick and ill-tempered. The diaphragm gave me cystitis. Condoms made me sore. I'd heard horror stories about the IUD but when my doctor suggested I try it, I did. It's brilliant. I've had no problems with contraception since."
>
> Sally, 36, health worker

Two types of IUDs are available in the States. The ParaGard Copper T 380A can stay in place for up to ten years. Progestasert works by continuously releasing a small amount of progestin, so must be replaced annually.

Scientists aren't entirely sure why the IUD prevents fertilization of the egg. It may be that it prompts the egg to move through the fallopian tube too quickly to be fertilized and/or that the copper (in ParaGard) changes the environment in the uterus by affecting the behavior of enzymes in the lining. Experts suspect the progestin in Progestasert thickens cervical mucus, providing a barrier that prevents sperm from entering the uterus. Whatever it is, it's incredibly effective. The IUD's protection against pregnancy is beaten only by Norplant and Depo-Provera.

Most trained clinicians will insert an IUD in their consulting rooms. First, they'll explore your medical history and then do a pelvic and bimanual exam (inserting one or two fingers inside) to ensure your vagina and cervix are normal and the size, shape, and position of your uterus and ovaries is suitable for this method.

IUDs can be inserted at any time but it's usually more comfortable during a menstrual period, when the cervix is softest. You might be asked to take an over-the-counter painkiller before insertion and could be given antibiotics to protect against infection afterward. Most women find insertion a little uncomfortable but certainly not painful. (If you have a sensitive cervix, you can request an injection of local anesthetic.)

You'll need to schedule a checkup following the first period after insertion to check the IUD is still in place but can check yourself between annual checkups by feeling for the plastic strings that are left on the device for this purpose. (The string can't be seen outside the vagina but is long enough to be felt by a finger pushed inside.) Once it's inside, neither you nor your partner is aware of the IUD.

What's good about it
It's cheap, long-term, maintenance-free once inserted, and highly effective because you don't need to remember to do or take anything before having intercourse.

The bad news
If you've had previous pelvic infections, abnormal Pap smear results, or a heart condition, you'll be advised against this method (your clinician will discuss these, and other conditions, with you during your medical history check).

After insertion, many women adjust to their IUDs pretty quickly. Others aren't so lucky, experiencing heavy bleeding and cramps in the first few months. There may also be some spotting between periods and quite a few women find their periods are permanently heavier and longer than usual. If you change partners frequently and (very stupidly) plan to ditch condoms once fitted with an IUD, forget it. It offers no protection against STIs.

Serious infection from an IUD is rare but you're more likely to develop a pelvic infection during the first four months. In one to three out of 1000 insertions, the uterus is accidentally punctured, though it's usually discovered and corrected immediately. Sometimes IUDs come out, usually with the first few periods, so it's imperative to check the strings each month after your period. During the first few months after insertion, check every few days.

Best suited to
Women who haven't had pelvic inflammatory disease, gonorrhea, or chlamydia within the last year, who aren't at risk of contracting an STI, and aren't breast-feeding. It's a great alternative if the Pill doesn't suit you or you have other medical conditions that prevent your taking it.

Effect on future fertility
Because untreated infections associated with IUDs may make it impossible or difficult for you to get pregnant, they're not usually recommended to women who've never had children, want more, or have had trouble conceiving in the past.

Most pregnancies happen when the IUD falls out without your realizing. If you become pregnant with the IUD still inserted, there's a 50 percent greater risk of miscarriage. Get it taken out as soon as possible and the risk drops to 25 percent.

Protection against HIV and STIs
None.

The failure rate
Only Norplant and Depo-Provera are more effective. Eight out of 1000 women using copper IUDs will become pregnant during the first year of use. Less than 3 in 100 will get pregnant using an IUD with progestin.[6]

Do I need to see a doctor?
Yes. To find out if it's suitable for you, for insertion, and subsequent checkups.

How easy is it to use?
After insertion, you simply need to check it's in place by feeling the strings. IUDs are available from Planned Parenthood centers, your HMO, or doctor.

Is it expensive?
The cost of the exam, insertion, and follow-up visits ranges from $250 to $450 (though some centers price according to income and are covered by Medicaid). Pretty cheap when you consider the one-time insertion cost of $400 (for a copper IUD) lasts ten years!

How enthusiastic will he be?
The IUD is inserted deep inside so he won't feel a thing.

The combined oral contraceptive (the Pill)
How it works
The Pill has been around for more than twenty years and is the contraception chosen by most young women. The Pill gives a daily dose of synthetic hormones, estrogen and progestin, which act like the natural hormones in the body. When there's a certain level of these hormones acting on the brain, the ovary does not get stimulated to produce an egg—and if there's no egg, there's no pregnancy. There are lots of different Pills on the market, each containing various combinations of progestin and estrogen. They come in twenty-one-day or twenty-eight-day packs; the latter includes sugar pills, which you take during your period so you don't get out of the habit of taking a pill every day. Usually you'll be started on a low-dose Pill or a triphasic Pill (one that varies the amount of hormone taken throughout the month) but if breakthrough bleeding occurs and doesn't settle down within three months, a higher dose is prescribed. It's quite normal to try a few different Pill brands before settling on one that suits you.

The Pill is almost 100 percent effective if you take it at around the same time every day and don't have any health problems that may affect its absorption. If you miss a pill or are late by more than twelve hours, take it as soon as you remember; take the next pill at the usual time and you'll still be protected. If you miss more than one dose, use other contraception for seven days while continuing to take the Pill. Because it's designed to be swallowed and absorbed at a certain rate, vomiting and diarrhea, some medication (including some antibiotics), and extraordinarily high doses of Vitamin C can interfere with its effectiveness.

What's good about it
It's easy to use and highly effective, and there's another great spin-off for women who hate having their periods—there's really no need to have one. Manufacturers believed women wanted periods (and some do like the reassurance that they're not pregnant) so they included the sugar pills to allow a break from the hormones, which brings on a period. But lots take the pill continuously (just

skip the sugar ones and continue to the next packet), or break for a period every three to six months or so. If you do choose to still have periods, chances are they'll be lighter, less painful, and nearly always on time. The Pill may also help cure acne and reduce PMS—and there's scientific evidence that it may have other benefits: there's less chance of getting serious pelvic infection, cancer of the ovary, cancer of the endometrium (the lining of the womb), anemia, noncancerous breast lumps, and cysts on the ovary.

The bad news

Some women shouldn't even consider taking the Pill. If you're over thirty-five and smoke, steer clear—the Pill makes smoking even more dangerous. The hormones in the Pill slightly increase the blood's natural tendency to form clots; combine this with an unhealthy diet, excessive drinking, and smoking and you're asking for trouble. Before it's prescribed, your doctor will go through a long list of health problems and your family health history to check if you're a suitable candidate. Women who have had liver problems or breast cancer, for instance, will probably be advised to use another method. Minor side effects may include chloasma (a slight pigmentation of the skin which makes it look brown and blotchy) and some minor fluid retention (though it's a fallacy that the Pill makes you fat). Some women complain of mood changes and depression but changing to a lower dose or a different brand often solves the problem. Years ago, women were advised to take breaks from the Pill because they were high-dose formulas; today's newer, low-dose Pills are fine to take continuously.

Best suited to

Women who don't smoke and have no serious health problems or a family history of health problems.

Effect on future fertility

Contrary to common perceptions, the Pill doesn't "build up" in your body and there's no need to wait a few cycles to get it out of your system before trying to get pregnant. Usually, you'll revert to a normal cycle within a month or two, with most women getting pregnant within six months after they've stopped taking it—about the same fertility rate as women who've never taken the Pill.

Protection against HIV and STIs
None.

The failure rate
When used properly the Pill has a tiny failure rate—only 5 pregnancies per 1000 women per year. Forgetting to take it every day is the most common cause of failure.

Do I need to see a doctor?
Yes, for the initial prescription and for subsequent health checks when you renew it.

How easy is it to use?
Simply swallow a tablet daily. If you're the forgetful type, work it into a routine (maybe keep the packet on your bedside table so it's the first thing you see when you open your eyes in the morning).

> **❗ Feeling sexy? It could be your Pill, not him! Women who take triphasic Pills, with varying levels of hormones, appear to be more interested in and enjoy sex more than women on fixed-dose Pills.[7]**

Is it expensive?
The cost varies depending on which Pill you're on, but most work out to be between $15 and $25 per cycle (per month), often less at family planning clinics.

How enthusiastic will he be?
Over the moon. There's practically no chance of pregnancy if you take it every day.

The progestin only pill (the Mini Pill)
How it works
The Mini Pill contains about one-third to one-fifth of the dose of progestin that's in the combined oral contraceptive and it doesn't contain any estrogen. It's slightly less reliable than the regular Pill but useful if you can't take estrogen because it makes you feel sick. The Pill works by delivering a daily dose of synthetic hormones that act on the brain and stop the ovary from being stimulated to produce an egg. The Mini Pill works differently: its

dosage of progestin increases the mucus plug at the cervix, making it thick, tacky, and difficult for sperm to penetrate. It also changes the lining of the uterus (the endometrium), making it less "friendly" to fertilization, and it can have an effect on ovulation. It's taken every day without a break so it always comes in a twenty-eight-day pack and it's essential that it's taken at around the same time every day. Its contraceptive effect is greatest three to twenty-one hours after each tablet is taken, so if you have sex at night and/or in the early morning, take your tablet between midday and the early evening.

What's good about it
Unlike the combined Pill, the Mini Pill can be taken by women who have a history of blood clotting, stroke, heart attack, or who smoke heavily.

The bad news
It's imperative that you take it at the same time every day and do not miss any pills. As with the combined Pill, if you're vomiting, have diarrhea, or are on any other medication, take extra precautions. Unfortunately, the Mini Pill doesn't have the advantage of cycle control, so you can't skip periods or manipulate your cycle to have a period at a certain time. You may experience spotting (bleeding in between periods) or mood changes like PMS and depression.

Best suited to
Organized women who can't take the combined oral contraceptive Pill, who are breast-feeding, or who can't take estrogen.

Protection against HIV and STIs
None.

The failure rate
The failure rate is around 2 to 3 percent.

Do I need to see a doctor?
Yes, for the same reasons as the Pill.

How easy is it to use?
You take one tablet daily, but it must be at the same time.

Is it expensive?
Around $15 to $25 per month.

How enthusiastic will he be?
Extremely, if you're sensible and can be relied upon to remember to take it—nervous if you're not.

Depo-Provera, injectable hormonal contraceptive
How it works
The newest, widely available contraceptive, Depo-Provera works just like the Pill by stopping the release of an egg from your ovaries. The difference is that it's injected once every twelve weeks rather than being taken orally every day—which means a much lower failure rate because you can't forget to take it! The first injection of a progestin preparation is given into the muscle of your upper arm, rear end, or upper thigh during the first seven days of your period. You need a booster once every twelve weeks. Despite its obvious benefits, Depo-Provera isn't a common method of contraception, probably because it can wreak havoc with your periods and can delay fertility for between seven to eighteen months.

What's good about it
It's effective immediately and has an extremely low failure rate. You can forget about contraception for three months at a time. Depo-Provera is also used to treat endometrial cancers.

The bad news
You can't predict the effect it has on a period. Most women after two or three injections have no period at all, but you could experience erratic, unpredictable bleeding. You might get no period for two months, then bleed for eight to ten days. Depo-Provera has also been associated with weight gain, headaches, and depression.

Best suited to
Like the Pill, there are women who shouldn't use Depo-Provera—those with a history of depression and breast cancer, for instance—

but your doctor will discuss this with you. Otherwise, if you're constantly forgetting to take the Pill, this is a great alternative.

Effect on future fertility
This isn't the method to choose if you're planning on getting pregnant sometime soon. Depo-Provera takes a long time to wear off; most women will take seven to eighteen months from the last injection to ovulate and become fertile, with the average time being about ten months.

Protection against HIV and STIs
None.

The failure rate
Theoretically, it's the same as the combined oral contraceptive Pill; in practice it's more effective, because you can't forget to take it.

Do I need to see a doctor?
Yes. You'll need to visit your doctor or a family planning clinic once every three months.

How easy is it to use?
It's just a case of writing your appointments in your diary and sticking to them.

Is it expensive?
Around $30 to $75 per three months, plus the cost of the visit to the doctor's office.

How enthusiastic will he be?
Highly.

Norplant
How it works
Effective within twenty-four hours of insertion, Norplant offers protection against pregnancy for five years. Not surprisingly, it's becoming an increasingly popular contraceptive. This method involves inserting six thin, flexible plastic implants (around the size of matchsticks) under the skin of the upper arm. Each implant releases levonorgestrel, a hormone similar to progesterone, which

stops the ovaries from releasing eggs and thickens cervical mucus, which prevents sperm joining with the egg.

The implants are inserted through one small cut (don't panic, your skin is numbed with a painkiller first). The whole process takes about ten minutes, but you need to avoid heavy lifting and wear a bandage for a few days afterward. Some women find that the implants feel a little uncomfortable for the first few days. A follow-up visit is recommended three months later and annually after that. The implants are removed (and replaced, if you want) after five years or whenever you want to get pregnant.

Not everyone can use Norplant, so you'll be thoroughly checked by your clinician. He or she will discuss your medical history and do blood pressure checks, a breast and pelvic exam, and Pap smear.

What's good about it
It works within one day, is virtually painless, maintenance-free, and the contraceptive effect disappears mere hours after the implants are removed. You don't have to even think about contraception for five years.

The bad news
In return for all the benefits, you might have to put up with some irregular spotting and bleeding between periods. Some women may also experience headaches, nausea, depression, nervousness, dizziness, and weight gain or loss. If you're prone to scarring, there might be a scar or discoloration of the skin where it's inserted.

Best suited to
As always, certain conditions (in this case including diabetes, high cholesterol, and heart disease) prevent you from using the method. If you've ever had high blood pressure, unexplained vaginal bleeding, breast cancer, or other specific conditions (which will be explained to you during your exam), you'll probably be advised against it.

Effect on future fertility
A few hours after the implants are removed, you're capable of getting pregnant again.

Protection against HIV and STIs
None.

The failure rate
Fewer than 4 in every 100 women who use Norplant for five years will become pregnant (less than one a year). It's slightly less effective than sterilization—but not permanent.

Do I need to see a doctor?
Yes. To check for suitability, for insertion, and checkups.

How easy is it to use?
After insertion, the odd checkup hardly qualifies as difficult.

Is it expensive?
You'll pay between $500 and $600 for the medical exam, the implants, and insertion. That's around $100 per year over a five-year period. If you're on a low income, several programs may subsidize the cost (see your doctor or family planning clinician for details).

How enthusiastic will he be?
Couldn't be happier.

Emergency Hormonal Contraception, or the Morning After Pill

How it works
Despite its name, you can take the Morning After Pill (MAP) up to seventy-two hours after unprotected sex. Most regular users, according to a family planning study of 400 women, are in their twenties and used condoms that broke or a rather ineffective withdrawal method (that is, their boyfriends forgot to). This method of contraception involves taking two doses of high-dose combined estrogen and progestin twelve hours apart. It prevents pregnancy in one of two ways: if the pills are taken before you ovulate they can delay ovulation (which means you need to be particularly careful for the rest of the month because you may ovulate later than

usual). If they're taken after you've ovulated and an egg has been fertilized, the MAP prevents the fertilized egg from implanting in the womb.

What's good about it

While it shouldn't be relied upon as permanent contraception, it's ideal as a backup when condoms break or if you suspect your regular contraception has failed. Some women, who have sex *very* infrequently, use the MAP instead of using regular contraception.

The bad news

The major side effect isn't pleasant—about 50 percent of women feel sick and are. For this reason, you'll often be given antinausea pills to take as well. If you're sick within two hours of taking a dose, you may not have absorbed the hormones and need to start all over again. You may get other mild symptoms—breast tenderness, headache, or light bleeding—but these usually disappear within forty-eight hours and require no treatment.

Best suited to

Women who need an emergency backup.

Effect on future fertility

If you're already pregnant (if you conceived in a previous cycle or earlier in your present cycle), the MAP will not stop that pregnancy continuing or harm the fetus.

Protection against HIV and STIs

None.

The failure rate

About 2 to 3 percent.

> **Number of women who've failed to use contraception at least once: 87.1 percent.[8]**

Do I need to see a doctor?

Yes, the pills aren't available over the counter.

How easy is it to use?

It usually requires a hastily scheduled doctor's appointment and twenty-four hours time out if you feel ill.

Is it expensive?
Between $8 and $25.

How enthusiastic will he be?
Relieved that there's no unwanted pregnancy and hopefully sympathetic if the pills make you sick.

Permanent contraception

Forgive me for stating the obvious, but permanent contraception usually means *permanent*. Though some operations can be successfully reversed to make you fertile again, don't count on it. Proceed with caution. Are you absolutely, totally sure you're *that* serious?

Tubal ligation (or sterilization)

Commonly known as "getting your tubes tied," the fallopian tubes are cut, clipped, or tied to stop sperm going up the tubes and eggs going down. The egg is still released but it's harmlessly absorbed by the body. Usually done under general anesthetic through a laparoscope, it only requires a one-day stay in the hospital, though it will be a week before you'll feel normal. *Permanent* is the key word here; reversal is tricky and it's successful only 30 to 60 percent of the time, depending on the particular case.

Vasectomy

This is a simple twenty-minute operation that stops sperm traveling out of the testes and into the semen; sperm is still produced, but it's reabsorbed. Done under local or general anesthetic, the surgeon cuts the front of the scrotum, picks up the *vas deferens* (the tube that carries the sperm) on each side in turn and cuts and seals the ends. Though pretty hazard-free, it's not effective immediately: it may take as many as sixteen ejaculations to clear sperm that's still in the tubes. You must continue using contraception until he gets a negative sperm count. Having a vasectomy isn't a decision that should be

❗ Clever boy! The same guy who discovered the G-spot also came up with the world's first IUD. Ernst Grafenberg experimented with silkworm gut before designing a ring of coiled silver wire.[9]

made flippantly. Even if the reversal procedure goes smoothly, there's no guarantee he'll go on to father a child.

Coming attractions

RU486—Mifepristone

Some say RU486 is a better alternative to existing emergency contraceptive pills because it has fewer side effects, i.e., it doesn't make you sick. It may also be effective in treating fibroid tumors, endometriosis, and some types of breast cancer. But the struggle between antiabortionists and (among others) the Feminist Majority Foundation continues and RU486 is not yet available to women worldwide as a contraceptive method.

Available in France since October 1988 (the French Minister of Health declared it "the moral property of women"), RU486 has been approved for distribution in the U.S. but the French company that makes the drug has been unable to find a manufacturer and distributor.[10]

The vaginal ring

Dubbed "the contraception of the future," vaginal rings are as effective as the combined oral contraceptive Pill without the failure risk. This is what most of us will dump our current method for. A ring, smaller than the average diaphragm, is inserted into the vagina where it releases the same hormones that are in the combined oral contraceptive Pill. Once inserted, the ring stays there for three weeks—you remove it for a week only if you want to have a period or you can leave it in permanently and enjoy a period-free life for up to a year at a time. The obvious benefit? You don't have to remember to take a pill every day. Family planning clinics in Australia are also doing trials of a gel containing progestin, which is rubbed onto the skin of the abdomen each day, where it's absorbed like the Mini Pill.

Male contraception

Despite the occasional excited announcement that a male contraceptive pill is in the planning stages, effective male contraception (apart from the condom) is light-years away. It's not a conspiracy to keep contraception our problem; it's simply much easier to control our fertility than a man's—one egg per month as opposed to

50,000 sperm per minute that have taken three months to mature. A method involving a weekly injection of testosterone is in the experimental stages. If successful, it'll take the form of three-monthly injections or an implant similar to Norplant. Australian researchers are currently experimenting with implants using Depo-Provera. If successful, they may be available within three years. The problem is lots of contraception methods work on the pituitary gland, and if you stop its functioning in men the result is often impotence—effective contraception all right, but not quite what he (or you) had in mind!

SEX ON VACATION

The sun's shining, the waves are lapping, and the hardest decision you've had to make all week is which way to point your beach chair. That wonderfully relaxed mood can make it seem like real life doesn't exist. Unfortunately, AIDS, STIs, and unwanted pregnancies don't disappear just because you're feeling blissfully brain-dead. Vacations are danger time for many people. Make sure *you* don't come home with more souvenirs that you'd bargained on.

- Pack condoms, lubricant, and enough supplies of your chosen contraceptive to last the trip, plus "spares." (It's tough enough asking directions when you can't speak the language—try explaining what a flat-spring diaphragm is and why you need one *now!*)
- Don't rely on the calendar, mucus, or withdrawal methods. Symptothermal methods are notoriously unreliable at the best of times, worse on vacations. Time differences and long flights can screw up your menstrual cycle and it's difficult to keep track of fertile days. Heat, lounging around spas, a yeast infection brought on by pre-vacation panic, all can affect vaginal secretions. Use condoms and lubricant instead; they'll protect you against pregnancy, HIV, and STIs. Don't use the withdrawal method with weekend romancers. It's easy enough for a boyfriend to get carried away—can you trust a stranger to keep his word?
- It's Tuesday there and Thursday at home, so when should you take the Pill? Keep your watch on "home" time during the flight and take a tablet that morning or evening (whichever is usual for you), even if it means taking it early. Then take one

tablet per day until the flight back home. Keep your watch on vacation time on the flight back and continue taking the tablets. When you get home, repeat the process: take a tablet that morning or evening, then settle back into your old routine. Remember that the Pill's effectiveness is hampered by vomiting and diarrhea caused by a bug you picked up on vacation. If you vomit within an hour of taking it, it hasn't been absorbed. Use condoms or a diaphragm as backup.

- If you use a diaphragm, pack two and keep them in separate bags (in case you lose a suitcase). Flying, swimming in salt water, even scuba diving won't affect your diaphragm. Just remember it must stay in for six hours, so don't get confused with changing time zones. If you suffer a particularly bad bout of gastric, (or anything else that causes you to drop ten pounds or more), your diaphragm may be the wrong size and ineffective. That new, flat tummy won't stay flat for long if you're pregnant!

- Practice safe sex in all senses. What might pass as flirting back home may be interpreted as a blatant invitation for sex somewhere else. Quiz your travel agent on the customs and morals of the country you're visiting. And don't assume any guy you invite in for coffee will behave like a gentleman—no matter what country you're in.

THE (DREADED) STIs

It's no wonder soap opera scriptwriters never write sexually transmitted infections (STIs) into the plot. Since the entire cast of *Melrose Place* have slept with one another—without so much as a *rustle* of a condom being unwrapped—"infecting" one character would have the whole cast on antibiotics. Hollywood isn't too fond of nasty little bugs and viruses, either. We don't see the Bond girls doubled up in agony, peeing razor blades, two weeks after James has swept suavely through, or Kim Basinger braving a whopping penicillin injection nine and a half weeks after having unprotected sex in sewers and kitchens.

Which leads some people to believe life really is like a glamorous, exciting action film where people dive under the covers looking fabulous, and emerge, makeup intact, wondrously infection-free and ready for the next love scene. If only it were true. In real life, orgasms aren't the only thing you can get through sex, so arm yourself with the facts as well as with condoms. Read this section *now* rather than frantically flipping through the pages searching for a symptom you have just discovered.

A sexually transmitted infection (STI) is any infection that can be passed from one person to another through sex. Unfortunately, there are a lot of them. Some are fairly harmless and are cured by a course of antibiotics, others can kill you. They're usually passed on at the beginning of a new relationship so every time you have unprotected sex (sex without a condom) with a new partner, you should be tested for STIs.

Now here's some *really* bad news if you're feeling smug about the half-empty family-sized pack of condoms in the bedroom drawer. While condoms will protect against STIs spread by the exchange of bodily fluids (like sperm, blood, and mucus), you can still catch herpes and warts because they can be spread simply by touching infected skin. And pubic lice or scabies won't care if he's wearing six condoms; they'll still merrily jump on the nearest strand of hair they can find. In fact, the only guaranteed defense against all STIs is not to have sex at all.

Right, now that you've spent a millisecond considering that option, what next? The next best thing is a monogamous relationship with an uninfected person (where neither of you sleeps with anyone else), the third is to only have casual sex in ways that are considered "safe" (like kissing, touching, and mutual masturbation), and the fourth is to sleep with whomever you like but to use condoms (and common sense) every single time.

Like most diseases, STIs aren't fussy and you can't pick out the people who have one. Avoid "dirty," "promiscuous," or "bad boy" types all you like but if you think you're safe having sex only with "sweet," "nice," "clean," or "innocent" people, you're being unbelievably naive. Ditto those who think they're okay because they have asked their partner if they have any symptoms. Let's face it, they're hardly going to look up and say, "Well, now that you mention it, I had these godawful blisters on my penis yesterday and now they've turned into pus-infested ulcers." Besides, they may not have noticed anything unusual because some STIs are alarmingly symptom-free.

If *you* notice any change in the discharge from your penis or vagina, pain or irritation during intercourse or when you pee, any blisters, ulcers, warts, lumps, or rashes anywhere on or around your genitals or buttocks, or any itching or irritation there, put this book down and go see a doctor or a sexual health clinician NOW. If you find you are infected, it's not only polite but essential that you pick up the phone and tell anyone else you've slept with. No, they're not going to be thrilled by the news, but they should be grateful. Left unchecked, many STIs can affect our ability to have children later in life. Others, like AIDS, are fatal.

Following, in no particular order, is a rundown of some of the most common STIs. I sincerely hope you never become intimately acquainted with any of them.

AIDS

What is it?

This gets top billing for obvious reasons—it's lethal. AIDS stands for acquired immune deficiency syndrome and HIV (human immunodeficiency virus) is the virus that causes the disease. It was first noticed in the early 1980s and it predominantly affected homosexual and bisexual men and people who injected drugs. They still make up the two biggest groups affected by AIDS. HIV is spread by sex (oral, anal, and vaginal through semen and vaginal secretions), by needles (sharing a needle that is contaminated), and can be passed on during pregnancy and childbirth. It's not spread by saliva (except in one or two rare and extraordinary circumstances), touching, kissing, drinking out of the same cup as an HIV-infected person, toilet seats, shaking hands, mosquitoes, sneezing, or swimming pools. HIV attacks the body's immune system, which is our natural defense against disease. Eventually, it becomes so weak the body can't fight against any infections or diseases and you can die.

How do I know I've got it?

There's no immediate sign. A few weeks after exposure about *half* of its victims get a glandular fever-type sickness (fevers, tiredness, swollen glands), which passes. At this stage you're "healthy" but carrying the virus—a condition known as "HIV-positive." Months or years later, if you get really sick, you then have AIDS or an AIDS-related illness. Persistently swollen lymph glands is a typical symptom of the later stage and you may experience fevers, night sweats, and a cough, lose weight, have chronic diarrhea, develop skin lesions (sores or raised red marks), and be constantly tired and weak.

What now?

A blood test around three months after the initial infection can identify if you're carrying the HIV virus. If you tested negative it's wise to get retested three to six months later. Obviously, count the three months from when you last had sex without a condom or shared needles.

Can it be cured and will it come back?

At the moment, AIDS is incurable. Researchers the world over are working on a cure but, at the time of publication, none had proven to be effective though several are looking promising. Usually, the inevitable bugs and diseases you pick up are treated as they arise, until late in the disease when the body has so few defense cells, it can't respond to antibiotics.

Have I infected my partner?

Quite possibly. If your result is positive, the news will usually be delivered by a crisis counselor who'll help you work through the pain, grief, and anger you'll feel. They'll also advise you on how to tell your current partner and any past partners you may have infected. It goes without saying that not telling them is paramount to sponsoring your own personal killing spree, especially if the person who infected you doesn't know he or she is a carrier.

Your best defense against the virus?

Take it seriously, use condoms and lubricant (unless both of you have tested negative and you're 100 percent certain there's no chance of unprotected infidelity), and don't share needles. Oral sex is considered low-risk.

Will it affect my chances of having children?
AIDS can be passed from mother to child, an important factor to consider if you're planning a pregnancy.

Gonorrhea
What is it?
It sounds dreadful—and it can be. Caused by bacteria passed on by an infected partner, it turns into an infection that sometimes spreads via the bloodstream. Gonorrhea isn't common, but it's still out there.

How do I know I've got it?
The incubation period (the time it takes to develop symptoms or show signs of exposure) is anywhere from two to ten days and the first symptoms are often so minor, you may not notice. Men may find peeing painful or notice a white or yellow discharge from their penis. Women may also find urination most unpleasant and/or that their vaginal discharge is heavier than usual. You can catch gonorrhea in the anus or throat as well.

What now?
Your doctor will take a swab (a sample) from the pus discharge and test it. Gonorrhea is usually sensitive to penicillin and you may be given a single, high dose by tablet or injection. Sometimes, it's resistant to penicillin and you'll need other antibiotics. You'll probably also be treated for chlamydia, since the two often go (miserably) hand in hand.

Can it be cured and will it come back?
That's usually the end of it, though repeat tests will be ordered to make sure it's totally gone.

Have I infected my partner?
Gonorrhea is spread through vaginal, anal, or oral sex. If you've done all or any of those and not used a condom, it is possible they've got it too (or gave it to you in the first place).

Will it affect my chances of having children?
Not if it's treated promptly.

Genital herpes

What is it?

Pre-AIDS, it was the most feared of all the STIs. Post-AIDS, coping with a little cold sore suddenly seems bearable. Herpes sounds bad, but it's not serious and just means you get cold sores on the genitals rather than on the mouth. It's an infection caused by the herpes simplex virus and it comes in two types, 1 and 2. It's the same virus that causes cold sores on your lips, so if your partner has one and gives you oral sex, he may leave more than just a nice memory.

How do I know I've got it?

Your first warning may be an odd, "tingly" sensation on or around your genitals. Then—what a fabulous surprise!—one or several blisters form on or around the genitals around two to twenty days after exposure, rupturing to form ulcers. It's pretty hard to miss if you have a severe attack. In women, the sores or "lesions" usually appear on the vulva or the entrance to the vagina, though you may develop some on your cervix. In men, they'll appear on the penis, sometimes on the testicles. The initial infection is often the worst and can last up to twenty horrible, sickly days. You may feel feverish and achy, your lymph nodes may swell and feel tender. The sores heal in about twelve days but—sorry—haven't disappeared forever. Further attacks usually occur in the same place but are less severe and heal quicker (around four to five days). You are more prone to attacks when you are run down, tired, stressed, or have been drinking too much. The latest research has shown it's quite possible to pick up herpes and not get a lesion for several years afterward. Bear this in mind if your partner suddenly shows symptoms but swears he or she has been faithful—it might well have been picked up way before meeting you.

❗ What's the single most effective cancer screening tool in the history of modern medicine? The Pap smear test.

What now?

Your doctor will take a swab from one of the sores and analyze it. You may be given local anesthetic jelly to apply and aspirin or codeine for the pain. Some experts believe there's a link between herpes and cervical cancer; more recent research indicates it's unlikely. Either way, it's another good reason to have regular Pap smears if you've been infected with any STI.[11]

Can it be cured and will it come back?
Herpes is manageable but not curable. The virus remains in the body, lurking in a nerve fiber, ready to come back out and party if *you* party too hard. Some people find taking relatively new antiviral drugs, which shorten the length and severity of attacks, helpful (your doctor can give you a prescription), others simply treat each outbreak by bathing the area with salty water or antiseptics and taking painkillers. The better your general health is and the less stress you're under, the less prone you'll be to an attack.

Have I infected my partner?
Herpes is spread by vaginal, anal, or oral sex or direct skin-to-skin contact with infected areas. As a general rule, you're unlikely to infect someone if you avoid sex from the moment you're warned of an attack (by the "tingling" sensation) right through until the blisters have formed, dried up, and the skin has returned to normal. However, some people have "asymptomatic shedding" (the virus is present but there are no symptoms) or sores that are hidden from view and not noticed. It's rare but you can pass it on unawares during this time. Condoms help to stop transmission and, so long as the part that's infected is covered, provide 100 percent protection if there's an active sore. Despite this, it's not recommended you have sex during an attack, simply because it's painful.

Will it affect my chances of having children?
If you have an attack at the time of birth, they'll deliver the baby by caesarian to ensure you don't pass it on to the child.

Pubic lice (crabs) and scabies
What is it?
Pubic lice are tiny little crablike insects that are spread through any intimate contact (in bedding, towels, etc.), not just intercourse.

Scabies are a mite and spread the same way.

How do I know I've got it?
If you've got crabs, your pubic hair will be itching like crazy. Look closely and you'll discover it's not your imagination: there are tiny little insects scurrying around. Scabies cause red, itchy lumps in all the same places.

What now?
Race to the nearest pharmacy, swallow your pride, and ask for a lotion to kill pubic lice and/or scabies. They're sold over the counter and come with instructions.

Can it be cured and will it come back?
Simply apply a lotion to the affected areas (no, you don't have to shave your hair off) and that should be it.

Have I infected my partner?
If you've had close contact, yes. They should be treated as well.

Will it affect my chances of having children?
Not unless you're so put off by the experience, you never have sex again.

> "I've had herpes for years and I tell all my future sex partners. Some of them freak out and assume I'm a male slut. It's so unfair since I caught it from a much-loved girlfriend, who'd been infected when she was really young."
>
> Craig, 25, laborer

Syphilis
What is it?
In the old days, anyone who was anyone had syphilis (artists, kings, queens, you name it); today it's very rare in the heterosexual population unless you've been traveling through Southeast Asia (and not used condoms) or your partner has (flashing red light alert if the unprotected sex he had was with a prostitute). Syphilis is spread through intercourse and goes through three stages.

How do I know if I've got it?
The first sign may be a painless sore on the penis, vagina, rectum, or throat that sometimes develops during the *primary* stage,

anywhere from three weeks or three months after exposure to the disease. The infection reaches the bloodstream and spreads during the *secondary* stage, causing a fever, painful ulcers in the mouth or throat, rashes, and sometimes warts on the genitals. Stupidly ignore the symptoms and you may think it was all a bad dream because the body's defenses now get to work and the symptoms fade away for anywhere from two to fifty years. Unfortunately, it's hidden, not eradicated. About one-third of sufferers go on to the *tertiary* stage, developing large ulcers that can damage the heart, major blood vessels, spinal cord, and/or the brain or prove fatal.

What now?
If you've experienced any of the symptoms or fear you've been exposed, you'll need a blood test to identify the disease. If it's positive, you'll be given a course of high-dose penicillin injections and carefully watched for several years to ensure it hasn't progressed.

Can it be cured and will it come back?
If it's treated before the tertiary stage, it's completely curable.

Have I infected my partner?
Syphilis is spread by vaginal, oral, or anal sex. If you test positive, you must inform as many previous or current sexual partners as you possibly can.

Will it affect my chances of having children?
Not if it's treated promptly.

"I went to the bathroom one day and felt this intense stinging sensation. When I took a look, I saw a tiny little blister inside my vagina and knew I had herpes. I just couldn't figure out how the hell it had happened since I'd been in a monogamous relationship for years. My boyfriend was as horrified as I was. We went to an STI clinic, both eyeing each other very suspiciously, to find out he'd probably transmitted it to my genitals from a tiny cold sore on his mouth."

Trina, 20, student

Trichomoniasis
What is it?
It's a common infection, caused by a one-celled organism of the same name, with ghastly symptoms. It incubates for between one and four weeks though some researchers claim women can carry the germ for years before showing symptoms. Trichomoniasis is usually passed on through intercourse.

How do I know if I've got it?
You'll know it if you're a woman and showing symptoms! A thin, revoltingly smelly, greenish-yellow and sometimes frothy discharge appears from your vagina. Most men have no symptoms, though some notice a slight discharge and need to pee more often.

What now?
A smear (sample of the discharge) will be taken and analyzed. If it's positive, you'll be put on a course of antibiotics—either one, strong single dose or a week's worth.

Can it be cured and will it come back?
Yes it's curable and, unless you're reinfected, it won't come back. A good home remedy to relieve symptoms until you can see your doctor is to soak a tampon in two tablespoons of white vinegar, one drop of baby shampoo, and a pint of warm water. Insert (which is easier said than done—tampons tend to explode to EXTRA-large size after being soaked) and leave in place for up to four hours. Don't do it immediately before seeing a doctor because it can affect the swab results.

Have I infected my partner?
It's spread by vaginal sex, so quite possibly. Both of you should be treated simultaneously.

Will it affect my chances of having children?
No.

Human papilloma virus (HPV) or warts

What is it?

In fairytales, the princess kisses the warty frog to turn him into a prince. In real life, having sex with a wart-infected person will simply get you warts. HPV is a virus that causes warts in the genital area.

How do I know if I've got it?

It's common—about 70 percent of women (and most likely a vast majority of the population) carry the virus—but only a small percentage go on to develop warts on their genitals.[12] They're small, painless lumps that look like tiny cauliflowers, and they appear on the vulva, vagina, penis, or anus. They can take weeks or years to develop after exposure and you may not even notice very small lesions which, nonetheless, shed virus particles and make you infectious.

What now?

There are fifty-two different strains of the HPV virus.[13] Numbers 6 and 11 cause genital warts; numbers 16 and 18 are the ones most likely to be associated with cervical cancer—but they don't cause warts. The reason I'm dazzling you with statistics is because lots of people think having genital warts puts them at risk of cervical cancer. It usually doesn't (though regular Pap smears are still a very good idea). If you have visible warts, a doctor will paint them with an acid solution, which causes them to dry up and fall off after a few treatments. Alternatively, you may need to have them removed in a hospital through diathermy (burning), cryotherapy (freezing), or laser treatment.

Can it be cured and will it come back?

Recurrence is common, especially if you're stressed, smoke, or use steroids. As with herpes, the better you look after yourself, the less likely you'll be plagued by attacks.

> "When I was sixteen, I was terrified of catching a disease but when I got to college, everyone's attitude changed. It was like, 'I've got a dose of the clap, I've got to see the doctor.' You boasted about it. It was a bit of a hero thing; proof you'd been screwing girls."
>
> Nathan, 21, student

Have I infected my partner?
In adults, HPV is spread by having vaginal or anal intercourse with an infected partner. Condoms *help* prevent the spread but even they aren't 100 percent protection against infection. Avoid having sex while one of you is having warts treated.

Will it affect my chances of having children?
No.

Hepatitis A, B, and C
What is it?
Hepatitis is inflammation of the liver caused by a number of things, including alcohol, chemicals, drugs, and infections by viruses. Hep A is usually transmitted by contaminated food or drink and through anal sex; it's not transmitted through intercourse but may be by oral sex. Hep B is passed on via semen, mucus, or blood through intercourse (vaginal or anal) or needle-sharing. (In fact, you're more likely to pick up Hep B than you are HIV through heterosexual sex because of the nature of the bug—it can survive for longer in less ideal environments.) Hep C is similar to Hep B but mainly blood-borne and usually transmitted through sharing needles. Whether it's transmitted sexually or not is unclear at the moment. Both Hep B and C are associated with liver cancer.

How do I know if I've got it?
Hep A usually lasts a couple of weeks (causing vomiting and diarrhea) then disappears spontaneously, leaving no lasting effects. The incubation period for Hep B and C is anywhere from six weeks to six months and you may show no symptoms or very serious ones. Yellowing of the skin and eyes (jaundice), unusual tiredness, darker than usual urine, and paler than usual stools are some symptoms.

What now?
If you suspect you've been exposed to any of the three types, get a blood test (even if you aren't showing symptoms). As with AIDS, there's a window period—which means you should be retested several months later. Unfortunately, there is no effective cure.

Because it's a virus, it doesn't respond to antibiotics, though some drug treatments have proved helpful.

Can it be cured and will it come back?
Hep B and C sufferers can be lucky—your body fights the bug, it goes away, and you're no longer infected or infectious. Other times (for reasons unknown), the Hep B or C bug hangs around in the bloodstream and you're a carrier. Even if it doesn't make *you* sick (though it usually does cause problems like liver disease later in life), you can still pass it on to others. Hep B can be prevented with a vaccine that involves a course of three injections. If you inject drugs or have unprotected sex, it's worth getting vaccinated, (and therapy while you're at it, to stop you from doing either).

Have I infected my partner?
Quite probably. It's safest to have all sexual partners tested.

Will it affect my chances of having children?
No.

Chlamydia
What is it?
It's common—in the U.S. about 4 million women and men become infected each year—but it's a shy little bug and few sufferers realize they have it.[14] Nicknamed the "silent STI" because it causes mild or no symptoms, chlamydia can make a woman infertile very rapidly. It's picked up through intercourse with a person who's already infected, and the ramifications are serious.

Chlamydia can cause permanent damage to the tubes vital for reproduction in both sexes, making you infertile. It's one of the major causes of pelvic inflammatory disease in women and ups the chances of ectopic pregnancy (where the baby grows in the tubes instead of the womb).

How do I know if I've got it?
It's silent, remember, which means it's often symptom-free. If symptoms do occur in women, they're likely to be a thick, sometimes bloodstained discharge, pain when you pee (or needing to go more often), or pain during intercourse. Men may also have

a discharge, pain on urination, swelling of the testicles, or diarrhea.

What now?

It's tested by a swab taken from the cervix or inside the tip of the penis, or (more recently) by a urine test. Luckily, chlamydia is relatively easy to treat through antibiotics: either one high-dose pill or a ten-day course. You'll be retested after the course to make sure the disease is cleared.

> "He was the first guy I'd ever slept with, a doctor and twelve years older than me. He gave me hepatitis, and I was sick for months. I learned the hard way why condoms are a must."
>
> Flavia, 22, waitress

Can it be cured and will it come back?

If you test negative after treatment, you're cured.

Have I infected my partner?

It's spread through intercourse. Condoms help prevent passing it on but both of you should be treated simultaneously if you haven't used them *every* time, to avoid passing the disease back and forth. Avoid sex while you're taking the antibiotics and until you've both been given the okay.

Will it affect my chances of having children?

If it leads to pelvic inflammatory disease, yes.

Pelvic inflammatory disease (PID)

What is it?

It's something women should avoid like the plague if they plan on ever having babies. PID is an infection in the womb and tubes, often caused by bacteria passed on through sexual intercourse. As the name suggests, some or all of the organs and tissues in the pelvis become inflamed and sore. If you suspect you have it, see a doctor NOW. Left untreated, PID can permanently damage the tissue and affect fertility and/or increase your chances of ectopic pregnancy (pregnancy outside the womb). Chlamydia and gonorrhea are common causes. A termination (abortion), childbirth, and some gynecological operations can also trigger PID.

How do I know if I've got it?

It can cause no symptoms or quite severe ones, including stomach pain, vaginal discharge, pain on sexual intercourse, pain on passing stools or urine, bleeding between periods or heavy, painful periods, vomiting, and fever.

What now?

Your doctor will give you a pelvic examination (feel your abdomen and inside your vagina) and take vaginal swabs (samples of your discharge), particularly for chlamydia, which is a common cause. PID can be "acute" (you've noticed symptoms recently) or "chronic" (it's been there a while but gone unnoticed). Chronic PID can cause symptoms on and off over a period of months or years. Either way, once it's discovered, you'll probably be put on antibiotics, perhaps several types over a period of weeks. If it's a serious attack, you may need intravenous antibiotics in the hospital. It's important to rest and drink fluids during treatment, and you must avoid having intercourse until two weeks after the treatment has ended. Follow-up examinations and tests will give you a clean bill of health.

Can it be cured and will it come back?

It won't recur if it's treated properly, but if you're severely infected, you might well be in for bouts of chronic pain and general ill health before full recovery.

Have I infected my partner?

Condoms help prevent infection but usually your partner is treated as well, just in case, to stop passing the infection back and forth.

Will it affect my chances of having children?

Sadly, yes. Many women with PID have major difficulties getting pregnant. After one episode of PID, 10 percent of women have damaged tubes. If untreated or reinfected, two episodes leave 25 percent of women infertile, and after three episodes the figure jumps to 50 percent.[15]

FESSING UP—HOW TO TELL A LOVER YOU HAVE AN STI

Sarah got herpes when she was seventeen. At twenty-seven, she still had mild attacks about once every two years but avoided sex at those times and figured the chances of infecting her fiancé were pretty slim. Five years later, her now-husband found out—as she was about to give birth to their first child. The stress of pregnancy brought on a massive herpes attack and the child was at risk of being infected.

"We have to do a caesarian," the obstetrician explained to the anxious father, "because Sarah's infected right now."

"With *what?*" he answered. What should have been a gloriously happy event was marred by angry arguments about why he hadn't been told.

Lots of people don't tell their partner they've got an STI because they're worried they'll be branded "cheap," "slutty," or "dirty." And sometimes they're right—some sexually naive, uneducated, or extremely narrow-minded people *will* judge you. But the way I figure it, if you explain the facts and your lover still thinks you're trash, surely it's better to find out early on that he/she's a righteous bigot? *Anyone* who's sexually active is at risk of getting an STI. If you've used condoms with the person you're about to tell, the most they can justifiably accuse you of is having unprotected sex in the past, though even *that* isn't true in some cases.

Here's some pointers to help guide you through a tricky discussion. (If you're carrying HIV, see "Should I have an AIDS test" on page 189.)

- If you've just found out you've got an STI, had unprotected sex recently, and think you may have infected your partner, there's nothing to do but tell them immediately. (I'm taking it for granted no one in their right mind would *knowingly* have sex without a condom if they knew they were infectious.) Say you had no idea you were carrying anything but are worried sick you may have inadvertently passed it on. If they're angry and accuse you of all sorts of irresponsible behavior, calmly point out that the decision not to use a condom was made by both of you. You both took risks and who knows who gave it to whom, anyway?

- If you have herpes or an STI—other than HIV or AIDS—that can't be cured, you don't need to tell every person you sleep with. If transmission of the STI is prevented by condoms, you use one, and you aren't currently having an attack, it's unnecessary to tell casual lovers. They're not at risk so it's none of their business.

- Pick the moment carefully to tell long-term partners if you have herpes or an STI that can't be cured. The time to confess a long-standing STI is when you decide the relationship is serious, or has the potential to be. A good relationship is based on trust and if you leave it too long, your partner will feel understandably "had." Pick a time and a place where you're both relaxed and won't be disturbed but . . .

- Prepare first. If you don't already have books or leaflets explaining the STI you have, get some (family planning clinics usually have great info you can take with you). Your partner can then read the facts for themselves. Rehearse what you're going to say so it doesn't get all mixed up on the way from your brain to your mouth. Imagine how you'd like to be told if the roles were reversed.

- Speak calmly. Say you have something to say and would appreciate it if they don't interrupt until you're finished. Then simply tell your story—how you got the disease, how upset you were when you found out, how you deal with it now. It's a very good idea to explain early on that because you've been using condoms, there's no chance you've infected *them*. That way, they'll listen to what you're saying rather than sit there thinking, "Oh my God, now I've got it too." Tell them you're confessing because you trust them not to judge you, can see a future together, and want to be completely honest. Now's the time to bring out the literature to back up the facts you're presenting.

- Refuse to be judged. Unless you got it from screwing their best friend behind their back, it's nothing to be ashamed of. Expect a little uncomfortableness (if they like you, they don't even want to *think* about your having sex with someone else, let alone what you got from it), but don't let anyone put you down. Once you've told them and worked out any effect the news will have on your sex life, drop the subject.

- Ask that they keep it confidential. It should go without saying, but protect yourself anyway. Even if you are healthily undisturbed by others knowing you've got an STI, it's for you to tell people, not them. If they breach the agreement and blab to all and sundry, send him or her back to the nursery and get them out of your life.
- If they can't accept it, reconsider the relationship. If your partner has read all the facts and can't deal with the news, tell them they've got two choices: either talk to a counselor (try an STI clinic) to get over any issues it's thrown up or leave. Do you want to be with someone who constantly reminds you of how "bad" you are or makes hurtful jokes at your expense?
- If someone's given you an STI, treat them with the respect you'd hope they'd show you. It's rarely deliberate, so don't point the finger and blame them; just get the facts and get on with your life—with or without them.

SHOULD I HAVE AN AIDS TEST?

Anyone who's ever had unprotected sex (in other words, pretty well all of us over the age of twenty-five) has had those terrifying moments when we're convinced we've got AIDS. Even if it was one, stupid encounter, we huddle under the bedcovers, stare into the darkness, and think, "I bet I've got it, I know I've got it." Health workers call us "the worried well"—usually infection-free people in a low-risk category who take the test more for peace of mind than anything else. (That's not to say we *haven't* been infected, it's just pretty unlikely.) Others have been infected or are in a high-risk group. They've injected drugs, are homosexual men, have had sex with bisexual men who haven't used condoms, or they've had lots of heterosexual unprotected sex with a number of people. Whichever category you fall into, having an AIDS test is well worth considering. It's not scary, no one will look at you "funny" or think

> ❗ *More than 40 percent of AIDS cases worldwide are among women, with nearly nine million HIV-infected. There are currently 85,500 cases of women with AIDS in the U.S.[16]*

you're promiscuous, and they don't allow Big Brother cameras in clinic waiting rooms, honest.

Where do I go?
First, wait three months from the last time you had unprotected sex or shared a needle, then head for a sexual health clinic (most major hospitals have them), family planning clinic, or your doctor. You can then be tested for *all* STIs, many of which have no obvious symptoms. The clinics are legally bound to ensure confidentiality, so they can't tell your parents, your partner, or your boss (though they may suggest *you* tell them if you do test positive).

What will happen?
You'll be counseled first and asked about your sexual history, drug use, and general health. The counselor will ask why you want the test, how much you know about the disease, and how you would react if you tested positive (they need to be satisfied you won't throw yourself off the nearest cliff immediately). Then, you'll be taken to an examining room and a doctor will take some blood (and swabs if you're getting a thorough checkup). The blood test will detect the antibodies produced by your body when it encounters HIV. Few clinics give results over the phone, so you'll need a second appointment to find out the verdict.

What happens if it's negative?
Say a "thank you God" prayer. Now's the time to make a personal pact to practice safer sex always.

What happens if it's positive?
Some people don't go further than pretest counseling because they aren't prepared to deal with a positive result. Others take the punt. Remember that if the news is bad it still doesn't mean you have AIDS—it could be ten years before you experience symptoms. A counselor will tell you the result and help you decide if or how you'll tell family, lover(s), friends, and your employer. It's advisable to get regular counsel-

❗ *Number of women who say they've changed their sexual behavior because of AIDS: 53.6 percent.* [17]

ing for at least a few months after; as you can imagine, being HIV-positive isn't something that's easy to deal with. Your reaction to the news will vary over the next few months and years and it helps to know people in the same situation. The clinic will give you phone numbers of the many support groups available as well as explicit instructions on how not to pass it on.

OTHER THINGS THAT CAN HAPPEN "DOWN THERE"

The human body is an amazing thing and awfully efficient when it's well oiled and whirring along happily. But let's face it: if we were a car or a CD player, we'd have been recalled by now due to machinery faults. One microscopic, *teeny-weeny* bacteria or bug and the whole thing can fall apart. Even if you're one of those sickeningly health-conscious, never-do-a-thing-wrong types, you'll still get sick occasionally. And while we'll all happily trot along to the drug store or doctor for help getting over the flu, we're not so quick to find out what's causing problems "down there." Many people, particularly women, get embarrassed—which is a bit silly when you think about it. Your doctor or gyne-cologist has seen vaginas, penises, and breasts before. Granted, maybe not yours, but they're all pretty similar, don't you think? Then you have to admit you have—*What? SEX!*—to explain your symptoms or worries? I suspect this won't come as a horrible shock to your doctor either—she might even have it herself every now and again.

In other words, there's no need to be shy, red-faced, or self-conscious. If you suspect you have any of the following common infections, get professional help. Unless you're a seasoned sufferer (and your doctor's given you the go-ahead), don't attempt to cure yourself. I've listed some home remedies to tide you over until you get to see your doctor and things you can do to avoid future attacks, but they're not substitutes for medical attention.

Cystitis and other urinary tract infections (UTIs)

Inflammation of the bladder can affect men, women, and children. In adults, cystitis is the most common complaint (62 percent of women will get it at some point).[18] It's caused by germs entering the urethra, and—guess what?—one of the most effective ways to get it is to have lots and lots of great sex, hence the nickname "honeymoon disease." (If you've had a big session, pee immediately after intercourse to flush out any germs; using lubricant during sex helps.) Classic symptoms for both sexes include an urgent need to pee (then nothing comes out when you get there), intense pain on urination, or blood in your urine. Given that the symptoms are truly miserable, most people are begging their doctors for the first available appointment, which is just as well because it can lead to more serious things if left to fester. Once you start treatment—usually a course of high-dose antibiotics—it is wonderfully, immediately effective. The problem doesn't disappear that quickly (you need to take a full course), but the symptoms do.

Do-it-yourself relief until you can see a doctor
Drink a solution of ¼ teaspoon of baking soda in a cup of water once every eight hours, and a glass of plain water once every two hours. Over-the-counter UTI remedies are also useful for mild attacks. To prevent future infections, drink cranberry juice (it helps stop bacteria from latching on to the bladder walls), shower regularly, use mild soap, dry thoroughly, and wipe front-to-back when you go to the bathroom. Drink lots of water regularly to flush out germs and pee immediately after sex.

Yeast Infection (candida)

This is a relatively harmless fungus infection. Why, then, do some women run screaming from the room at the mere mention of it? Because it can be a living hell if it won't go away. As persistently annoying and as stubborn as a two-year-old, recurrent yeast is single-handedly capable of ruining sex lives, good moods, and underwear without very much effort at all. In short, it can leave you feeling as hot for sex as a tub of ice cream.

Candida is a yeast that most of us have growing in our vagina all the time. It's generally kept under control by the natural acidity of the vagina but things like the Pill, antibiotics, heavily perfumed soaps and bubble baths, vaginal deodorants, sex, pregnancy, diabetes, stress, and general ill health can cause an imbalance. It's not new—candida was found in the tombs of Ancient Egypt—and men get it too, but to a lesser extent (even so, he needs to be treated as well).

Symptoms include itchiness, a white, cheesy-looking discharge, vaginal swelling or redness, and pain during sex or peeing (usually caused by urine or sperm stinging the tiny cuts you've made by scratching wildly in your sleep). Your doctor will prescribe antifungal vaginal suppositories (you insert them and they "melt" inside your vagina) or cream (with an applicator to insert inside). There's also a new, single-dose, oral antifungal tablet. A man can use the cream or the tablet.

Do-it-yourself relief
To prevent further infections, up the "good" bacteria in your body by eating yogurt with live lactobacillus cultures daily or go on a course of acidophilus tablets (available from drug stores and health food shops). Eat less sugar, yeast products, and alcohol. If you're plagued by it, pick up one of the many books on the subject which list umpteen theories on getting rid of it for good.

Gardnerella vaginalis
More common than candida, it's something that normally lives in your vagina, keeping to itself until you do something to upset its home environment—like take the Pill. The first symptom may be a fishy smell (especially after intercourse) or a discharge, either thin and watery or frothy. It's cured with antibiotics and not passed on sexually, so he doesn't need to be treated.

Do-it-yourself relief
Alter the pH balance of the vagina using a gel or vinegar douche (one-third vinegar to two-thirds warm water).

Endometriosis
This is a condition where the endometrial (lining) cells of the uterus grow in places outside the uterus like the ovaries, fallopian tubes, bladder, or large intestine. It's not understood why but it affects women in their reproductive years (most commonly women in their thirties and forties). Endometriosis doesn't always cause symptoms but it can stop you from getting pregnant easily, or at all. Symptoms may include pain in your abdomen or while going to the bathroom, during sex, or during abnormally heavy periods. The most common symptom is severe pain just before or during

your period that feels like a dull, dragging ache rather than the usual period cramps. It's diagnosed through an operation called a laparoscopy, where the surgeon looks for evidence inside. Treatment depends on how severe it is and whether or not you've had, or would like to have, children. You may be given medicine to relieve painful symptoms or hormonal drug therapy, which is designed to cause the tissue to disappear. In some cases, the tissue needs to be removed surgically. In severe cases, the surgeon will remove your uterus, tubes, and/or ovaries as well.

EVEN IF EVERYTHING'S WORKING JUST FINE . . .
Look after your body and watch for changes
Get some info on how to examine your breasts for lumps. (He should examine his testicles for lumps on a regular basis, also.) Wash regularly, using mild unscented soap, try really, really hard to wear cotton panties most of the time, and if you notice any abnormal lumps, discharge, or redness, see a doctor.

Don't use feminine hygiene sprays or "freshening" douches
For a start you don't need them, and second, they alter the delicate pH (acidity) balance of the vagina and can lead to infections, like yeast. If you're worried about being "smelly," get a checkup to rule out infections, then shower regularly, use mild unscented soap, and wear cotton underwear. It's that simple.

Get regular checkups and Pap smears with a gynecologist or your doctor
If you're sexually active, go every time you notice something unusual (or visit an STI clinic instead) or once every six months to a year. You'll probably be advised to get a Pap smear yearly or twice-yearly. They don't hurt and the payoff is enormous: a Pap smear not only can detect cervical cancer in its earliest stages, it picks up any cell changes that may be caused by infections you don't know you have.

First, your doctor will visually inspect your genitals and may do an internal exam (put his or her fingers inside to check for swelling or pain). Then he or she will use a speculum to look at your cervix and a cotton swab or cervical brush to scrape off a few cells. The sample is then sent to pathology to check for abnormalities. You may be offered the services of Papnet for an extra fee. If you've had abnormal smears in the past, it's well worth considering because it's the latest in high-tech screening. If they've all been clear, it's probably unnecessary.

7

Performance Problems

Some of the reasons sex goes wrong and how to get it lustily back on track

•••

As a writer who specializes in sex, I discuss penises, clitorises, and the pros and cons of G-spot orgasms as often as other people talk about where to go for lunch. I've done stories on dominatrixes and drag queens, prostitutes and premature ejaculators; I've visited bondage and discipline parlors, a sex addicts' club, and sat around with a group of naked women armed with vibrators big enough to build houses with. All that experience makes me a popular dinner party guest—but it freaks penises out big-time (not to mention the men they're attached to).

Add a tendency to forget not everyone's as open about sex as I am, and you can see why some men find me too hot to even think about handling. "So, you can help me out with a story I'm doing," I said to one guy on a first (never-to-be-repeated) dinner date. "Oh really?" he said nervously, Adam's apple doing an Irish jig. "It's an easy one," I continued. "All I need to know is this. When you're giving a girl oral sex, have you ever noticed if any fluid comes out? See, this story's on female ejaculation." I scooped up a mouthful of pasta and beamed an encouraging, cheerful smile. "Ummm . . . how's your meal?" he answered. Later, he told a mutual friend the only guy who'd be confident enough to sleep with me answered to the name of Bond.

No matter how much I tell men the pressure's on *me* to perform in bed, some still give me this watery, wan smile and continue to think, *Oh God, she knows so much, I'm bound to do something wrong*. And, of course, they do. Which probably explains why I can't really understand all the fuss over genital malfunctions. So our body parts don't behave as we want them to occasionally. So what? Genitals are like expensive electrical equipment—they act up now and again. Leave it until the next day and the problem often magically cures itself. Penises, vaginas, and clitorises might be part of your body but they're not always within your control. Accept this one simple fact and you'll avoid the psychological head games that turn a lot of isolated technical hiccups into chronic sex problems.

As for other sex- or relationship-related trouble zones, again you'll notice the same advice given over and over. Talk to your partner. Discuss the problem. Tell him or her you're not happy. Your mouth is great for a lot of things to do with sex but its most important function in the bedroom is for talking. Good communication can solve lots of problems and make them *all* easier to cope with. Talk is cheap, cheaper than sex therapy.

This chapter looks at the common physical and emotional reasons why sex goes wrong and suggests practical solutions to the problems.

PENIS PROBLEMS

Personally, I'd hate to have a penis—it's so humiliatingly obvious when things go wrong! Because female parts are hidden, we get away with all sorts of things. We're *dying* to have sex but our vagina's as dry as a piece of unbuttered toast? No problem. A quick trip to the bathroom, a scoop of K-Y and our lover's none the wiser. Not so for men. A limp penis stands out like . . . well, it *doesn't*, and that's pretty obvious to both of you. As for coming too soon, I've yet to

"You never, ever talk about penis problems to other guys. It's almost like your penis is you. Guys are so ego-oriented and sex-oriented. If I confessed to a friend, he'd have one up on me. I actually find it easier to talk to women about it than men—women you're not sleeping with, that is."

Christopher, 23, music rep

hear a man complain if his girlfriend hits the target within three minutes (more like *hallelujah*!). The pressure on men to perform is enormous, even if nothing else is.

If you're a guy, chances are at some point in your life you'll find yourself in one of the following situations. If you're a woman, it's pretty obvious you could be the one he's with at the time. Men take their penises very, very seriously, so it pays for both of you to be prepared. How you react to the problem initially very often dictates how long it remains one.

He can't get it up (impotence)

Sometimes, penises and brains have different ideas of what's fun. You want to ravish her, but your penis wants to snuggle up into your Calvins and have a nap. Nearly every man will have had problems getting an erection by the time he reaches forty. It's *normal* and usually explicable. Maybe you drank too much, work pressures are stressing you out, or you're simply tired. Dismiss it as a one-time-thing and chances are that's what it will be. Worry yourself sick

❗ Only one-third of impotency cases are due to physical problems, and almost all are treatable.¹

about it, and it may well happen again. The more wound-up and anxious you are the next time, the more nervous poor old Willy's going to be and the less likely he'll be to rise to the occasion. Your worst nightmare will

be confirmed and you will be officially (if only temporarily) impotent.

Why did it happen in the first place? Too much booze can do it, so can recreational drugs, physical exhaustion, pressure, stress, and guilt (your penis may try to be faithful, even if you don't). Usually, it's psychological but there may be a medical reason. It's easy to figure out which category you fit into: if you have an erection when you wake up in the morning or during masturbation, it's probably psycho-

"The first thing that women do is grab your penis, and when they're used to grabbing firm erections not limp ones, they often visibly flinch. That makes me shrivel even further."

Ethan, 35, mechanic

logical. You're not getting one with your partner because you feel anxious, embarrassed, or ashamed—maybe she's made you feel that way by being critical.

FOR HIM

Real men don't always get erections whenever they want to. I'm not being kind, it's true. I asked every female who called the day I was writing this and out of ten only one had never encountered the problem (my niece, who's five years old). Accepting that you're not the only one is often the solution to the problem. Many of you get horribly upset because you think of sex as intercourse—which needs an erect penis. Illogically, you'll think you're a dud in bed even if she's had ten orgasms through oral sex. That's really silly. Take it from me, women don't think like you do. We'll go for the guy who gives us great head over an erect penis every time. So first up, change your mind-set.

"It first happened when I was nineteen. I'd just met a girl and couldn't get it up. I thought it was a bit strange but put it down to the fact that I was really into her and wanted things to go really well. The second time it happened, I became obsessive—wound myself up into a complete state. The girl kept saying, 'It must be me,' and that made it worse. After her, I slept with a few girls casually with no problem, then I met my next long-term girlfriend and was back to square one. I finally figured it only ever happens with women that matter so I warn them and once I'm relaxed it goes away."

Tony, 28, teacher

Talk to your girlfriend and confess that you're going through a weird time. Don't avoid sex, just have it without penetration; use your tongue, hands, and mouth to pleasure her instead. (She'll be praying you stay impotent forever.) Rule out any medical reasons for the condition. Take a break from drugs, alcohol, and cigarettes and rethink your health and lifestyle generally. If you're on any prescribed medication, ask your doctor about possible side effects. If it's happening a lot, ask your doctor for a referral to a urologist for a physical examination or make an appointment to see a sex therapist. Think about why it's happening. Is it with all women or just this one? If it's just her, maybe you're mistaking friendship for lust or love. Sometimes, if you're really crazy about her, you're scared limp because you're so desperate to please her. Relax a little. If she's going to leave you because you can't get an erection, she wasn't worth the effort in the first place.

(F) FOR HER

- **Don't take it personally.** It doesn't mean your tummy is too big, he doesn't like your underwear, or he fancies the blond in accounts.
- **Don't pretend you don't notice.** Talk to him about it. Say, "I know how that feels. Sometimes I want sex, but I don't get wet." Ask him if he'd like you to try to arouse him or whether he'd prefer to get some rest. Talk to his penis as well. Say, "Poor thing, you're tired" or "Too much beer, eh?"—anything to lighten the situation. The worst thing you can do is ignore it. Gently stroke it from base to tip or give him oral sex but don't labor the point. If he doesn't become hard in a few minutes, shift to another area— his nipples, his mouth, his testicles.

- **Turn it around. Say, "Fantastic! This means I get you all to myself."** Let him use his hands and tongue to bring you to orgasm. Masturbate for him. Relax and enjoy yourself—an orgasm each doesn't necessarily have to be the goal of love-making.
- **Have intercourse anyway.** If you can push it in (with his or your fingers), he'll often become erect inside you.

> "The relationship was great, except we still hadn't had intercourse and it'd been six weeks! He'd give me these amazing, passionate kisses out in public, but while I couldn't wait to get home and rip our clothes off, he'd avoid it. Then I found out why: he'd been impotent for months. Of course, I was convinced I could solve it. When I couldn't, I thought, 'Oh shit, this guy really does have problems.' I'm a really sexual person and I need to have sex and orgasms. If he'd taken the time to satisfy me with his hands and mouth, it wouldn't have been such a problem, but he seemed so caught up with it, he forgot about me."
>
> Carla, 24, secretary

He can't come

What's going on? You've been at it for so long she's not only planned the menu for tomorrow night's dinner party but the shopping list and what to wear as well. Rapid thrusting usually does the trick, but this time, though you're close to orgasm, you can't quite get there. Usually it's because sensation in your penis is deadened by too much alcohol, drugs (especially speed), or (lucky you!) she's worn you out from too many previous climaxes. Women are used to having sex without the ultimate reward of orgasm—you're used to quite the opposite.

If it's not the result of overdoing it, it could be psychological. Have you just swapped girlfriends and are too shy to tell your new lover what you need to tip over the edge? Some men can only orgasm if their partner squeezes their testicles; others want her to insert a finger into their anus. If you've just split with someone and always orgasmed the same way, your body and brain may be waiting for the signal to let go. Alternatively, you might be feeling emotionally upset. Are you worried about losing her, having work hassles, or generally going through a stressful time? You're having trouble because your mind's not on the job.

Ⓜ FOR HIM

A good night's sleep is an instant fix if the problem's related to drugs or alcohol. Telling her what you need to orgasm is another issue altogether. Communication is nearly always the key. Unload those problems by talking to her or another sympathetic friend, and ask her if she ever has trouble coming (she does, believe me). A problem shared is a problem halved and all that. Are you spending too much time giving her foreplay and not enough on yourself? Encourage her to pull out all the stops, pull on the sexy underwear, tell you a fantasy while you're making love, or just to let you know how horny she's feeling. Also get her to stimulate your anal region, massaging the area between your testicles and your anus. A well-lubricated finger up your anus can work wonders.

Ⓕ FOR HER

- **Get wet.** You're not the only one who's sore—he is, too. Add some K-Y (not too much) and it'll instantly feel more delicious for both of you.

- **Let him know how much he's turning you on. Appeal to all his fantasies.** Dress up, masturbate for him, do a Kim Basinger style striptease. Get him to bring you to orgasm as many times as you can stand it (a bore, I know), turn up the volume on the groans and the *"Oh yes"*es. Seeing you come can have a domino effect.
- **Use your mouth.** If you've been having intercourse for ages, your vagina's as worn out as you are. It's overstimulated and probably not gripping his penis as hard as usual. Switch to oral sex or mutual masturbation, using firmer pressure than usual.

He comes too soon

Premature ejaculation is the most common sex problem of all. During the 1940s and 1950s, Kinsey found 75 percent of men ejaculated within two minutes of penetration. Recent research suggests men today last ever-so-slightly longer (like one minute more) but what's more important is lots of men climax before they, or their partner, want them to.[2] As a teenager, you probably didn't worry too much (if indeed, you knew there was anything to worry about). Even when you're older, there are some situations that seem excusable (like living out a highly erotic fantasy, first-time sex with the girl of your dreams, or sex with anyone if you haven't had it for a while). But when it happens every single time? Let me put it this way: even if you don't notice, she does.

❗ *Any man, even the strongest, most competent, and most virile, however old he is, will at some point in his life experience impotency.[3]*

Defining a premature ejaculator (the technical term for it) is difficult. There's no set time period that you can measure yourself against, no "test" to pass. Some couples think premature ejaculation is his coming after an hour of thrusting, others are quite happy with (or used to) three minutes of intercourse. But if you feel out of control when it comes to coming, it's worth looking at for both your sakes.

Some men ejaculate when they touch breasts. Others get a little further but blow it on the very first (and undeniably the best) thrust. It's got a lot to do with the lessons you learned when you were young. If, as a teenager, you rushed through sex because you were worried you'd get caught, you've conditioned your penis to rapid ejaculations. Usually, age and a regular lover solve the problem—if they haven't, there's still lots you can do to fix it.

Ⓜ FOR HIM

Most sex therapists boast they can solve the problem within six weeks. Therapy usually revolves around learning to relax and relieving the pressure of performance. "Homework" includes sex without penetration (taking the focus off intercourse through oral sex, mutual masturbation, and generally exploring each other's bodies) and continuing to have sex even if you do ejaculate. Masturbation is one of the most effective means of control. The more you masturbate the better (it desensitizes your penis), especially if each time you do you "hold off" (try counting backwards, starting from 500).

The stop/start technique is 90 percent successful if followed for a few months. Either you or your partner stroke your penis until you get an erection, you start having intercourse, then stop and withdraw the minute you feel close to coming. Stimulation stops until you start to lose your erection, then the whole process is repeated three or four times before you're allowed to ejaculate.

The squeeze technique—you or she grasps the penis just below the head and presses hard when you're close to orgasm—is another alternative.

Generally, the aim is to stop feeling so turned-on. The more "unsexy" your thoughts, the more control you're liable to have. Using distraction techniques, like mentally composing your résumé, can help; so can keeping your eyes closed so you can't see how sexy she looks. If the problem's really bad, zero foreplay for you and minimum for her; if necessary, don't touch her genitals at all. Use lubricant, put the penis in the vagina very carefully, avoiding too much stimulation, and keep thrusting to a minimum. Stop and hold perfectly still or withdraw if you're losing control.

Ⓕ FOR HER

- **Get him to give you an orgasm first.** It takes the pressure off. Initiate nonpenetrative sex like massage, oral sex, and masturbation as well as intercourse.

- **Keep still.** This is one time he'll thank you for lying back and thinking of England. No groaning, moaning, or raking your fingers down his back. Remain as passive as possible—don't contract your vaginal muscles or move your pelvis at all.
- **Keep going.** The more often he comes, the longer he'll last the next time. Try not to lose your temper or act bored (yawning is a no-no). Sure, it's frustrating not being able to touch him, and lying there like a stuffed dummy isn't anyone's idea of hot sex, but (hopefully!) it's not forever. The more you have sex, the better it will get.

He doesn't feel like it

The honey-I've-got-a-headache line sounds awfully odd coming out of *his* mouth. Blame it on society (Hollywood or the soaps), but a *man* turning down sex? Gosh, something must *really* be wrong. Not true, of course. These days, it's just as likely to be her ripping off your suit and your complaining you're too tired. And as women become more comfortable with sex, men are becoming less secure. Sex is demanded of you more often—and it's a massive blow to your ego if she wants it more than you do. The sheer pressure of trying to be the perfect 90s man can make sex seem more of a chore than a pleasure.

❗ Men the world over are becoming less and less fertile. The average man's ejaculate has declined in sperm concentration and number per ejaculate at the rate of 2 percent a year over a decade. What's to blame? Everything from smoking to women having children later in life.[4]

Your desire could also be dampened by outside pressures. Men aren't sex robots; they're human and affected by stress and feelings just as much as women are. You're also individuals. Which means some of you have a high sex drive (or libido) and some don't. In an ideal world, we'd all find our libido equivalents. If you only want to have sex every two months and that suits her, it's not a problem. Hook a horny hedonist and it's a huge one.

Are you simply bored by sex and happy to let other things in life take precedence? Most of us move out of the can't-get-enough stage after those first few, fervent months. Unfortunately, it's often replaced by lovemaking that's as predictable as Grandpa's war stories. Physical tiredness is often to blame for temporary lack of interest. Are you trying desperately hard to establish a career, with not much energy left over for anything else? Working long hours (or partying too hard with too many drinks and smokes) can mean sex is the last thing you feel like when your head hits the pillow.

Ⓜ FOR HIM

Vacations can do amazing things for a lagging libido, which means reducing stress is an obvious place to start. Sexual desire appears to originate in the brain. If you're juggling so much your brain feels like an amusement park, there aren't many cells free for fantasy. Make time for sex. Deliberately focus on it; read erotic books or watch some films. Get back to basics and spend more time on foreplay than intercourse. Let her massage you; rediscover sensuality and the simple delight of kissing and touching each other.

Ⓕ FOR HER

- **Help destress his life.** Schedule in "pamper time"—an hour or two per week when you massage and stroke all his stress away. Don't panic and think that it's your fault (that you're obviously not sexy enough) and resist the urge to jolt him out of it by tying yourself naked to the hood of his car. He'll feel like a complete failure if you have to go to those extremes.
- **Have lots of "quick" sex sessions.** If he's tired, he'll be much more interested in a quickie than in marathon sex. Get him to give you oral sex if he's not interested (you'll feel satisfied, he may find it the turn-on he needs), and return the favor on other occasions. Every sex session doesn't have to last an hour.

HOW TO GET YOUR LOVER TO SEE A SEX THERAPIST

Telling anyone it's time to seek professional help is tricky; getting your lover to see a sex therapist is even more delicate. Resist the temptation to blurt out "You really should get help" immediately after (yet another) failed lovemaking session. Best to have this conversation outside the bedroom. Wait until you're both relaxed, then gently explain that although you love them and your sex life, you think a third party could help solve the problems you're both having. Use words like "both" rather than "you" when talking about the problem—it'll seem less attacking and more like you're making the suggestion for the sake of the relationship rather than pointing the finger.

Many people still think that only "crazy" people see therapists, so have the old "you see an expert for every other problem, why not this one" argument ready. Once they agree to see someone, choose a sex therapist/psychologist carefully. Your doctor can usually help with a referral or look up "psychologists" in the telephone book. Call the American Psychological Association (APA) for referrals. They'll be able to provide you with a list of professionally trained counselors in your area who specialize in sexual problems. If someone recommends one or you get a name from an ad, call the APA to check they're certified. If your partner refuses outright to see an expert, you might want to rethink the relationship as well as your sex life—if they're not willing to compromise on this important issue, what about future problems?

FIVE WAYS TO HELP HIM THROUGH A ROUGH TIME

1. **Don't overreact.** If he's having problems *most* of the time, he needs to see a doctor, possibly a sex therapist. But if it's only occasionally, what's the big deal?
2. **Have orgasms from oral sex and masturbation.** Show him that an erect penis really isn't necessary.
3. **Sympathize but don't lie.** Don't tell him he's hard if he isn't, don't tell him it was great if it wasn't. Pretending he doesn't have a problem will only make things worse.

CAN'T, WON'T, SHOULDN'T: THE THREE MOST COMMON FEMALE SEX PROBLEMS

Psychologists recently did a word association test on a group of college students. They were given a subject (like *family*), then asked to instantly list any other words they associated with it (children, mother, stroller, park, etc.). Guess what happened when "sex" came up? The male students smiled broadly, rubbed their hands over grubby Levi's, and launched gleefully into a long list of words like *blond, fun, legs, boobs, bed, orgasm, penis,* and *sweat.* The girls paused, foreheads crinkled, put their hands between their knees, and came up with *guilty, wrong, bad, babies,* and *tears.* To say they honed in on the negatives is an understatement. The study conclusion? Men focus on the in-out physical act of sex, women on the emotions associated with it. *Puhleeze!* They could have hopped down to the nearest bar to find out that little gem of information.

Yet it's that fuzzy, emotional side that's at the root of most female sex problems. We worry too much about what people think. We won't let go in case he judges us, we don't tell a godawful lover he's hopeless in case we scar him for life. Head of the class for being polite and caring; flunking grade for sexual enjoyment. We tend to take everything our mother, the church, our friends, or ex-lovers have said in the past to bed with us. Even the neighbors get a look in—that planned Saturday afternoon orgy of lust turns into a reluctant rendezvous if they're home ("Shhhh! They'll hear you!"). Hell, if the *dog* wanders in and looks at us the wrong way, it can stop us from coming. All a bit ridiculous, don't you think? So stop worrying about everyone else during sex. The dog can't blab your secrets, and Aunt Fanny's not peering in through the blinds.

She doesn't feel like it

It's easiest to divide sexual disinterest into *permanent* and *tempo-rary*. At some point, all of us have found the thought of having sex about as appealing as cleaning the toilet. The lifestyle of a typical 90s woman isn't conducive to great sex, for starters. Overloaded sched-ules leave us feeling stressed, unhealthy, and unattractive. We don't feel sexy, so we don't want sex. Stress and tiredness affect our hor-mones, blocking those that give a lovely libido lift, increasing oth-ers that make us anxious. Taking time out, making priorities, and planning time for sex can solve the problem in a flash. Medication can also affect your sex drive. Antidepressants like Prozac can make you feel great from the waist up, but dead from the waist down.

Relationships are a common culprit—like being in the wrong one. Hooked up with a nice guy who does little for you sexually or hanging on to one who treats you badly? Sex slumps aren't usu-ally just about sex; they're a sign that your relationship's gone awry. If you have problems outside the bedroom they'll filter through eventually. A bad lover is a common cause of sexual disinterest, par-ticularly a selfish, inexperienced, or incompetent one who's only interested in his own orgasm. If he's a bore in bed, why *would* you be champing at the bit to hop in?

If you've *never* enjoyed sex, have it only because "you have to" and it rarely satisfies or arouses you, there are deeper psycho-logical factors at play. If intercourse feels like being "speared" or you divorce yourself from the act (experiencing that weird, *this-is-happening-to-someone-else* feeling), you could be reacting to an ear-lier traumatic experience or a strict religious upbringing. Possibly, you've decided not to bother with relationships at all. (Read "If you're hung up about it" on page 10 and "If you've never had an orgasm" on page 113.) Consider seeing a therapist. It can be a sign of childhood abuse combined with repressed memories (see Chap-ter 8, "Serious Sex-Related Issues").

F FOR HER

If it's temporary, consciously concentrate on feelings and sensa-tions when you are having sex, and don't get too hung up on hav-ing an orgasm. Reacquaint yourself with your own body, learn what it responds to. Talk to your lover; tell him what turns you on, what doesn't, ask for more foreplay and use extra lubrication if you're dry. Deliberately focus on your erotic self. Do you *feel* like a sexual person? One therapist I know claims she can pick people who enjoy sex by the way they dress, walk, and behave. People who like sex focus on their appearance, walk with confidence, and like touching. People who don't aren't as aware of their bodies. Have sex more—the more you have it, the more you'll usually want it, so indulge whenever you feel remotely turned-on.

If your problem's long-term, you may have grown up feeling guilty about sex and may never have been "woken" erotically. In other words, you simply don't know how to respond to sexual sensations in your body. A *sensate focus program* is what sex therapists use to help you "learn" how to give and receive pleasure. The idea is to reawaken your sexual feelings gradually by using sensual massage to explore first your own, then your partner's, body. Intercourse is banned—you give and get pleasure through touch alone. Start by exploring *your own* body through massage. Have a bubble bath, use soap in the shower, or oil your body and lie on the bed. Experiment with different strokes (soft, firm, fast, slow) to find out what feels good and arouses you. Don't just concentrate on the genitals and breasts; explore all of your body. Stage two involves massaging each other with oil in much the same way, this time avoiding the sex organs. In stage three, you're officially "allowed" to touch more sexually sensitive parts with one proviso: you must talk constantly, keeping up a running commentary of what stroke and pressure feels best. When you've explored each stage thoroughly, you have permission to have intercourse. It helps if you also reduce stress as much as possible, opt for less "threatening" sex (like massages and oral sex), and make a "date" for sex at least once a week if you both have busy schedules.

Ⓜ FOR HIM

- **Don't make her feel guilty.** Pressuring her into having sex when she doesn't want to will kill any desire she may have. Make it clear you won't get upset or offended if she says "no" to sex. Remove the pressure.
- **Talk to her.** Say you've noticed she doesn't seem that keen (lately or always). Ask her why. Is she just tired or do your techniques need improving? Does she need more foreplay? Would she like a massage?

- **Support her if her disinterest is caused by a painful past.**
  Encourage her to get professional help if she needs it. Don't
  insist she tells you every sordid detail of what happened but let
  her know you're there if she wants to talk. Don't judge her and
  don't offer advice. Instead, listen and give her lots of (nonsexual) hugs.

She can't come

Hands up if you expect to have an orgasm every single time you
make love. Great! An optimistic attitude alone will guarantee you
more climaxes. But it's a tad unrealistic all the same. The mood
you're in, what's happening in your life and relationship, the
amount and type of foreplay—all these can affect whether we'll
come or not and a lot are out of our control.

Inhibitions stop us feeling relaxed enough to orgasm with a
partner. Inexperience—not knowing our own body—doesn't
help either. But again, the biggest obstacle between us and the Big
O is a partner who's just plain hopeless in bed. If his idea of foreplay is "Are you awake?" the chances of orbiting into erotic ecstasy
are pretty slim.

If you've never had an orgasm at all, there's a section devoted
exclusively to you in Chapter 4, page 113. Here, we'll deal with
women who have trouble coming with their lover.

F FOR HER

First up, look at how you orgasm when you're on your own. Are
you addicted to your vibrator? Learn a more couple-friendly technique by learning to climax with your fingers. It's then simply a
matter of showing him the right buttons to push by doing some
serious communication, both in and out of bed. Use a bridge technique if you have no trouble coming while masturbating. While
he's inside you, get him to stimulate your clitoris with his fingers;
or bring you to the brink through oral sex, then use your own finger to continue stimulating your clitoris during intercourse. Try
the "fake it till you make it" technique (act as if it's happening and
it might).

Some women subconsciously stop themselves going over the
edge with a partner because they're worried they'll lose control or

get too attached to him. If this rings true, ask yourself, "What's the worst thing that could happen if I did come with him?" He'll think you enjoy sex? (How awful!) You might fall in love? (He might feel the same way—and if he doesn't, you'll survive.)

Only 10 percent of women have never had an orgasm by any means, and most therapists agree (rare physical problems aside) that all women can be taught to orgasm with a partner through sex therapy.[5] All it takes is time, patience, a relaxed and open attitude, and (most important) a skilled, sensitive lover. (Remember, sex can be "taught.") If you need professional help, get it. Call the American Psychological Association and ask for a referral to someone in your area. Why miss out on one of life's most pleasurable experiences?

Ⓜ FOR HIM

- **Stimulate her clitoris.** Add extra lubrication and use your fingers to stroke it gently throughout intercourse.

- **Become a better lover.** Read some good sex books, rent a few how-to videos (I don't mean porn—try Andrew Stanway's *The Lover's Guide* series), ask her for feedback.

- **Give her time.** Women take longer to reach orgasm than men do. If you only masturbate her or give her oral sex for a few minutes, you might as well not bother. Settle in and tell her to take as long as she likes.

> "I can masturbate to orgasm within a minute. With my boyfriend, it takes at least fifteen minutes of skilled stimulation. I don't know why, but it's always been that way for me."
>
> Ellen, 27, advertising executive

Sex is painful

Almost all of us have occasionally let out a loud *"Ouch!"* at some stage during sex, particularly if we're trying a new position that goes too deep. But if it's hurting on a regular basis and you're mainlining martinis to cope with the pain, it's a warning something's wrong.

Painful intercourse is officially called *dyspareunia*. The pain may be deep and aching, sharp, a momentary twinge, or intensely uncomfortable. It can be selective (it's only painful at certain times) or permanent (all the time) and the causes are diverse. It could be the result of an infection (even a flare-up of candida can make us dry and sex painful), constipation, a sexually transmitted infection, a disorder of the reproductive system (like endometriosis), a urinary tract infection (like cystitis), or again (sorry guys!) clumsy or rough technique on the part of your partner. If he doesn't spend enough time on foreplay (or isn't very good at it), your vagina doesn't expand and lubricate in preparation for penetration. Instead, it stays tight and dry, which makes intercourse uncomfortable or shoot-through-the-roof painful.

Not being wet is one of the most common causes of painful sex. Our natural lubrication is affected by the menstrual cycle, stress and tiredness, age—a million things! The best way to increase lubrication is to have more (good) foreplay, the second best way is to add a water-based lubricant at the beginning of making love. It'll make sex more pleasurable, encouraging your natural secretions to kick in. The Pill can cause vaginal mucosa, a thinning of your natural lubrication; fix it by switching to a pill higher in estrogen or change contraception. Hot tubs, vaginal deodorants, and scented soap all also rob moisture.

If the pain is severe, you may have *vaginismus*, which causes the vaginal muscles to go into spasm, stopping penetration entirely. It may start from the first time you have sex or occur later, usually after a painful infection or unexpected pain from a deep thrust. (It's a little like impotence: dismiss it as a one-time thing and you may be okay; worry about it and you'll get tense and start to associate intercourse with pain.) The causes are usually psychological, and it's not something you can control because it's a reflex.

In almost all extreme, chronic cases of vaginismus, the woman has had a frightening early experience with intercourse—been raped, sexually abused, or always suffered pain. (If you suspect or know this has happened to you, get professional help. At the very least, read Chapter 8, "Serious Sex-Related Issues.") If your parents saw sex as wicked, the mere mention of the word can leave you feeling terrified and tense.

Ⓕ FOR HER

First things first. Call your gynecologist or your doctor. If a chronic
infection or urinary tract disorder is
responsible, a course of antibiotics
may be all you need. Your vagina
tenses up on the odd occasion? It
could have to do with relationship
fears. Are you frightened of getting
pregnant or an STI? Don't trust
your partner? Maybe you're just
not in the mood for sex and your
vagina is telling you so. If you've
ruled out medical reasons and it's a
major problem, consider therapy.

> "Guys seem to think if they can hump away for hours, it makes them a stud. The fact is, after five or ten minutes, I'm bored. If he's still thrusting after twenty minutes, I'm sore and also thinking, 'He can't be that turned on by me or he'd have come by now.' "
>
> Robyn, 24, dental assistant

A sex therapist will concentrate on two areas to solve your problem: how you feel about sex generally and your lover's sexual technique (or lack of it). In the meantime have more foreplay to make sure you're lubricated, add extra lubricant, spread your thighs wide and bend your knees to aid penetration, bearing down (pushing out) as your partner enters you to relax the muscles of the vagina.

If you have vaginismus, try these self-help exercises. Do them daily for several weeks and avoid intercourse until you're ready.

1. Start by taking a bath or simply lying quietly for a little while. Then look at your genitals in a hand mirror. Touch the entrance with a lubricated finger, then try inserting it when you feel relaxed, bearing down slightly.

2. Leave the finger in place for a few minutes, then push it in a bit farther. If you start to tighten up, stop, then *deliberately* tighten the muscles around your finger, to a count of three then release. Repeat until you feel in control; aim for at least twenty con-tractions. These are called Kegel exercises. Keep practicing until you can push a finger all the way in without spasming.

3. Try the same thing with two fingers, using lots of lubrication. Then . . .

4. Repeat the exercise with a trusted partner. You set the pace. When you feel ready for intercourse, try a woman-on-top posi-

tion. Get him to lie still, lower yourself on and let him penetrate when you feel ready. Deliberately tighten and relax your vaginal muscles as he penetrates.

Ⓜ FOR HIM

- **Encourage her to get a check-up.** Make sure she rules out medical reasons, then suggest she sees a therapist if you think it's psychological.
- **Triple the foreplay.** The more relaxed and aroused she is, the less likely it is to hurt. Don't attempt intercourse if she feels dry and/or tight.
- **Always use lubricant.** It's the single most effective way to reduce pain.

"My ex-boyfriend was totally hung up on the fact that his penis was slightly smaller than normal. Every time I touched it or looked at it, he'd say, 'You're disappointed aren't you?' I wasn't, but I was sick of having to give constant reassurance. I mean, get over it!"

Carla, 20, nurse

FIVE WAYS TO HELP HER THROUGH A ROUGH TIME

1. **Vary your lovemaking as much as possible.** The more effort you put into making sex fun and erotic, the more likely she is to want it. Educate yourself. You can't be sexually experienced without being sexually educated.
2. **Don't be negative.** Accuse her of being frigid and she'll retreat even further. Do quite the opposite. Shower her with compliments (sexual and otherwise), lift her self-esteem to the sky, spoil her with (nonsexual) massages, say you don't mind just cuddling if that's what makes her happy. If you feel frustrated, masturbate.
3. **Talk to her about it.** Take on the problem as if it were your own. The more she opens up to you, the closer you'll both be to hitting on the cause.

EMOTIONAL TIME BOMBS

A sex therapist friend of mine estimates that for every ten times a couple has sex, one or two sessions are fantastic, about five are mediocre, and the remaining three are boring or disastrous.[6] I agree with her. *No one* has great sex all of the time and one reason is this: It's not just the two of you in the bed. Getting in beside you both are your ex-lovers, your mothers and fathers, sisters, brothers, the horrible teacher you had in fifth grade, the man who "flashed" you when you were two, his grandmother, and the girl in the corner shop he kissed when he was ten. In other words, by the time you're ready to settle down, both of you are products of numerous small and several significant life events. You can't turn him into a sexual or emotional version of you or vice versa. There will always be points of difference both in and out of the bedroom.

A lot of the way we relate to our partner is dependent on our parents. Psychologists believe most of our emotional programming happens when we are very young: 50 percent between the ages of zero to five years, 30 percent between five to eight years, and 15 percent between eight and eighteen. So, by the time you're eighteen, you're 95 percent programmed—which leaves 5 percent to work with. Horrified? Don't be. That teeny

❗ A case of getting the milk for free, so no need to buy the cow? Psychologists found couples who live together are less enthusiastic about marriage than singles who still live at home with Mom or Dad. Cohabitating couples also want fewer children and are more tolerant of divorce.[7]

5 percent can turn around most of your programming if you want it to.[8]

The secret to a happy, successful, long-term sex life is compromise and communication. Here are some solutions to common couple sex problems.

What do I do if I'm bored with sex? I've been in the same relationship for years and we've done just about everything already. Is it inevitable that sex dies?

Nothing gets my blood boiling more than when people say to me, "It's natural for sex to die. There's nothing you can do about it." The sort of people who feed me that drivel take great offense at my standard reply of "Actually there are lots of things you can do to keep sex hot, you just have to work at it," because they're lazy. The only advantage new lovers have over long-term ones is newness—the thrill of conquering unknown territory—pretty insignificant when weighed up against the positives: feeling comfortable with each other, talking openly, and enjoying a total lack of inhibition because you trust each other implicitly. Believing sex always fizzles out eventually is like not applying for a job because you're convinced you won't get it. Who knows what might happen if you make the effort? It's the same with your sex life. It's *common* for couples to lose the sexual fizz but it's *preventable*. This whole book is devoted to suggesting ways to make sex varied and better. Forgive me for not believing you've done "everything" already, but I don't.

Why do I find sex less exciting once I fall in love?

When we sleep with someone purely for sex, we can be as wanton and wicked as we like because we don't really care what they think of us. Once we decide we like them and do care, it's like a bucket of freezing water is poured over any and all sexual fantasies and desires that aren't considered "normal." Will he think I'm slutty? Will she think I'm weird? We switch from horny lover role to what we think is Husband or Wife material. Talk to your partner next time you feel like this, hopefully sharing a laugh about how silly your fears are. If they do expect you to act differently in bed now that you're an item, I'd be considering whether I wanted to be.

I'm always the one to initiate sex, and I hate the fact that she doesn't.

When you initiate sex, does she enthusiastically respond or seem halfhearted? If it's the first scenario, she may feel she needs "permission" (your suggesting it first) because good girls shouldn't really like it *that* much. Or perhaps you have a much higher libido than she does and simply want sex more often (she doesn't get a *chance* to get horny because you're always jumping in first). If she's lukewarm to your suggestions, she probably doesn't enjoy sex (with you or at all) and does it just because she has to. Ask her why. Maybe you're a bad lover, and she's too shy to tell you. Ask her if there's anything you can do to make it more enjoyable. Wine and dine her, massage her, give her lots of foreplay and see if that makes a difference. If something feels good we *like* doing it often.

How come I always end up having sex his way?

I don't know. Presumably you can speak. Get a grip, girl! Tell him you want to try something new or just take control and jump on top of him. If you lie back like a receptacle, can you blame him for assuming you want him to call the shots?

My girlfriend loves sex but hates "quickies." Why?

It could be something as simple as this: it takes her a while to lubricate. Buy some lubricant and see if that helps. Lots of women get turned on rapidly mentally, but it takes a while for their body to follow (and "dry" sex isn't fun). Ask *her* why she doesn't like them. Quickies are a great adjunct to leisurely sex but if you opt for one every second session, I don't blame her for not being thrilled.

Who sleeps in the wet spot?

One night you do, the next he does.

How do I say no to sex without upsetting him?

Here's a novel concept: don't worry if you do. Most men would prefer you say no than have sex when you don't want to. If he does want you to perform on demand, change partners. The fact is, you don't need his permission to refuse. If you're polite and he's a nice guy, he might roll over huffily and sulk for a while but, hopefully, he'll be aware he's acting childishly. How best to say thanks but no thanks? That really depends on the guy. Try telling the truth. "I'm exhausted and just feel like sleep" or "I don't know why, I just don't feel like it. Let's cuddle instead." Make it clear you're rejecting sex not him, and he should handle it okay.

Is it ever okay to fake it?

No (most of the time), maybe (sometimes). See "Faking it" (page 96) for answers to these cryptic clues.

How do I tell a much-loved partner he's abysmal in bed without using words?

Try using body language to get the message across. When he does something you do like, exaggerate your response: moan loudly, move closer, kiss him harder so he can't help but get the message you like what he's doing. If you don't like something, make that abundantly clear as well: twist away, lift your body away from his touch, or (better) redirect his hand/mouth or penis. Most people do to their partners what they'd like done to them. If you like having your ear licked and bitten, you'll lick and bite his. Slip this into a conversation as a bit of interesting trivia then give him the attention *you'd* like the next time you're in bed.

If he still doesn't get the hint, you've got no other option but to talk to him. You really are better off using words than actions anyway. Just about every woman has lain there thinking, "If I just hang in there a bit longer, he's *bound* to hit the right spot sooner or later." But squirm all you want, sometimes it just isn't going to happen unless you say something. Sadly, you're not alone in wanting to stay silent. A lot of people don't say anything in bed, let alone "Let me have it harder and a little to the left." But how's he to know you think he's boring unless you tell him?

I like doing "kinky" things but get the feeling my current lover would be horrified. How do I feel her out about this, without embarrassing myself or scaring her off?

It really depends on what you—and she—define as kinky. No matter how broad-minded your lover is, I wouldn't suggest striding into the bedroom, dressed in her underwear, without giving her a little warning first. But if "kinky" simply means trying something new, try using the third-person perspective to introduce a tricky topic. Say "I heard a story about a friend who" or "I had a dream about" and see what reaction you get. Or say you've got a fantasy about such-and-such. That way, you're insinuating rather than directly propositioning, which can be erotic anyway. If she nervously starts wringing her hands, there's your answer. If she looks interested, follow it up with "Why don't we try it next time?"

> "I was doing a girl doggie-style once and really getting into it, but all she could talk about was how big her butt must look. It was a turn-off! We don't notice your flaws, so there's no need to hide them. When we stare at you walking around naked, we're appreciating the good parts, not focusing on what you think are the bad."
>
> Jeremy, 18, bartender

Will he think I've "been around" if I suggest something unusual?

Again, it depends on what it is but I'd imagine most guys would be ecstatic rather than horrified if you'd like to try something new. If he thinks you're not a "nice girl" for wanting to experiment, you're probably mismatched anyway. Do you want to spend the rest of your life acting like a nun?

> "You can't help but love women who can achieve that up-but-falling-down look with their hair or put on a show and parade their new underwear. The sight of her, lying deliberately arranged on the bed in my underwear gives me an erection so hard, I could carve my initials in it."
>
> Phillip, 23, photographer

Often, I don't orgasm during intercourse even though my lover always does. I know I could come if he gave me oral sex afterward. Is it fair to ask?

Is it fair that he has an orgasm and you don't? Of course it's fair to expect to feel satisfied at the end of making love. Just bear in mind that men aren't as blasé about body secretions as women are (they've never had to cope with things like periods) but a quick one-minute wash in the bathroom is likely to change his mind until he loosens up a little. Alternatively, have an orgasm before intercourse through oral sex, or ask him to manually masturbate you with his fingers afterward. Better still, get him to stimulate your clitoris *during* intercourse.

If he/she gives me an orgasm through oral sex, do I have to give him/her one, too?

You probably are expected to reciprocate, but it doesn't have to be immediately. Take turns. Lots of couples plan sex sessions where one partner concentrates on the other. One day, he can massage you, finish with oral sex, and let you drift straight off into a delicious sleep; the next time, you do the same for him.

> "I always feel vulnerable after sex—I think all women do. I don't want poetry, just some sort of acknowledgment that you enjoyed it and I wasn't just a notch on the bedpost."
>
> Katherine, 25, chef

He wants me to try anal sex, but I don't want to.

Many men and women find anal sex a turn-on; lots of others would rather have pins stuck in their eyes. It's a personal decision, and while his suggesting it doesn't make him secretly gay or a pervert, he shouldn't pressure you if you don't want to. If you do decide to give it a try, let him insert a finger into your rectum to see if you like the sensation before inserting his penis. See "Anal stimulation" (page 80) for more details.

My lover wants me to masturbate in front of him. Am I being a prude by not doing it? Is this now considered normal behavior?

Ten to fifteen years ago, women didn't even admit that they masturbated, let alone put on live floor shows. Men, on the other hand, have always masturbated—a lot—and this is why he thinks it's no big deal to ask. There's a very good reason to go along with the idea—he'll have a front-row seat to watch how you give yourself pleasure. (See Chapter 1 for hints on doing it in front of each other.) Don't let him pressure you, but consider trying it: we should always push ourselves a little sexually. Stay in the comfort zone all the time and you won't grow.

Should I share my fantasies with my partner?

It depends on how well you know and trust your partner. A friend of mine once confessed to a new lover that she'd always fantasized about sleeping with another woman. The next time she saw him, they had company: an escort girl he'd hired. Lizzie, understandably, wasn't as impressed with his "little surprise" as he thought she'd be. Kept secret or told to the right partner, most fantasies are harmless, terrific sex-boosters. Told to the wrong person, they become revenge material for the dumped and bitter. Personally, I'd save them for a long-term, committed, and sexually liberated partner. (See "Lights, camera, erection!," page 264, if you do decide to share.)

Why does she hate it if I look at porn mags? Do I give up now on her ever watching porn *with* me?

Ever since Hugh Hefner launched *Playboy* in 1954, women the world over have gotten their panties in a wad over pictures of women not wearing any. The fact is, the *majority* of men don't watch porn for the sinister reasons women think they do. They do it because it's fun. Most men are turned-on by mainstream porn (which doesn't include material involving children, animals, or extreme violence). Because men are better at separating love from sex than women are, they consider porn films an innocent "boy thing," and most can't understand why girlfriends take offense. Quite frankly, neither can I if we're talking about

"A bed is good for two things, and the other one is sleeping. Why do women turn it into a cross between an analyst's couch and a confessional by wanting to talk about 'us' in those post-sex, pre-sleep moments? Where do you get the energy? If you want to talk about the relationship, save it for dinner. Even worse, is the guilt tripper. 'I wish I hadn't done that,' you'll say. What we really want to hear is 'That was great. Let's do it again tomorrow night.' "

Alex, 36, musician

the odd copy of *Playboy* or *Penthouse* or an occasional X-rated video. Just don't *expect* her to watch or read it with you unless she wants to—and if she's extremely antiporn, yes, give up now on ever sharing it with her.

It's a different story, however, if you're obsessed with porn. Do you subscribe to *all* the porn mags, including the hard-core ones? Have you given up work to sit by the TV? Do you use it as a substitute for sex with her or can't perform without it? Then you've got problems best dealt with by a sex therapist. But research shows that the infrequent porn user is your average guy. It doesn't mean you don't love your girlfriend or find her sexy if you look at porn mags. It doesn't mean you're comparing her to the girl on the page or screen or that you particularly want her to act like that. Men are turned on by pictures, women by words. You don't get upset when she curls up with a steamy novel, do you?

Why don't women like giving oral sex?

Some women think penises are unclean, "yucky," or "disgusting" because that's the place you pee from. Others have had a bad experience: some guy forced their head down until they gagged or maybe he didn't wash his genitals properly (particularly nasty if he's not circumcised). Some women don't like giving fellatio simply because they're frightened they'll gag and be sick, others don't like swallowing the semen at the end. If you shower regularly and thoroughly, let her control the position and depth, don't put your hands on the back of her head, and don't make a fuss if she doesn't swallow, a lot more women would be converts. Let her know this is how you'll behave. Also tell her even if she's a novice, you don't really care what she does, it'll feel great. Men love oral sex because their girlfriend appears to be worshiping what he's worshiped since he discovered it—his penis. Plus, he gets to do nothing, while she becomes the aggressor.

Must I swallow?

Most men are so happy to have their penis in your mouth, not swallowing at the crucial moment is a small part of the whole process (only a handful think it's like watching the Superbowl without a beer). So long as you don't abandon him completely as he's about to climax, chances are he won't really care. Some women don't swallow but simply hold the semen in their mouths for a minute until they can spit it out in a tissue or the sink. Others switch to using a hand or let him thrust between their breasts.

I'm more turned-on during my period than at any other time of the month. Should I warn a new lover or just continue having sex?

Definitely warn him—looking down to see blood isn't pleasant even when you are expecting it; when you're not, it's run-out-of-the-room stuff. If you have your period and want to have intercourse, all you need to do is have an old towel handy (and hopefully a shower close by) and say something like, "I've got my period but I don't want to wait. It doesn't bother me if it doesn't bother you." Don't get too huffy if he balks at the idea. Blood makes lots of us squeamish and remember, he's had a lifetime of women saying, "I can't. I've got my period." He may just need a little time to get used to it. For some women, the thought of having sex during their period is unthinkable; others can't see what all the fuss is about. It depends on your mood and the heaviness of your flow.

> "Some men think if a woman's experienced and really gets into it, she must have slept with the Foreign Legion. I think there's nothing *worse* than a girl who lies there like a sack of potatoes. If she doesn't seem interested, I'm not, either. Moan, move, spout Russian—do *something* to let us know if you're enjoying it."
>
> Alex, 32, architect

He wants to know how many lovers I've had. How many should I admit to? Must I tell the truth?

What you did before you met him is your business, what he did before meeting you is his. There's no obligation to tell him anything at all about your sexual past unless it could directly affect his health. If you do decide to bare all, be aware that you will be judged—and not necessarily by the same rules he judges himself. If he confesses to fifty lovers, your fifteen may still be five too many.

The most commonly cited statistic is ten lovers for the "average" female. Just who she is, is anyone's guess. It also depends on your age—a twenty-five-year-old would reasonably be expected to have had more lovers than an eighteen-year-old. Plenty of women sleep with just one or two people, others clock up more than fifty guilt-free, and lots hover around the twenty to thirty mark. Instead of reducing your sexual history to a number, why not let the truth slowly emerge over the years? As the relationship deepens, you soon figure out each other's significant previous relationships. The rest don't count.

OTHER RELATIONSHIP WRECKERS

Unless that's *all* you're in it for, you can't separate sex from your relationship. Here are some common couple "love" complaints and how to handle them.

My boyfriend cheated on me when we were going through a rough patch, and I can't forget about it.

Don't try because you won't. Some couples do survive infidelity, most don't. A lot depends on his reason. The fact that he was drunk and it just happened isn't acceptable to most people. Did he wear a condom? If he was together enough to get it out of the wrapper, he was lucid enough to spare you a thought. Could he get an erection? He wasn't that drunk. Saying sorry isn't enough. You need to find out why he did it and why he thinks he won't do it again. If he's remorseful for a few weeks then gets tired of discussing the subject, ditch him now. *He* screwed up, you're the one trying to live with *his* mistake, so it's up to *him* to make you feel better. If you've only just started going out and you still can't look at him months later without feeling angry, let him go. If you've been going out for years and intellectually understand why

> "I appreciate that lots of women aren't obvious when they orgasm, but does he have to ask if I've had one every five minutes? I'll just be starting to enjoy oral sex when his head pops up to ask the question. It puts me off and I feel like I have to hurry. I wish he'd shut up and get on with it."
>
> Erica, 19, journalist

he did it (even if it still hurts like hell), hang in there for six months, maybe even get some counseling. But it's up to him to earn back your trust. Sometimes an affair can unearth problems and something good comes out of it. Most of the time it simply means he can't control himself and doesn't respect you.

I love my fiancé but I can't honestly say I lust after him. Am I being too picky to want chemistry when everything else is so perfect?

No. A relationship without sexual attraction is friendship. If you don't lust after your boyfriend, he's your best friend, not a prospective husband. This is hard to accept and there are plenty of people out there who will tell you to ignore my advice and marry him anyway. If you do, I hope you have a happy, contented life together, but I fear you'll spend most of it eyeing waiters, flirting with the butcher, and probably having a series of affairs. Living a sexless life isn't fair to you and it's not fair to him. He might do nothing for your libido but there's someone out there who thinks he's sex-on-legs. Let her find him. If you're lucky and treat the situation sensitively, your fiancé could well end up being what he should have always been: a very special friend.

My partner constantly eyes other women. How do I stop him?

There's a difference between noticing and admiring good-looking people and that creepy undressing-with-their-eyes lecherous leer some men have perfected. The first is normal, the second disrespectful. He'll probably say you're paranoid, jealous, or insecure when you confront him. Some women *do* overreact, so do a reality check first. Ask a well-trusted friend (even better, a well-trusted ex) if they think you have a history of imagin-

❗ What do men rate as most essential in a female sex partner?
Stamina: 9.1 percent
Large breasts: 10.3 percent
Good oral sex technique:
  11.9 percent
Good body: 19.2 percent
Sense of humor:
  20.2 percent
Being clean: 24.5 percent
Willing to try anything:
  33.3 percent[9]

ing things. If they don't, you're convinced you're viewing the situation objectively, and you really like the guy, start by telling him calmly how much you dislike him looking at other women while you're with him. Ask him to stop it. If he denies he behaves that way in the first place, simply say, "Great. But I just want you to know it upsets me." Wait until you've been out a few times to see if there's an improvement. If there isn't, sit him down again and say that unless he stops now, you're not interested in being with him. If he changes his tune immediately, give him *one* more chance. If he doesn't and you find it intolerable, leave.

My partner is smothering me. She wants to be with me every second, calls (the few hours) when we aren't together, and sucks every last drop of energy I have. I love her, but when I ask her to give me space, she gets upset.

Relationships guru Barbara De Angelis calls people like this "emotional vampires" and that's exactly what they are: desperately needy, scared of being alone, feeding off your energy, your *life*. The constant attention is tremendously flattering to start with but quickly becomes tremendously irritating. The fact is, no matter how much time or love you give her, it will never be enough. Someone or something has hurt her in the past—and you're not her therapist. Don't hang around out of pity (or fear that she'll do something silly).

Do suggest she seek professional help to unravel why she's so insecure. People who love themselves aren't leeches—they enjoy their own company and draw on their own resources rather than always relying on others.

My old boyfriend/girlfriend hurt me badly. I'm taking it *very* slow with my new lover, but am frightened I'll never love again.

Good for you. It's prudent and sensible to take it slowly. You really *shouldn't* wear your heart on your sleeve: it belongs where nature put it—protected inside. Keep your eyes wide open, look at your new partner objectively, and don't rush things. Make sure you've learned from old mistakes. Why did the relationship break down? Did you pick the wrong person or were you also at fault? Work on your self-esteem. You deserve to be treated well—don't settle for anything less.

I've been seeing a girl for months but still never met her friends or family. What's the story?

Pretty much what you fear, I suspect. There are some situations that could explain it: like she's married (do you ever meet at her home?) or recently separated (she doesn't feel the people close to her are ready to be introduced to a new lover). Alternatively, maybe her friends and family have given her previous boyfriends a hard time and she's protecting you. But if she appears to adore them, refuses to discuss the problem, and simply doesn't include you, she either doesn't think you're good enough to parade in public or can't see a future together. Ask her outright, don't be blown off, and have pride.

> ❗ *19 − 5 = happy:*
> *Count the number of times you and your partner had sex last month, then subtract the number of arguments you had over the same period. A positive number means your relationship is strong. A negative number means you've got a lot more to solve than just this equation![10]*

THE THREESOME THAT WORKS: UNHAPPY COUPLE PLUS COUNSELOR

Lucky I'm not in charge of granting wedding licenses—I'd refuse to hand one over until all in-love couples had counseling. Look at it this way: would you go and see a doctor if he didn't have qualifications? Then why commit to live with someone for the rest of your life if they don't have good relationship skills? Counseling isn't just a way to repair the past, it's great preparation for the future.

There are psychological questionnaires now available that test your relationship IQ. You can't pick one up at your local newsstand but most good psychologists have one. Usually based on twelve major areas (like communication, children, sex, and conflict resolution), the questionnaire can predict what parts of your relationship you both need to work on and which are coasting along nicely. Do it *before* you move in or get married and you'll know what you're up against. The counselor will also give you practical tips on handling the problems before you hit them. Makes sense to me.

Already in a serious relationship that isn't great? You've got two options: walk out or work it out. If counseling can't save the relationship you're in, the next will benefit from it anyway!

Get help if you're:

- arguing about the same things over and over.
- feeling irritable and moody, bored or frustrated.
- finding excuses not to be together and spending less time with each other.
- not having regular sex.
- feeling like you're "beating your head against a brick wall" when you talk to each other.
- noticing (and fancying) others.
- feeling more like roommates than lovers.
- considering ending it—or having an affair.

FOUR THINGS MEN WISH WOMEN KNEW ABOUT SEX

1. We hate pillow talk.
2. We love it when you're obviously sexy.
3. We hate it if you just lie there.
4. The only lumps we notice on your body are your breasts.

FOUR THINGS WOMEN WISH MEN KNEW ABOUT SEX

1. We don't want to sleep with King Dong.
2. We don't want you to go on all night.
3. Asking "Have you come yet?" stops it from happening.
4. Saying something nice afterward is a good idea.

What will happen if we go to a counselor?

It depends on what state your relationship's in and how good your communication skills are. Most troubled couples have between six and twelve hour-long sessions, starting off once a week, then spreading them out over a longer period. During the first session, the counselor will talk about your problems and get an idea of the relationship dynamics—your personalities and how you relate to each other. After that, they'll start problem solving, put some action plans in place, and teach skills. Don't be surprised if the problem you went for doesn't turn out to be the real issue. While his not helping around the house is driving you nuts, it could be his refusal to even consider marriage that's *really* bothering you.

! *It seems absence does make the heart grow fonder. Two-thirds of separated couples polled said they missed each other more, not less, as time went by.[11]*

A good therapist will tailor a program to suit you both, but make no mistake, it will be incredibly demanding. For a start, you'll be given lots of homework (no point learning skills unless you practice them) and it's hard to break old habits, even if you know they're getting you nowhere. (P.S. The counselor won't tell you if it's best you split, but they will guide you in that direction if they honestly think you're beyond help.)

Counseling works for couples:

- who get help early. The sooner you go, the less damage the problems will cause long-term.
- who want the therapy to work. If one of you has fallen out of love or is under duress, the odds aren't tipped in your favor.
- who have a sense of humor. If you can laugh together, you're off and running.

Counseling doesn't work for couples:

- in the middle of a crisis. By the time you've sorted out the mess, you're too exhausted to work on change and you settle back into your old habits.
- who use it as a last resort. If one of you has already decided to leave, counseling just softens the blow.

- if one (or both) of you is having an affair and has no intention of ending it. Do I really need to explain why?
- who think the therapist will solve all their problems. They can only help you help yourselves.
- who aren't prepared to change. If you're so addicted to work/your friends/Monday night football and refuse to put the relationship first, the prospects aren't great.

How to find one

Call the National Board for Certified Counselors at 336-547-0607 (they also have a Web site at www.nbcc.org with a state-by-state listing) and ask for a list of recommended counselors in your area. You can't get a rebate from Medicare, though some private health providers do cover it. Some community groups offer free counseling, and some private psychologists will charge you pro rata on what you earn.

THE EX-FACTOR

Sometimes, sex problems stem from an unhealthy obsession with an unfairly intoxicating ex who seemed to steal your libido along with that favorite CD. If you're still fantasizing about an old lover months or years later (come on—no one's that good!), try the following.

1. Write down why sex was so great with that person: what you did (be as specific as possible), where you did it, why it felt sensational. It'll lean heavier on one of two sides: you'll discover the physical act was irrelevant and it was the person that turned you on *or* you did things with them you haven't done with others.

2. Can you re-create it? If it was the person, think about the circumstances of your life at the time. You can't compare dating Bill in hum-drum, daily life to screwing Brad while vacationing in Bali. Put Brad in your *real* life and sex would seem just as mundane. Utterly convinced it was a case of chemistry? Fine. If it's that important to you, hang out until the sparks fly with someone else. If you're pining over what

you did during sex, what's stopping you doing it with your new partner? Don't tell him how great it felt when Brad teased your clitoris with his tongue, tell him how great it would feel if *he* did it.

3. Do a reality check. Still convinced they're the only person who can ever make you feel like that again? You're not only being unrealistic, it's futile. For a start, you've idealized it: *no one's* that good in the sack. Go back to the start of the exercise, work out what it was that made sex so earth-shattering, then find someone to re-create it with.

4. Look hard at the relationship you're in. Is it a bandage? Are you having sex to dull the pain? Or are you so blinded by the past, you can't see that what you've got is actually better? Decide which category it falls into, then do something about it. Leave or give it 100 percent. Get some therapy if you seriously can't let go on your own.

8

Serious Sex-Related Issues

Coping with the aftermath of abortion, rape, and incest

•••

There are some sex-related problems that no one likes to talk about; consequently information is scarce and myths abound. This chapter is for women and men who have suffered the devastation of sexual abuse, either as a child or an adult, and I've also included a section for women who are contemplating having, or have had, a pregnancy terminated.

I've only scratched the surface of the emotions you may be struggling with, but hopefully you'll find helpful, practical information and answers to your most commonly asked questions.

HAVING A TERMINATION

About 65 million abortions are performed worldwide per year, and around 1.5 million of those are in the U.S.[1] Despite the fact that safe abortion is readily available, most women would probably prefer not to think about it, let alone have one. Unfortunately, you may need to at some stage in your life. This is what to expect if you do.

What should I do if I think I'm at risk of an unwanted pregnancy?

If you've had unprotected sex, go to a doctor and get the Morning After Pill. Taken within seventy-two hours, it will stop the pregnancy from happening. Having an IUD inserted within five days of conception is another option. If it's too late for either, pick up a home pregnancy test from a pharmacy (they're almost 100 percent accurate) and test two days after your missed period. Family planning clinics also offer on-the-spot pregnancy testing.

What are my options if I am pregnant?

You have three: have the baby and keep it, put it up for adoption, or have an abortion. Deciding which is best for you isn't easy. For some women, getting accidentally pregnant is a blessing in disguise. For others, particularly young women or those not in a serious, long-term relationship, it's devastating.

Some of the questions you need to ask yourself include:

- Do I want to bring up a child with the father? Would I have stayed with him if I wasn't pregnant?
- If I go it alone, do I think the child will suffer from not having a father? How will I cope as a single parent?
- Am I emotionally mature and able to cope with a child and all the associated responsibilities?
- How would I cope with the emotional fallout of putting my baby up for adoption?
- Will having a child affect my earning capacity? Will I feel resentful later because it detrimentally affected my career and my lifestyle? Can I/we financially afford to support a child?
- Do I have a good support network—family and friends who will help out if I decide to have the baby?

You may also struggle with moral issues. For obvious reasons, abortion is a highly emotional subject. Some religions, cultures, and antiabortion campaigners (like the Right to Life organization) believe it can't be justified under any circumstances (though some will make allowances for pregnancy resulting from rape). If you do decide to proceed with a termination, you may have to pass through protesters on the day of the procedure. If this concerns you, try to get it done during the week. (Most protests are scheduled for the weekends, particularly Saturdays.)

If adoption appeals, consult with a religious counselor or look in the Yellow Pages under "Adoption." Explain that you're considering putting your child up for adoption and ask for counseling.

Should I tell the father?

Advice from the experts varies here. Some say, barring exceptional circumstances (you were sexually abused or fear the father may become violent), he should be told. If he has trouble fathering a child in the future, it's important for him to know he was fertile in the past. Others say, if it's a casual relationship, you'll gain little by confessing. But if the relationship is serious and you plan to continuing going out after the termination, it's probably advisable to share the burden. It takes two to get pregnant and telling him means you can support each other throughout the trauma. Despite the rare case where fathers have taken women to court in a bid to stop them from having an abortion, the father can't legally stop you having an abortion.

Who do I call to arrange a termination?

There are specialist termination clinics in most cities, run privately or through public hospitals. Many private gynecologists also perform abortions; simply get a referral from your doctor. Otherwise, call Planned Parenthood, consult a friend who's had one, or look in the Yellow Pages under "Abortion." Be aware that some right-to-life groups list their numbers under these headings. How do you know you're not calling one? You don't, but it will become obvious. Explain that you want a termination, ask how much it costs, and a few medical questions (about things like physical complications) and it will soon become clear whether the group performs abortions or wants to counsel you to change your mind.

You can make an appointment over the phone. Terminations aren't horrendously expensive, but if you can't raise the money, tell the clinic when you make the appointment. You can usually get an insurance rebate if you're covered by a plan—and women are also eligible for the procedure through Medicaid.

Is it legal?

In the United States, abortion is legal, thanks to the 1973 Supreme Court decision *Roe* v. *Wade*, which affirmed women's right to privacy—and the right to choose to have an abortion. But each state can still pass laws regarding how and where a woman can terminate a pregnancy. Even though abortion is legal nationwide, there are some places where it's made more difficult (if you're a minor or live in a state where public opinion is antiabortion, for instance). In other words, even though the ultimate choice is yours, it's worth checking with a local women's clinic or your doctor to find out how you'd fare if faced with an unwanted pregnancy.

When is it too late to have one?

The best time is between your sixth and twelfth week of pregnancy; they can't operate before the sixth week because the fetus is so small it's easily missed. Some clinics will operate up to eighteen weeks, but the more advanced you are, the more it costs, the more complicated and unpleasant it is, and the higher the risks. If you're eighteen weeks or over, it's a two-day procedure. On the first, you have counseling, an ultrasound, and dilators are inserted into your cervix which stay in overnight; you come back the next morning for the actual operation. A few clinics will perform terminations on women who are twenty-five weeks pregnant, but that's usually the cutoff point.

What will happen to me on the day?

In most clinics, counseling and the procedure are done on the same day with the whole process taking between three and four hours. You'll fill out some paperwork on your arrival, then be taken in for a counseling session to ensure the decision to have a termination was yours and that you're happy to proceed.

The counselor will ask questions like: Did someone else pressure you into having the abortion? Did you consider having the baby? How do you think you'll feel afterward? If the counselor is not totally convinced it is your choice, they won't give permission for the operation. They'll also send you away to think things through if you're not certain you're doing the right thing. If you haven't told anyone about it (you're too embarrassed or worried people will judge you), the clinic may arrange for support through community or private counseling.

Counseling will also focus on the reason you're there in the first place: ineffective (or no) contraception. They'll help find a method of birth control that suits you, perhaps give you a Pill prescription or Depo-Provera injection (which covers you for three months). They'll also go through your medical history, check that you get regular Pap smears, and talk about general sexual health (like the importance of using condoms).

If the decision is made to go ahead with the abortion, you'll be seen by two doctors or nurse practitioners: one who will sedate you, and one who will perform the procedure. Then you'll be asked to change into a T-shirt or nightie (which you will have been told to bring with you) and taken into the operating room. Most clinics use intravenous sedation as well as injecting local anesthetic into the cervix. The sedation ensures you won't feel pain during the operation and you may not even remember it.

There are various methods of performing an abortion but all involve removing the products of conception from the uterus: the placenta, the sac, an embryo (up to eight weeks after conception) or fetus (after eight weeks). The technique is called *suction curettage* and it's similar to the dilate and curette (D and C) procedure sometimes used to investigate abnormal bleeding. The cervix is numbed with a local anesthetic and gently dilated, allowing a fine tube to be inserted into the uterus. The contents of the uterus are then suctioned out and the walls gently scraped with an instrument called a curette. The entire procedure takes between five and ten minutes.

Afterward, you'll be taken to a recovery room to rest for an hour or so and given something to eat and drink. A nurse will check the bleeding, take your blood pressure and pulse, and ensure you're coping emotionally. It's wise to rest when you get home and to take it easy for a few days, since you'll feel physically tired and emotionally drained.

What if I change my mind?

Some women decide they've made the wrong decision as they're taken into the operating room. This is totally acceptable. You'll simply be sent home and told to come back if you decide to go ahead with the termination. (About 50 percent of women return.)[2]

How will I feel afterward?

Physically

Many women experience a cramping pain on the first day, and most bleed. Some bleed heavily for a few days, then it lightens and should stop completely within seven to ten days. Intercourse, swimming, and baths (though you can shower) are not allowed for at least two weeks until the cervix returns to normal. You're also not allowed to use tampons (use pads instead) for the same period. The clinic will give you a week's supply of antibiotics to avoid infection. After two weeks, you'll need a checkup either at the clinic or with your doctor to ensure there's no infection and the uterus has returned to its normal size.

Complications are rare because most abortions are performed by experienced doctors. But there are two things that can go wrong: infection (make sure you take the full course of your antibiotics and alert the clinic of abnormal bleeding and/or pain) or "retained product." Retained product means they missed some of the fetus. Emotionally that can be hard to cope with, but physically it's easily fixed. Persistent bleeding, passing blood clots, or cramping pain (similar to a really heavy period) are all warning signs. If this happens, you need to go back to the clinic for another curette.

One termination won't usually affect future pregnancies. Some doctors claim ten won't either, as long as they're all performed by experienced doctors and you have no complications. Others say frequently dilating the cervix can make it "incompetent" (unable to support a fetus) or cause scar tissue.

> "I got pregnant when I was fifteen and my mother wouldn't let me have an abortion. I was forbidden to tell anyone and sent away to a home for unmarried, pregnant women when it started to show. My baby was taken from me and given to adoptive parents immediately after the birth. I didn't even get to hold her. It screwed me up for years and I've never forgiven my family. Why couldn't they have just organized an abortion rather than put me through all that pain?"
>
> Wendy, 35, housewife

Emotionally

Judging by the latest research, the vast majority of women who've had an abortion don't suffer long-term emotional trauma. But the best clue to how you'll cope is your mental well-being before the termination. One recent report, which focused on an ongoing study on more than 5000 women who'd had an abortion, found those with high self-esteem were able to put the event behind them and get on with their life.[3] In other words, those who found the procedure traumatic were troubled long before they showed up at an abortion clinic.

Having said that, there is obviously some emotional fallout. Almost all women experience a bewildering mix of relief and grief afterward. Even if you know it was the correct decision for you, you may mourn the loss and need to work through feelings of sadness, anger, or guilt. (Don't confuse regret with sadness—just because you feel sad, doesn't necessarily mean you've done the wrong thing.) It's important that you talk through any feelings you're experiencing, either with a counselor or a nonjudgmental friend or relative. Try keeping a diary for a few weeks or months afterward. Record how you feel about the loss of the baby as well as the man who fathered it. If he left you, it's a good way to vent anger; if you didn't tell him, write him a letter (even if you don't send it). You'll also experience hormonal changes (like depression) because you've gone from being pregnant to not pregnant. It can take up to a week to readjust hormonally.

How will the father feel?

You're not the only one who may struggle with guilt and grief and *both* of you may view sex differently. Some men are so fearful of it happening again, they'll avoid sex, have trouble getting an erection, or not want to orgasm inside you. You may also lose enthusiasm for obvious reasons. Usually, time heals; if it doesn't, get professional counseling.

CHILDHOOD SEXUAL ABUSE

As a child, you were probably told not to talk to strangers. In reality, you're far more likely to be abused by someone who's a member of or well-known by you and your family. Usually it's a close relative. More than 10 percent of men and 23 percent of women are believed to have been sexually abused at some stage of their life.[4] In 1995, local child protective service agencies identified 126,000 children who were victims of either substantiated or indicated sexual abuse. Nearly 30 percent of child victims were between the ages of four and seven.[5] Most people are horrified by these statistics but it's a sad fact that abuse, particularly childhood sexual abuse (like incest), is common.

Unfortunately, that doesn't make it any less emotionally devastating for its victims. If you were abused as a child, or suspect you might have been, please seek professional help rather than simply read this section of the book. It's designed as a starting point only. Obviously, this information is aimed at adults who've been abused in the past, not at the children tragically suffering now.

When is child abuse usually "found out"?

In the vast majority of cases, abuse is not discovered at the time it is happening because incredible pressure is put on the child to keep quiet; usually, the abuser tells the child they'll harm them or someone they love if they tell. Occasionally, an astute teacher or parent will notice sexual knowledge that seems inappropriate for the child's age, or unusual or sudden depression, aggression, or even suicidal tendencies. Or the child gets pregnant or picks up a sexually transmitted disease. Sometimes, if the memory of abuse is buried, it can burst out later in life through some significant experience—perhaps when you have your own children or your kids reach the age when you were abused. Even watching a program or reading an article about abuse can trigger the memory and cause someone to seek help.

"My father sexually abused me from age four to twelve but refuses to acknowledge it because he didn't penetrate me with his penis. I confronted him when I turned twenty, after confessing to a close girlfriend. I said I remembered him making me perform oral sex and him doing the same to me and all he said was, 'Don't be silly. That was just a game we played.' My mother doesn't believe me, and the police said I didn't have a strong enough case to prosecute. But he knows I remember and I tell everyone what happened. I don't care if they don't believe me, at least I'm planting doubt in their mind."

Shirley, 32, nurse

What emotions and feelings usually result from abuse?

At the time of the assault, regardless of your age and sex, you felt totally terrified or shocked, possibly disoriented. Immediately after, you were in crisis: you experienced anything from hysteria and tears to feeling cold and cut off from your emotions. You may have fluctuated between the two. Older girls may feel ashamed, disgusted, and blame themselves. A few people are furious (this is a good sign as it shows your sense of self is intact); lots of others kick into denial or *minimization*. They think, "I can't deny it happened but it wasn't so bad. I'll put it behind me and won't let it drag me down." This head-in-the-sand approach usually doesn't work because it's very difficult to work through the aftereffects of abuse without facing up to them.

Other people develop *post-traumatic stress disorder* (PTSD), a condition where you're susceptible to reliving the event whenever a *trigger* sets off a memory (something reminds you of the event). War veterans who dive to the ground when they hear a car backfire like a bomb are suffering from PTSD. For you, it might be the bristles on a man's face, the smell of aftershave, the feel of a naked body, or the act of penetration itself.

A common reaction is to feel responsible for the abuse, that somehow you "asked for it." Rape victims think, "It was my fault for walking down that dark street." Childhood abuse victims think, "Maybe I acted like it was okay; maybe I didn't make it clear enough that I didn't want to do it." Because of this, you keep your mouth shut and suffer guiltily and silently.

What about people who remember years later they've been abused? Can memories be put into people's heads by overenthusiastic psychologists?

Most therapists are adamant that at the age of thirty you can suddenly remember what happened to you when you were twelve. This is because our psychological defenses, through a process called *disassociation*, sometimes don't allow us to experience or remember "bad" things. In extreme cases, particularly if you were very young, you may have felt like you left your body while you were being abused (as though it was happening to someone else, not you, and you were watching).

People can disassociate in four different ways: from the sensations (you can't remember the feeling of the person touching you), the behavior (you don't register what the person actually did), the emotions (you take away your emotional reaction of fear, terror, or sadness), or the knowledge (you deny the experience ever happened). You can disassociate from all four things or any combination of them. So it's quite possible that you have no conscious memory of what happened to you, particularly if the abuse was violent or ongoing or by someone very close to you. You may sense *something* bad happened—feel depressed and fearful your entire life—but not know why. Later, at a time when your brain decides you're strong enough to remember, something can happen to bring back the memories.

Needless to say, discovering you've been abused as a child is intensely shocking. Therapists who specialize in abuse say the emotional aftereffects are something you wouldn't wish on your worst enemy. So it's unlikely they'll "plant" memories in your head or encourage you to remember things that didn't actually happen.

How can I tell if I've been abused but "forgotten" it?

Common signs of past abuse are often caused by events other than abuse, so don't jump to conclusions! But some things to look for are difficulties in forming and maintaining relationships, and problems with sex. If you were repeatedly abused as a child, how you dealt with the abuse can be carried through to your adult life. Feeling like it's not really happening to you, feeling numb or weirdly uninvolved during sex could be a sign. You may also feel extremely vulnerable. Vaginismus (when the vaginal muscles spasm and prevent penetration) is a common reaction; so is pain during intercourse, and not being able to orgasm or get aroused at all. Alternatively, so is being overly promiscuous: you may be trying to "prove" there's nothing wrong with you. High achievers, people who strive to be perfect, and "good" people are also possible victims. Abuse often leaves you feeling like you're a "bad" person, so you try, often unrealistically, to be as pure as the driven snow.

Childhood abuse is a gross betrayal of trust, and trust is central to almost all human interaction. Children don't just trust those who are close to them; we start out with an inherent belief that people in general won't hurt us. So feeling abnormally cautious and paranoid may also be a warning sign.

Where do I get help?

The surest route to ridding yourself of the effects of abuse is through counseling. Your doctor can refer you to a psychologist or you can call any major hospital—most have assault units. Alternatively, look in the Yellow Pages under "Counseling," "Counselors," or "Psychotherapists" for help. For therapy to work, it's imperative you feel you can trust your counselor (check they're qualified and certified by the American Psychological Association or its equivalent for a start). Even if you haven't got a logical reason not to trust or like a particular therapist, keep searching until you find someone you do feel comfortable with. If you feel more comfortable speaking to someone anonymously at first and would like to find a counselor in your area, I would recommend calling RAINN (the Rape, Abuse, and Incest National Network) Hotline at 1-800-656-HOPE.

What will happen if I accuse or charge the person?

Most people spend the first half of their life trying to deny they've been abused, and the second half acknowledging it happened and trying to get over it. Therapy drags up feelings you've buried for years and you may feel incredibly angry at the person who did it to you. It's often at this point that the truth finally comes out: you decide to accuse the person, perhaps take them to court, or confess to the rest of your family what happened.

In 1996 in the U.S., only 31 percent of rapes and sexual assaults were reported to law enforcement officials—less than one in every three.[6] And, of those reported, a lot of charges are withdrawn or there's insufficient evidence to proceed to trial, though, according to most therapists, very rarely is an allegation made that isn't founded on truth.

One reason you may decide not to proceed is family pressure: other members may be terrified of the scandal it will cause. If you're accusing your father and he's still supporting your mother and other children, it could mean she and they will lose their income if he's convicted. In the vast majority of cases, however, victims are supported by their families. A child is easily silenced and often accused of "telling tales." An adult is more powerful, able to articulate what happened, and a lot more likely to be believed. (Your therapist won't recommend you tell your family because it's *you* who has to deal with the consequences. If you feel they are pushing you to do so against your will, report them to the American Psychological Association and change counselors.)

Sadly, most perpetrators of sexual abuse aren't arrested or charged. Often, the person is dead or (thankfully) no longer in your life and you don't know how to find them. Of those that are charged, relatively few are found guilty. Your chances of winning the case are higher if you told people along the way: maybe a girlfriend, sister, or your mother. Repressed memory—discovering later in life you were abused—is still a bit of a hot potato in the courts but a competent lawyer can advise you on the strength of your case.

What will a counselor do?

The road to recovery is different for each person. It depends not only on the degree of damage done but also on practical things like your finances, how much time you have, and how you're able to handle the emotions it unearths. Usually, you'll be counseled at least once a week for between two and five years, talking during these sessions about things you'd still rather avoid remembering. It's a painful and draining process and humans are oddly resistant to change: part of us is more comfortable with the way things are now, even though it's horrible. There's no short-term cure, though you'll progress faster if you're highly motivated and attend more than once a week. It's also acceptable to take breaks rather than do it all in one stint.

The counselor will talk about your life, the abuse, and how it's affecting you. It may take a long time before you're able to talk through a lot of what happened but that's normal—and far preferable to leaving the memories smoldering away inside. Some people aren't interested in counseling and find *doing* something helps restore their sense of power. Taking the person to court or helping someone else in the same situation by joining an action group are common reactions. At the end of the day, however, most victims find they need to sit down with another human being to work things through. And the best person for that job is a professional counselor.

ADULT SEXUAL ASSAULT

Outdated, ridiculous, and largely offensive myths still surround rape. Some of the more common ones include:

- Women attract rape by the way they dress and behave (only certain types of women get raped).
- Women secretly enjoy it.
- Men who rape are sick and can't help or control themselves.
- Rapists don't look like normal people.
- It's a woman's responsibility to control a man's behavior.
- When a woman says "no," she sometimes means "yes."
- Rape always involves violence or the use of a weapon.
- Unless you can show physical injury, don't bother reporting it.

All of the above are false. Rape or sexual assault is when a person is forced into any kind of sexual activity with someone, known or unknown to them, without their consent. In other words, *no one has a legal right to touch any part of your body unless you want them to.* Let me reiterate two points because these are myths many women still believe. Rape doesn't always include physical force—verbal threats are just as (if not more) effective. Rape doesn't always include him putting his penis in your vagina. You can be raped with fingers or objects; you can be orally or anally raped. Don't believe anyone who tries to tell you this isn't true. Rape is now officially called "sexual assault," though victims and workers in the field still usually refer to it as rape (which is why I have done so in this chapter).

As with childhood abuse, rapists usually know their victims in one way or another. We think they only hang around dark alleys, but they don't. Quite often they're someone we trust, even like. Family members, friends, acquaintances, and colleagues count for about half of most offenders. A further one-fifth are people the victim met that day for the first time. More than half of all sexual assaults occur in the home—yours or his. In many cases, the victim let the rapist in—not surprising, given that she usually knows him. Outdoor areas like parks, the street, and parking lots are second favorites. Most assaults happen on Fridays and Saturdays between 6 P.M. and 6 A.M. rather than during the day, with about 60 to 80 percent of rapes happening at night.

Almost always, it's a man raping a woman. According to the U.S. Department of Justice, somewhere in America, a woman is raped every two minutes. But while nine out of ten rape victims are women, men and boys are also victimized. In 1995, 32,130 males aged twelve and older were victims of rape, attempted rape, or sexual assault.[7] Adult male rape isn't common, though it's becoming more so, particularly for gay men. If a man is sexually abused it's usually when he's a child or serving a jail sentence and the abuser of a man is nearly always another man. For these reasons, I've slanted this section toward female rape victims, though men will experience similar feelings and (hopefully) receive the same treatment by police.

> "When I was in the tenth grade, a girl at my school pressed rape charges against another student. She was very academic and pretty, he was the quintessential good-looking school athlete. It divided the school: the girls believed her, the boys sided with him. But when he was found guilty, everything changed. We all knew how hard they'd been on the girl in court and we looked at her with a new respect. His reputation was shot. 'Why did you do it? You could have any girl you wanted,' I asked the guy. He answered with, 'Dude, she asked for it and she wanted it.' He had no guilt whatsoever."
>
> Tony, 26, electrician

What should you do immediately after the attack?

Your first priority is safety: get yourself somewhere safe as fast as possible. If the rape happened in your home, lock all the doors and windows then call a friend (or family) and the police on 911 or call your local police station. The police *prefer* you to call them first but totally understand that your first reaction is to call someone close to you. (Besides, they can be used later to testify if you take the matter to court.) If you don't want to call the police, contact a local sexual assault center.

> "I met this guy in a nightclub and he ended up coming back to my place for coffee. He'd spent the entire evening telling me how upset he was because his girlfriend had been raped recently and he didn't know how to handle it. I thought it was obvious we were just going to be friends and thought he'd be the last person to try anything. Wrong. The minute the door closed he pushed me back onto the couch, held me down with one hand and ripped my pants off with the other. I was terrified but kept my head. I told him I had to go to the bathroom to put my diaphragm in and when I came out, I walked straight to the phone and dialed 911 before he figured out what I was doing. The police answered immediately but he'd already bolted."
>
> Annette, 24, PR consultant

It's crucial that you don't wash your clothing. By all means change, but put the clothes straight into a bag to hand over to the police. Don't wash yourself or treat any physical injuries and try not to smoke, eat, or drink, particularly if you were orally raped (all could affect swabs that will be taken from your mouth, vagina, and anus). Try not to go to the bathroom until after your medical examination: that will also hinder the collection of forensic evidence. If it happened in your home, leave everything as it is—don't clean up. (If you're extremely distressed and do all of these things, don't panic—the police will be well aware you're not thinking straight.)

Emotionally, you'll react in a number of ways. You'll no doubt feel terrified the person will return, feel you've lost control and may go into shock. Some women feel (rightfully) furious; alternatively, you may feel guilty and blame yourself. You could be a confused, hysterical, blithering mess by the time the police arrive or feel strangely calm, unemotional, and cold. Quite often, rape victims are rude to police (a male raped you, the police that investigate are usually male). All reactions are common and normal; there's no "expected" way for you to behave.

What will happen after you call the police?

If you live in a major city, generally two of the closest available police officers will come out followed by an investigator who specializes in sex crimes. If you live in a rural area, your local police officer will attend. They will question you and take a brief statement about what happened, examine and preserve the crime scene, and ask if you want (or will agree to) a medical examination, which needs to be done within seventy-two hours.

Even if you're not sure if you want to press charges, get the medical examination done. You'll also be asked if you want to meet with a sexual assault counselor.

When you're up to it, they'll take you to a hospital, where a doctor will do a medical examination (usually using a specially designed sexual assault investigation kit). The police will take a full statement and fill you in on what will happen if you press charges. The police won't push you to charge the rapist; it's up to you if you want to proceed formally. (If you don't, that'll be the end of it though they'll usually arrange some sort of follow-up counseling.) You're then allowed to go home and the police will start investigating the matter if you have chosen to press charges.

Usually, you're not needed again until your case is scheduled for court, though you might be asked to identify the attacker from pictures or a lineup if you didn't know them.

If you know your attacker, the police can enforce strong bail conditions or file an order of protection on the suspect with specified conditions (like not to assault, molest, or harass you).

Unfortunately, you won't be assigned your very own police officer to protect you like they do in the movies, so you might consider moving in with your family or friends, or getting someone to live with you for a while if you live alone. It's generally a myth that attackers come back—they usually don't. Having said that, you'll understandably feel an intense need to be somewhere safe and it's wise to take precautions. Going straight home to an empty apartment isn't advisable.

What are the pros and cons of going through with the charge?

A very large number of sexual assaults are not reported to the police. According to Sexual Assault Support Services of Eugene,

Oregon, 68.4 percent of adult rape victims did not report their attack to the police. Male victims are even less likely to report rape because of the stigma attached. So why don't we? Two common reasons are "the police can't or won't do anything about it" or "the incident is too 'trivial' to make a fuss over" (especially if you're a date rape victim). Other reasons include feeling guilty or ashamed, worrying the police won't believe you, or that the court case will be too stressful.

If you do report the crime, the majority of you do want to take it to court, especially if it's happened recently. (You can charge someone years later but lack of hard evidence, like a medical report, can decrease what could have been a strong case.)

Don't kid yourself if you do decide to press on: rape cases are very unpleasant for the victim. The rapist's defense team will use whatever they can dredge up to discredit you and paint a shining picture of their client. Technically, it's not legal to drag your past sexual history, what you were wearing, or your character into the case, but that doesn't mean they won't try. All will be alluded to and used against you by a clever lawyer who's aware of loopholes. You have to be pretty tough to get through it. The police and a counselor will support you, but at the end of the day, the witness box is a pretty lonely place. You'll be asked to recount, in minute detail, the whole traumatic experience, possibly several times over. His lawyer will ask you questions that will make you feel that you're not believed, that you somehow "asked" for it and that you said "no" but your body language and behavior screamed "yes." Stick to what happened and think before you answer seemingly innocent questions. I'm not telling you this to put you off, just so you know what you're in for.

Only fourteen percent of all reported rape cases that go to court end in conviction.[8] If you win, it can be one of the most empowering moments of your life. If you lose, it's possibly the worst. You'll think people didn't believe you, but this often isn't the case. It simply means your attacker bought himself a good lawyer or, for some reason, your case was hard to prove. Some rape victims make better witnesses than others: they sound and look capable, are articulate, and are very composed. Others are so traumatized they can do little more than cry.

How might people close to you react?

No two families are the same. Some will rally around and want to wrap you in blankets, others may not believe you or say things like "I told you wearing miniskirts will get you in trouble." Friends are usually shocked, female friends frightened, both for you and themselves. Sometimes people won't want to believe that you're telling the truth because it means that they, too, are in danger. Because of this they may imply there was something you could have done to avoid it.

Your male friends, boyfriend, father, and brother will probably experience feelings of intense anger and hatred toward the rapist. Lots will plot revenge, though few follow through with it. This isn't your problem. Make it clear this won't help your case, then stay out of it. Sometimes family and friends will push you into pressing charges when you don't want to; other times the opposite occurs. It can depend on who the rapist was: a friend or neighbor or a stranger who grabbed you on a dark street. Regardless, make your own decisions and don't be swayed by others.

According to the police I have spoken to, most boyfriends are supportive of their girlfriends (but that obviously depends on what sort of guy he was *before* the attack). If he loves you, he'll be angry at the rapist and tremendously concerned and supportive of you. He may also feel responsible, that it's his fault for not being there with you.

How might it affect you in the future?

Rape can (and usually does) have a profound effect on the lives of victims for many years after. It's a violating and traumatic experience. How *you* react depends on what sort of person you are, the seriousness of the attack, your feelings about yourself and your sexuality, your age, your cultural background, maybe your religion. There are a wide range of psychological symptoms that just about all victims experience. Fear, anxiety, depression, anger, shame, sleep or eating disorders, and a feeling of powerlessness are all common. But by far the biggest effect will be on your sexual relationships. You may feel that you never want to have sex again. The thought of being touched, being naked, of someone just kissing you may make you feel physically sick. Again, this is normal and best solved by professional counseling.

You may feel a burning need to be believed and listened to. Psychologists call this "validation" of the experience: you want others to appreciate how serious, horrible, and terrifying the assault was and for it to be seen as significant. Long-term counseling is recommended for *all* rape victims; being treated for a few months after the attack usually isn't enough. Don't try to struggle alone with the issues. You might come out okay on the other side, but you'll do so a lot quicker if you talk to someone with experience in helping victims of sexual abuse. The police, any sexual assault service or center, or RAINN (see page 242) can refer you to a qualified counselor. You survived the attack—counseling can help you move on and get back to enjoying your life.

Who should I call if it happened a while ago?

Threats, feeling ashamed, not being able to talk about or face up to what happened—a lot of things can stop you from seeking help immediately after an attack. Maybe you thought you could cope with it yourself but now find you need help. It doesn't matter if you were raped one month or ten years ago, you can still file a complaint, press charges, or seek counseling. Contact the police or a sexual assault service attached to a hospital or community health center for referral to a counselor. Many are open twenty-four hours a day. Check out sexual assault resource sites on the Web, or look in the Yellow Pages under "Social & Human Services" to find a rape crisis center or support group.

How can you lower the chances of being raped?
When you're out
- Don't overload yourself with parcels or wear clothes that will stop you from running.
- Wait for public transportation in well-lit areas. If possible, avoid catching buses and trains late at night or very early in the morning.
- Sit near the bus driver or in the conductor's station on trains.
- Leave your car in well-lit areas, not deserted backstreets.
- Stick to main, well-lit roads at night and avoid walking through parks or other large, dark areas.

At home

- Install a peephole and deadbolt lock on your door.
- If you have the cash, install an alarm and a panic button near your bed.
- Don't answer the door unless you're sure you know who's there, and it's someone you trust.

On dates

- Be assertive and clearly communicate what you do and don't want to happen sexually.
- Think twice before inviting him back for coffee or going to his house—especially if one, or both, of you is drunk.
- Some men think that if they pay for your meal you owe them sex. If you have doubts, consider paying for yourself until you know them better.
- Take your own car the first few times. It's not uncommon for "dates" to drive their victims to an assault site on the way home.
- Trust your gut reaction. If you're out with someone who seems weird, go to the bathroom and on the way tell the waiter or bartender to call you a cab. Warn them that your date seems odd. Tell the guy you feel ill and have called a cab to take you home. Refuse his offer to drive you.

If you are attacked

- Running away is often the best solution. If you can, do it.
- If you can't run, make as much noise as possible. Carry an ear-piercing whistle and blow it; scream and shout. Use your legs to kick, your mouth to bite, and hit him where it hurts (in the testicles, throat, stick two fingers in his eyes). Use your keys or handbag as a weapon.
- If you think you can carry it off, try talking your way out of it. Tell him you're pregnant and he'll kill the baby by raping you, say you're HIV-positive, have an attack of herpes—anything to dissuade him.

9

Fantasies

Drop the but-I-thought-you-loved-*me* stuff—steamy fantasies make for even steamier real-life romps

● ●

I had my first sexual fantasy when I was seven years old and I'm ashamed to say it was about Engelbert Humperdinck. My father was crazy about this singer, who looked twice as dorky as he sounds and was at least 100 years old even back then. Brylcreamed hair styled into rippling, Elvis-like waves, swarthy skin set off by shiny suits, eyebrows a girl could tangle her fingers in—I thought he was sex-on-legs. Trouble was, I really didn't know what sex *was*, a fact that becomes rather obvious from the fantasy. I used to imagine that I'd kidnap Engelbert and keep him around the side of our house. (For some reason, he was quite happy to do nothing but stand on a concrete path for days on end.) I'd sneak out to visit him and then he would—wait for it—*roll bacon rinds up my arms*. What a turn-on, eh! Why the thought of this produced such a pleasant, naughty shiver up my girly spine is utterly beyond me. I've examined those record covers a million times since but still can't figure the connection between Engelbert and bacon fat—except maybe that they're both slimy.

You'll be relieved to hear my subsequent fantasies haven't come close to matching the oddness of that little gem but, like millions of others, I still thoroughly enjoy letting my imagination run wild. Just about everyone fantasizes: men, women, and (obviously) children, and there are lots of reasons why. In fantasy land, there are no rules. No one can accuse us of being right or wrong, nice or nasty, perverted, dirty, or plain revolting because (thank God) no one's invented a device to read minds. So, we're free to invent idealized situations that are totally impractical or unattainable in real life. Pimples, cellulite, cramps, periods, pissed-off girlfriends or boyfriends, smelly genitals, and children wanting cookies—they all magically disappear in fantasies. Our dream lovers know exactly when, how, and what to do to make us giddy with desire because *we're* directing the show.

No two people conjure up exactly the same fantasy, but there is a unifying thread to them all: a longing to escape from what's socially acceptable. In real life, ripping off your secretary's skirt and bending her over your desk will land you a sexual harassment suit. In your fantasy, it gets you the blow job of your life. Fantasies are a welcome escape from the stress of day-to-day living. Daydreaming about some gorgeous Jamaican delivering more than a cocktail on a sun-drenched beach is infinitely more appealing than worrying where next week's rent is coming from.

Most of the time, our fantasies revolve around things we'd never want to try in reality—some would *horrify* us if they actually happened. (Arriving home to find your girlfriend in bed with six workmen is a hell of a lot different from aimlessly daydreaming about it.) But their effect on our libido and sex life is immense all the same and, in some instances, our fantasies *would* delight us by coming true. The more you fantasize, the higher your libido. What came first, the chicken or the egg, is anyone's guess, but it's pretty well established that the more you think about sex, the more you want it. That makes fantasies the cheapest, most effective sex aid around. Even better, they're tailor-made to suit the user. We can turn them on or off at will and they introduce variety into our sex lives without the complications and devastation of real-life affairs. They add the spice of infidelity without a price to pay for it.

Fantasy and masturbation go together like bacon and eggs and lots of people have one favorite that always guarantees an orgasm. Studies show almost 60 percent of us fantasize every time we make love with our partner. Sexperts estimate the *real* figure (that is, when our partners aren't watching over our shoulder to see what survey box we check) to be much higher.[1] Of those that do fantasize during sex, all report a much more satisfying love life than those who don't. And our fantasies aren't necessarily about other people or other situations. Often, we'll imagine how we look or picture what our partner is doing to us as they're doing it, because we can't "see" with our eyes because of the position.

Whatever the motivation and whatever *your* brain conjured up, you'd be hard-pressed finding a sex therapist who didn't include fantasy in a recipe for hot sex. Here are a rundown on our most common themes, some real-life confessions, and hints on how to use them to enhance your sex life, both in and out of bed.

IN HIS DREAMS: THE 10 MOST COMMON MALE SEX FANTASIES

"What are you thinking, darling?" she asks, snuggled up romantically on the couch, one head on your shoulder. "Er . . . um . . . how much I love you." "Oh, how sweet!" she gushes. What was really running through your head was any of the following . . .

1. Fantasies about your current partner

No kidding. This is the number one sex fantasy for most men: things you've done, or would like to do, to your girlfriend. (It's her top fantasy too, by the way). Forget big-breasted blond Swedish women begging for more—scenarios featuring your girlfriend are far more frequent and likely. Why? Because available flesh-and-blood is sometimes more of a turn-on than the unattainable—there's a good chance it could come true or has already.

2. Having sex with a woman other than your partner

Often, she's a past lover, a friend of your girlfriend, perhaps a celebrity. The psychology behind this one isn't too difficult to work out: lots of people long to have sex with someone new and fantasy is a great way of indulging this longing without losing your partner in the process. If the woman in the fantasy is a virgin, you've cast yourself in the teacher role, initiating her into hedonistic pleasures through your skillful lovemaking. If she's got big boobs, choose from a variety of psychological theories. Freudians would say you haven't cut the apron strings; breasts (i.e., sucking on Mom's) are a symbol of your childhood. More sensible thera-pists would say you're one of those guys who equate big breasts with the ultimate sexy women.

3. Giving or receiving oral sex

This is near the top of the list for both sexes. Fantasy fellatio has one vital ingredient: the woman doesn't do it to *give* pleasure. She does it to *get* pleasure—worshiping your mighty penis, slurping, gobbling, begging you to let her take it into her mouth, giving long, lascivious licks. She accompanies the blow job with comments like "God, it's huge" and (of course) not only swallows every last drop of sperm but licks her lips afterward. This one's heaven for just about all men (and a very easy one for her to turn into reality).

Fantasies about giving her oral sex aren't surprising either. Many women are more obviously turned-on by oral than inter-course and as the ultimate pleasure-giver, this is what you *know* will drive her *craaazzy*. Plus there's still a part of us that secretly thinks of oral sex as "dirtier" than intercourse, hence the huge turn-on factor.

4. Sex with two or more women

This is the adult male equivalent of the childhood fantasy of being accidentally locked up in a candy store. If having sex with one woman feels good, having sex with two *must* be double the fun. Throw in some lesbian lovemaking and this one sends most of you drifting off into la-la land with an if-only expression on your face. In your fantasy, you're superstud: capable of bringing both women to screaming orgasms, over and over. In reality, lots of you worry (consciously or subconsciously) whether you're truly satisfying just one, so it's not surprising this is dream-fodder. Studies show the vast majority of men don't want (and actually couldn't cope with) such sexual demands in real life.

Orgy type fantasies not only

> **❗** *Fifty-seven point five percent of women feel good about the idea of having sex with another woman; 33.4 percent have done it, and out of those 92.9 percent enjoyed the experience.*[2]

remove real-life logistical problems ("Umm, would you mind moving your leg? Your toe's going right up my nose"), but you can magically orgasm time and time again. Watching two women make love (especially women you know—your partner is often one of them) is another common male fantasy. The classic version has you arriving home from work unexpectedly to find your partner, dressed in some wispy thing, curled up on the bed with a divine-looking "friend/goddess." Hands, handcuffs, and definitely tongues feature, but the climax is always them begging you to join in, so they can experience "the real thing."

5. Watching others have sex and/or being watched

It's called voyeurism (watching) and exhibitionism (being watched). In reality, few people would be able to stop themselves looking at a couple having sex if they were guaranteed not to get caught, but voyeurism is a fantasy, of both sexes, because sex is private and mostly hidden. Sure, we watch couples do it on TV, but it's rare we get to see *the real thing*, and there's also a narcissistic appeal: we imagine we're one of the couple because we can't *see* ourselves when we have sex. Even if you do it in front of a mirror, all angles aren't covered and you tend to forget to watch the good parts because you're too carried away by the sensation. Some of you are turned-on by the thought of watching other men make love to your partner—she's a creature of such savage sexual appetites, you alone can't satisfy them. Not surprisingly, few (brave or stupid) individuals actually take that one through to real life.

Exhibitionistic fantasies often revolve around others admiring you. You put on a fine show (of course) and the voyeur is usually envious of your sexual skills, desperately wishing they were the person you were making love to. It's an ego-boosting fantasy.

6. Having her masturbate for you (or watching her without her knowing)

Watching her "play with herself" is up there on most men's wish list, possibly because it reassures you that we're as into sex as you are. Secretly spying appeals to your curious side: what is she really up to when you're not around?

7. Anal sex

It doesn't mean you've got "gay tendencies," because the anus is undeniably an erotic zone, especially for men. A lot of you would love her to penetrate you with a finger—or want to have anal intercourse—but worry she'll think you're gay if you suggest it. So you fantasize instead.

8. Bondage (tying-up fantasies)

Being tied up is her favorite, tying someone up is usually yours—which works out rather nicely if you play this one out in real life! Bondage fantasies are usually about power—having it or relinquishing it, and both have their appeal. Sometimes, it can mean you want to tie her *down*, rather than up (you don't feel she's truly yours); most of the time bondage comes to mind because it's the subject of many scenes in erotic books or movies.

Sadomasochistic (S and M) fantasies are less common but certainly not rare. Sadism is getting off on inflicting pain on someone else; masochism is getting off on someone hurting you. Most mild S and M fantasies revolve around whipping and spanking. Pleasure and pain are inextricably linked in the minds of some people and, in reality, spanking increases blood flow to the genital area (and therefore turns us on biologically). Aggression is common in the animal world: some female animals only ovulate if the male bites them. Masochistic fantasies sometimes stem from subconsciously thinking sex is bad (you need to be punished for liking it).

! *Sex-line workers say these are the most popular fantasy requests from men who call them:*
- *37 percent want domination fantasies*
- *23 percent sex with schoolgirls*
- *15 percent anal sex with a woman*
- *9 percent sex with two girls*
- *5 percent to dress up in women's clothes*
- *4 percent sex with an older woman (often their mother-in-law!)*
- *3 percent an orgy*
- *2 percent sex with lesbians[3]*

9. Pretend rape

Contrary to what most women believe, when you fantasize about forcing a woman to have sex with you it's more about overpowering her through your amazing sexual technique and charisma than violence. She starts off saying "no," then can't help but say "yes" given the superhunk that you are. Often set in Disney dungeons, nobody really gets hurt and the victim enjoys it even more than you do. If she's forcing you to have sex, you're indulging in a submissive sexual role quite unlike the one you probably have in real life. Usually, it's just a release from the day-to-day responsibility of always having to be in charge.

10. Sex with another man

Same-sex fantasies or threesome fantasies involving another man are extremely common and don't mean you've got a secret wish to be gay; it just means you're sexually curious (see "Am I gay?" on page 292).

HER HEDONISTIC HEAD GAMES: THE TOP 10 FEMALE SEX FANTASIES

Thinking sexy thoughts make our tummies ache, skin tingle, and vaginas moisten. Women who rate themselves as good lovers fantasize more often. Not only that, those who prepare for future sex by fantasizing are more easily aroused and enjoy sex more when it happens.[4] While just about all of us use fantasy while masturbating, lots also do it during sex, particularly if we're having trouble tipping over the orgasm brink.

1. Fantasizing about your current partner

It's up there for both sexes, for all the reasons I've listed above.

2. Sex with a man other than your partner

For women, this is most often a past lover. Some feel adulterous or guilty reliving a particularly hot session from the past: don't. It's normal. We tend not to marry the person we were most sexually passionate with (most of us prefer to play it safe and settle for what we think are more sensible attributes). So, while you love your current boyfriend, an old one may have turned you on more.

If it's someone *new* you're fantasizing about, it's the old want-what-you-can't-have syndrome. Alas, morals and things like AIDS stop us from having sex with whomever we please. But being involved with a partner doesn't mean all other desirable men go away. So those adulterous feelings have to be dealt with in one way or another. The safest outlet of all is our imagination—and it's remarkably fertile. In it, we have sex—if we're white—with black men (he's got a prize penis and his different skin color makes him seem terribly exotic); boy toys (he's seen as more sexually active, gets harder, plus you're the experienced one who's calling the shots); and celebrities. In reality, stars are usually nothing like the public persona their publicity machine pumps out but, hey, they *seem* a lot more interesting than the average person. An extension of this is how famous you'll be if you get them: walking in with a Hollywood hunk on your arm is the quintessential ego boost and affirmation of your attractiveness.

3. Sex with another woman

We're more likely to have same-sex fantasies than he is, probably because it's seen as more acceptable. We're also far less likely to get hung up on homophobic fears that we're gay. The woman featured isn't usually one we know but she always knows exactly what to do to turn us on because she's got what we've got.

4. Something new you'd like to try

It's that dreadful "nice girls don't" stuff at work again. While many women are outrageously experimental and imaginative in their fantasies, not so many admit a desire for anything "kinky" to a partner for fear of being judged. Playing out the scenario in your head is the next best thing. For those who are open, fantasizing is also a form of rehearsal, upping the anticipation of experiencing it in reality. Included in this type of fantasy is being tied up, threesomes, group sex, and watching others. Having sex in public is another popular dream: we're turning on more than just our lover and our exhibitionistic side loves it.

5. Being given oral sex

It's the quickest, most effective (sometimes the *only*) way we orgasm, so it's not surprising it features heavily in our fantasies. The guy of our dreams doesn't just like giving oral sex, he's so enthusiastic, he'd actually like to climb inside and stay there for days. Often he's a sex slave: tall, drop-dead gorgeous, and muscle-bound. We order him to give us oral sex on demand (for hours on end) but he also feeds us, gives amazing massages, does the dishes, and makes the bed.

6. Fantasies involving romantic sex

This is the one most women readily admit to, probably because it's the most "acceptable." Somehow, it seems more ladylike to say "My fantasy is making love on a tropical beach at sunset" than "Being given oral sex by the Pope during high mass while the rest of the congregation masturbate." Romantic fantasies are sex with emotional attachment and most read like a Harlequin plot: gorgeous man, incapable of loving one woman, meets us, is knocked over by our looks and headstrong personality, *then* ravishes us on a moonlit beach. Personally, I don't know one woman who has romantic fantasies, but sex therapists assure me most "normal" women do (which I guess makes my friends deviants).

7. Being forced to have sex against our will

The "safe rape" is a very common female fantasy but it's such a far cry from the real thing it seems silly even calling it rape. Passionate and forceful but rarely violent and painful, the "rapes" in our head differ dramatically because we're always in control. Again, it's the good-girl thing: we relinquish responsibility as the man of our dreams overpowers us and "makes" us submit— we can relax because we are just a pawn in the sex game. On the opposite end of the spectrum are fantasies where we force him to have sex with us, often in male-dominated situations like a

> ❗ *Number of women who have sexual dreams: 76.9 percent. Number of women who enjoy and are turned-on by some porn magazines and videos: 71.8 percent. Women account for more than half of the 100 million porn video rentals in the U.S. Number of women who tell their partners about their fantasies: 60 percent. Those who go on to act them out: 33.6 percent.[5]*

courtroom or a business meeting. Being the aggressor or having physical power over him appeals because in real life it's usually the opposite.

8. Being found irresistible by a man
If you're so gorgeous/sexy/long-legged/stunning he can't help himself, you're absolved of responsibility once more. This is a favorite with women who still feel they need "permission" to let go but also a pleasant daydream for most of us. Who *wouldn't* want to be so beautiful they have men drooling at their feet!

9. Working as a prostitute
Again, this one's popular with women who may be inhibited sexually in real life. In the fantasy, they indulge their true sexual selves under the guise of being paid for it. It's sex for sale, free of commitment—and a marvelous chance to show off. Men paying to have sex with you is also reassurance that you're attractive: you have something men want so badly, they'll hand over cash for it. Stripping is a more common variation on the theme: you tease the men mercilessly, and they're popping their zippers they're so turned-on by your body.

10. Sex with a stranger
In reality, this sort of sex usually works out rather badly. In our fantasies, it's tremendously rewarding. Gone are the practical (often boring) needs of a relationship—this is sex for sex's sake and the reward is pure, unadulterated pleasure. You can be as wicked as you like because not only will you never see him again, he doesn't know who *you* are so can't spread any nasty rumors. Sex with a "faceless" man is even more of a turn-on. He comes up behind you, you feel rather than see him, and you can experience the sensations of sex without the intimacy of eye contact.

AM I WEIRD OR LIKELY TO END UP IN A RAINCOAT?
Relax! In pretty much all cases, strange but sexy daydreams are a sign of a vivid imagination, not deviant leanings. Here are answers to some common questions about fantasies.

Do men and women fantasize about the same things?

Yes, though there are differences. His fantasies are often more explicit, and men tend to center on things they've done rather than things they'd like to try, while we do quite the opposite. Men are also more active in their fantasies, focusing on the effect they're having on the imaginary partner. Women focus more on feelings and responses. While he often fantasizes when his sex life isn't great, we have more fantasies when it is, and while women who fantasize a lot tend to put at least some of their daydreaming into practice, he's not quite as lucky.

No two people's fantasies are identical, even if they are of the same sex, but a quick scan of the top ten favorites shows there are common themes. Why doesn't everyone fantasize about the same thing? It has everything to do with individual taste. Some people kill for freshly shucked oysters, others vomit at the thought. Same deal with sex.

Often, when I have sex with my boyfriend, I fantasize about someone else, and I feel guilty.

Fantasizing isn't just healthy for relationships, it can save them. It's natural to get jaded when you're sleeping with the same person night after night and playing a steamy sex fantasy in your head jazzes things up nicely without hurting anyone. Many sex therapists recommend it. Indulge your desires guilt-free—imagining isn't being unfaithful, living it out in real life is. I bet he's transformed *you* into someone else on more than one occasion, too. The only time you really need to worry is if you have to fantasize *every single time* and are never turned-on just by him. If that's the case, your sex life's in dire need of rescuing, or you've fallen out of lust with your boyfriend.

What if my fantasies are weird or completely out of character? Does it mean I'm a closet nutcase?

Most therapists say there's no such thing as an abnormal fantasy, *as long as the person can distinguish between fantasy and reality.* There's a big difference between thinking loony thoughts and wanting and intending to act them out. Deviant fantasies can be an indicator of true sexual deviancy, but for the vast majority of people they're not.

If there's a consistently violent theme, if all your fantasies center on a peculiar scenario that worries you, or if you find you now can't climax without thinking about the scenario, it could be worth checking it out with a sex therapist. It's rare that a person becomes so fixated on one particular scenario that he or she can't become aroused without it, but you might be the one in a million that it does happen to (in other words, you're probably worrying about nothing). Otherwise, think of your brain as a bus. You're the driver: drive it wherever you want, pick up as many passengers as you like, and tell them to hop off once you reach your destination. If a seemingly weird fantasy is arousing you, but you've got no inclination to do it in real life and it's not a fixation, what's wrong with it?

Should I tell my partner about my fantasies?

This is a tricky one. On the one hand, airing fantasies can zap your sex life through the roof. On the other hand, it can destroy it. You're definitely taking a chance, especially if you don't know your partner very well. What you think of as normal, he or she might consider perverted; it very much depends on individual views, upbringing, and morals. Don't assume that because something turns you on, your partner will feel the same.

Men often have problems accepting their partner's fantasies because they take it as a criticism that you're not happy with "just them." Women often feel jealous and insecure for the same reasons. I really wouldn't recommend sharing any fantasies about people you know (with the exception of a celebrity, who you're unlikely to meet) and I also wouldn't share any unusual fantasies unless I trusted and knew the person so well I was guaranteed a nonjudgmental, positive reaction. Be especially careful to ensure that your partner knows why you're sharing the fantasy. Spell out whether you want to playact it in any sense or are simply revealing intimate thoughts. (If you're female and share a rape fantasy, for instance, make it very, very clear that you're not asking for violence in real life.)

If someone shares their fantasy with you, treat the knowledge with respect. Don't be too scathing about their secret dreams, especially if their fantasy isn't one you were hoping for. Don't even think about telling your best friend and don't immediately launch into your theories as to why they're having *that* particular fantasy. He doesn't really want you to wear red leather with strategic cutouts next time you visit his parents. It's a fantasy, that's all. On the other hand, beware the date who reveals a weird or violent fantasy very early, particularly if you're female.

What if I don't have any?

You're not alone, though you do belong to a small subsection of the population. Those who claim not to fantasize usually have unconscious reasons for repressing them (such as they're unacceptable because of rigid morals or a strict upbringing). A few therapy sessions can work wonders for unblocking and unlocking your imagination.

Some people don't have any qualms about having sexual daydreams, they're just unpracticed at using their creative side. Maybe you aren't very creative generally, prefer working with facts and figures, or you think making up stories is a waste of time (something weirdos and children do). Loosen up a little and read other people's fantasies (start with the real-life confessions in this chapter; invest in Nancy Friday's *Woman on Top* or *Men in Love* if you want more). That's usually enough to get the brain ticking and trigger some of your own.

LIGHTS, CAMERA, ERECTION!

That lurid reverie about your elementary schoolteacher and raspberry jelly isn't first-date material. But sharing and acting out some fantasies is an excellent idea if you've been together a while, talk openly about sex, and, most important, know that your innermost thoughts won't be the subject of your partner's next boys' or girls' night out.

Literally thousands of us secretly use fantasies to orgasm during sex, so owning up and acting them out can be the lustiest sex game you've played in years. Provocative barmaids, nymphomaniac nurses, dominatrixes, and bootlicking boy toys, sexy slave girls and sultans, muscle-bound bikers and straitlaced career women: find the role that appeals to you and make like you're in the movies—though I strongly advise *against* turning it into one. "Of course it's for our eyes only," you both purr in the lovey-dovey stage. It's a different story when you ditch him for his best friend and a copy "accidentally" gets dropped in your mother's mailbox.

How do you suggest acting out a fantasy or finding out about theirs? Wait until you're both feeling relaxed and intimate, then say you had an amazingly sexy dream last night. Tell your partner about it and see what reaction you get. If they seem nicely titillated, confess that it's actually been a fantasy of yours for ages, and ask what are some of theirs. Once you're both talking, it's relatively easy to move into a line like, "Hey, I've just had a great idea. Why don't we act them out for fun?"

Try to choose fantasies that appeal to *both* of you, particularly the first time round, and work out the scenario together beforehand: what you'll each wear, how you want them to act and vice versa. Then use your own imagination to embellish the story, adding a few surprises to the screenplay, maybe taking it even further. You could also try each writing down three favorite fantasies along with instructions on how you'd like to act them out. Write them on separate pieces of paper and put them in a jar for either of you to fish out when you feel like playing. You won't know what fantasy it is until you open it, and neither will they.

Acting out fantasies doesn't have to be literal: symbolism is often all that's needed. Got an anal sex fantasy but don't want to actually do it? Pretend you are while having vaginal sex doggie-style. Use stockings and ties not rough ropes for bondage games; and there's no need to tie knots tight—the idea is to fake a struggle rather than to have a real one because your circulation's cut off. Lavishly expensive props aren't necessary (though they are worth thinking about for favorite fantasies): black stockings and high heels turn her into a prostitute; jeans, no shirt (and a suitably subservient expression) turn him into a sex slave.

Remember to set the scene using music and different rooms of the house (take it outside if it would work better) but don't stress about it. You don't have to be too literal—it's the "sense" of the fantasy that you're re-creating. Similarly, don't be surprised if the first time you do it, either (or both) of you nearly explode from trying to stop giggling. Laughing together is all part of it.

Keep going and you'll feel less ridiculous once you start getting into it.

Only one word of caution: work out an agreed "stop now" signal before starting anything. This is particularly important if your sex games include bondage or spanking. Part of the fantasy may be the person's begging for mercy, but how are you supposed to know whether it's real or feigned without a sign? Apart from that, the world is your stage and you're the superstars. Here is a fantasy each for inspiration.

 FOR HER

Playing the stern mistress

Reverse the traditional roles and become the master of his destiny (well, for about an hour, anyway).

If you own anything leather, put it on. Improvise—a leather jacket worn over black underwear (stockings, garters, push-up bra, and no panties) with knee-high boots will do the trick. Otherwise, anything tight, black, and short—the sexier the better! If you've got something in PVC (that horribly uncomfortable shiny stuff), drag it out from the back of the closet. His outfit's easy: nothing. Him naked while you're clothed sets the scene and makes him feel suitably helpless and vulnerable.

If you can't manage a thunderously threatening expression, go for no expression. Be as unflinchingly mercenary as you can. Show him who's boss by telling him he's misbehaved and you're going to punish him. *Order* him to sit or lie down, face turned away from you, blindfold him, and tie his hands together behind his back (pushing him forward into a submissive pose).

He's now naked, blindfolded, and bound—completely in your power! If he's really into this one, he may want you to hit him with a riding crop or wooden spoon. By all means make your strokes sting but you don't want to cause serious pain. (Now isn't the time to show the bastard how you really felt when he flirted with Rachel at that party.)

His begging you to stop is all part of the game. Refuse until you're either (a) so turned-on, you're frothing at the mouth for sex or (b) either of you are finding the late night movie playing in the living room more interesting than your own acting. Tell him you will show mercy but on one proviso—that he ravishes you NOW!

 FOR HIM

"Forcibly" seducing an innocent

It's forbidden sex for both of you and an easy role-play to start with. Don't panic, there's absolutely no violence or pain involved. This is a very mild version of the common "pretend rape" fantasy with a virgin element thrown in. Add more "struggling" and "force" to suit your taste!

She's naked, you're clothed (it doesn't usually matter what in, but dressing formally can add to the older man/younger woman element). She pretends to be discovering her sexuality privately by standing in front of a mirror, running her hands over her body. You come up silently behind her and cover her eyes with your hand. The feel of her naked skin against your rough clothes feels exciting because it's a new sensation. Be suggestive, speaking in a low voice and tell her you've been watching and fantasizing about her for weeks. If she likes you to talk dirty, here's your chance to let rip.

As you tell her what you intend to do with her and what she will have to do for you, begin to gently caress her body with your lips and hands. Just when she's starting to melt, turn on the tension and remind her she's in your power. You're still standing behind her, so pull her arms gently behind her back, hold them together at the wrists with one of your hands and use the other to continue exploring.

Now make good on your promises. She should resist any new advance initially, then be "overcome" and let you continue (pretending all the time that she's not enjoying it). You take the lead, pretending each touch is her first.

"Come on, you want it," you whisper finally. She halfheartedly protests, then surrenders and grants permission for you to penetrate her. Remember, she's inexperienced and this is her first time. Stop and ask if she's okay and once you're inside, thrust gently.

REAL PEOPLE REVEAL ALL

I asked four very different people to share their favorite fantasies and have faithfully recorded them in their own words. Be warned—there are a few four-letter words!

Catherine, 24, nurse

"I have lots of fantasies, but this one always gets me off. I'm walking past a building site and all these muscle-bound workmen start whistling at me. I'm so flustered I trip, fall over, and sprain my ankle (though it never hurts, of course). Two of the men rush over to pick me up and ask if I want to sit down. They take me into their lunch room (the rest of the guys conveniently leave for a diner), push beer cans, papers, and overflowing ashtrays out of the way, and lay me down on a big table. One kneels to start massaging my ankle.

" 'How does that feel?' he asks.

" 'Great,' I say enthusiastically.

" 'You look a bit tense,' says the other one. 'Would you like me to massage your shoulders? You've had a real shock,' and his big, powerful hands go to work.

"By this time, I'm horny, so say brazenly, 'Seems a shame to stop there.' They don't need any further encouragement and one guy runs his hand up my thigh and starts stroking my clit through my panties, which are wet through. The other guy takes off my top and starts sucking and biting my nipples. My panties are off before I know it and hands plunge inside me and diddle my clit, which feels like a marble in hot oil. The first guy is still licking my nipples and my neck, the second puts his head between my legs and gives me the best oral sex I've ever had. I come loudly, and the first guy unzips and fucks me while his friend watches and masturbates."

Karen, 21, student

"Every Tuesday night, my boyfriend and I and another couple go to see a movie. In my fantasy, I lock eyes with the cutest usher as we walk in: blue eyes, long hair, tall and well built. It's electric, that look, and we both know we're attracted to each other. Halfway through the film, I have to pee, and standing right outside is the usher. I stop, his eyes travel deliberately over my body. I'm instantly wet and start to throb. Without a word, he takes my hand and starts walking down a corridor. I follow like a lost little girl. He leads me into the projection room and I can see everyone in the theater—including my boyfriend. Then he lays me down on a table and runs his hand up the inside of my thigh. His thumb massages my clitoris, then his tongue excites it and my whole body explodes in his mouth. It's incredibly erotic—this guy's a total stranger and I can see my boyfriend innocently watching the film. I'm so bad. I get off the table and stand against a wall, my ass in the air so he can take me from behind. Without warning, he's inside me and I groan so loud a few people in the back row turn to look. We fuck hard and fast while I watch my boyfriend polishing off the last of our popcorn."

Jeff, 30, manufacturing manager

"In real life, I have to work with this fantastic-looking woman who does our PR. In my fantasy, I arrive early for our weekly meeting. She walks ahead of me up the stairs and I watch her ass moving underneath her short business skirt. She's wearing a blouse I particularly like, but this time it's open and she's got no bra on.

" 'We never seem to have time together and that's a shame. I'd like to get to know you a lot better,' she says, locking the office door and telling her secretary to hold all calls.

"I'm wondering why and hoping like hell it's what I think. She sits on the desk, motions me to a chair in front, then puts one high-heeled foot on either side of me. I can see she's not wearing underwear. She sits there, calmly talking about business and doesn't seem to mind me staring at her crotch, which is wet and totally shaved. Eventually, she takes pity, stands up, and unzips my fly. She takes out my prick then kneels down and sucks it expertly. I come a split second before her secretary knocks at the door saying the others have arrived. She straightens up, wipes her mouth with a tissue, and waits for me to get myself together before letting the others in."

Bruce, 26, electrician

"I've had the moves put on me by bored housewives before but never the ones you want. In my fantasy, I'm asked to install a light fixture in a bathroom. I knock on the door and this total babe answers. She's obviously just about to take a shower because she's got a robe on and a towel over one arm. My cock stirs. She shows me into the bathroom and asks if I'd mind if she took a shower while I'm working because she's running late. Who am I to complain? I pretend to fix the light but she's so close and in full view, soaping her tits and slipping her fingers into her pussy. She turns the shower off and asks me to pass her a towel. I say, 'No problem, let me dry you off.'

"So I start drying her shoulders and then get down on the floor to dry her legs. She puts her hands on my head and stands with her legs apart so I nuzzle her sweet-smelling pussy and lick that little knob until she's clasping her thighs so hard around my head, I can't stand it. It's mushy and wet and her juices are dripping down her legs. She begs me to fuck her, so I do. I bend her over the tub and fuck her from behind, thrusting so deep as I come, she has trouble keeping her balance."

> **!** *Of all our sexual fantasies, bondage (tying each other up) is the one we're most likely to act out. Twenty-three percent of men just fantasize about bondage, 27 percent have done it. Twenty-five percent of women just dream about it, 26 percent take it through to real life.[6]*

10

Sex Myths

Most couples do it 2.5 times a week, your best friend's getting laid more than you are, and other sex secrets and lies

● ●

It's funny the things we grow up believing about sex and our bodies. My friend Sarah was convinced for years that if men don't "use" their erections their testicles hurt for hours afterward. Todd still refuses to budge from his theory that some girls are so fertile *nothing* will stop them getting pregnant. My grandmother claimed she could pick a good girl from a bad one by the way she threw her leg over a bicycle. I, of course, being sexually superior, was able to effortlessly separate fact from fantasy. Well, that's what I'd *like* to tell you. In reality, I was the biggest sucker of all—thanks to my best friend Jenny.

Jenny knew everything there was to know about sex, all of which she made up. Gullible old me, eyes like saucers, believed it all. Penises have bones in them. You took the Pill vaginally. You could cut the finger off a rubber glove and use it as a condom. Men with big noses have big penises. Jenny was also the one who told me how to use tampons—you just lay them lengthways across the opening of your vagina. For weeks, I watched other girls lock themselves in the bathroom, armed with strange-looking cardboard cylinders, muttering about how they couldn't get the hang of tampons. I, on the other hand, was out and washing my hands before they'd even opened their instruction leaflets. Which is possibly what I should have done, since Jenny had no idea you were supposed to insert them *inside*. Those Playtex ads had me stumped. Girls swimming, surfing, and bouncing around in aerobics classes? All I could manage was a painful hobble, legs tightly closed to keep the thing in place. Silly when you look back (dumb, even) but also interesting how we cling to some sexual misconceptions for so long.

Some sex myths are simply outdated, reflecting different society values and morals. Times change, people change, and even the facts change sometimes when new evidence comes to light. But what remains truly astonishing is this: for a subject that's the number one obsession of the Western world, most of the general population still know little about sex. So, here's the truth, the whole truth, and nothing but the truth about all the things even the sexually educated have niggling doubts about. Jenny, this one's for you.

❶ *Does love at first sight really happen? Instant desire certainly does but experts say "knowing" right from the start is unlikely. That's merely knowledge after the event.*

THE TOP 10 WHOPPERS

Our parents had them (you'll go blind if you masturbate, good girls don't) and we've invented a totally new set of sex myths. Most of us are surprisingly naive when it comes to sorting fact from fiction—so let's dispel the real biggies once and for all.

They're great-looking so sex is going to be fantastic.

Not only is this untrue (there is a God after all), but neither sex has the foggiest what the other truly finds attractive. While you're sweating it out at the gym frantically working for a reed-thin body, the studies say he's eyeing "real women"—curvaceous, voluptuous creatures who probably qualify as "plump" by today's standards. Ditto the muscle-man working out beside you: we consistently rate nice smiles and a sense of humor as far more appealing than abs of steel.

Even if you *do* get to bed the best-looking guy or girl on the block, sex rarely lives up to expectations. Because their whole self-image revolves around their looks (that's all they ever get complimented on), the truly beautiful are often insecure, tense, and inhibited in bed. If they're not admired for anything else, it's essential they keep up the beautiful look at *all* times—not great when sex is messy, sweaty, and often unflattering at the best of times. A good lover doesn't notice sperm up their nose, pubic hairs in their teeth, and a roll of fat squashed between you both because they're so immersed in the sensation, they've lost conscious thought. Call me cynical, but if you're wondering if your Estée Lauder eyeshadow really has proved to be crease-free as he lines up for the final thrust, you're not into it. Ditto for men who worry about messed-up hair.

> ❗ **There's more to the term "settle down and get married" than you think. Men's testosterone level—the hormone that reputedly makes them aggressive—is high when men are single, goes down when they get married, and rises again on divorce.[1]**

Sex is the most important thing in a relationship.

You can only spend so much time in the bedroom. So if it's a love (not a sex) affair, you're forced to relate on other levels at least some of the time. Most people's needs in life divide roughly equally into spiritual (connecting with others), mental (brain stimulation), emotional (loving and being loved), and sexual. You can't (and absolutely shouldn't) discount sex because it's definitely important; on the other hand, it's only 25 percent of our lives. In my opinion based on surveys and studies on relationships I've read over the years, around 20 percent of you consider earth-shattering sex "crucial," the other 80 percent consider it "the icing on the cake" of a good relationship. According to the weighty *Kinsey Institute New Report on Sex*, bad sex isn't even a major cause of divorce (though it is certainly up there on the "why I want to leave" list). The general consensus from the experts seems to be this: when sex is good, or even okay, it's afforded the same importance we place on things like shared goals, trust, and love. It's when it's bad that it tends to become the focus of the relationship, insidiously destroying everything else.

Most couples have good sex most of the time.

"If John doesn't do it at least once a day, he goes crazy," your best friend reveals after a bottle of wine. "Oh, we haven't done it in bed for *years*," boasts Jane. Why is it that everyone else's sex life seems better than our own? One reason could be that you're at different stages in your relationships. You can't compare new sex with a four-year-been-there-done-that relationship; the human nervous system is programmed to become desensitized the more of the same stimulation it gets. That's not to say long-term sex can't be as good; it's just different. If your partner knows all the right buttons to push (and they should after all that practice!) orgasm is often guaranteed for long-time lovers and, with effort, you can still be *very* passionate. But cut-your-arm-off-to-get-it, out-of-control, raging lust *every* night, after years of sharing the same bed? Possible, but you'd be unable to hold down a job with the amount of energy it would take to sustain it. Life and all its pressures get in the way and many couples are too tired to have sex at some stages in their life (kids, new job, or skidding through a rough patch). So how come your sister still has mind-blowing sex after six years of marriage? She may think *you* have a great sex life and doesn't want to admit she doesn't. Or she really does have terrific sex—once a month. It's all subjective.

> ❗ Beware a lover who believes you were "meant" for each other. People who think romance is in the hands of destiny and fate tend to end relationships rather abruptly—the minute they discover you're less than perfect. (Human perhaps?)[2]

The average couple makes love 2.5 times a week.

We forget that an average statistic is just that—an average. Researchers have lumped in the couple who *shred* the sheets three times a day with Bertha and George who manage it once a year and all those who fall somewhere in between, added up their weekly totals, and averaged them all out. You could have sex every day for a month, then abstain totally for the next two and still make the average. Add to this that most women don't have sex during their period, most couples don't if they're sick, tired, or arguing, *and* that on vacation we make love three times more often, and you'd have a hard time trying to be Mr. and Mrs. Average. Besides, not all nationalities conform to the old 2.5 figure (though Americans are pretty close at an average of 2.6). Couples in Hong Kong only indulge in sex once a week; Italians (despite their image) do it 1.7 times. Americans top the global average for time spent making love—but don't feel too smug, it's still only 28 minutes. Pathetic when you consider the amount of time the average person spends watching TV![4]

> **❗ Americans have sex, on average, 138 times a year. The most sexually active people globally: Couples who live together but aren't married (146 times a year). Number of times singles have sex: 69 times a year. Married couples: 118 times.[3]**

Men sleep around more than women do.

A great deal of research has gone into solving the twentieth-century mystery of why men consistently report having three times more sex partners than women do. (If it's true there's an awfully sore woman out there.) It could be that, generally, men overestimate and women do the opposite. What's more likely is this: women tend to remember sex if it was part of a long-term relationship. We "forget" (somewhat conveniently) any one-night stands. Based on my research experience, I'd suggest the real total for women is about three times more than they say or admit. Oddly enough, that makes both sexes even.

If they're having an affair, they don't love me.

Wrong again. Affairs aren't about love, they're about sex, a certain *kind* of sex. It's the affair that's the turn-on, not the person. Sex on the sly, a bit on the side—even the expressions we use hint at the real reason people stray from home. It's the excitement of secrecy. One study found that not only were people more obsessed with past, secret relationships than those that were out in the open,

> **!** *Most of the things you and your partner argue about today, you'll still be fighting about a decade from now. Couples fight about the same issues 69 percent of the time—we don't resolve our problems because many of them are unsolvable. Swapping partners doesn't help either—you'll just get a different set of unresolvable issues!*[5]

but that the minute the forbidden relationship was revealed or (even worse) approved of, it fizzled out fast. The novelty of being with someone new is the other motivator. The thrill of the chase, the ego-boost—we're all suckers for a bit of attention. Having an affair doesn't mean your partner doesn't love you, but it *does* mean they don't respect you.

Most people now use condoms because of AIDS.

I'd dearly love to tell you otherwise but although people are buying and carrying condoms, they aren't actually taking too many out of the packet. Youth, booze, and hormones is proving a potentially lethal cocktail for teenagers the world over who regularly have unprotected sex. The newly single are another group who believe they're immune to AIDS: divorced, widowed, or separated people are five times more likely to have unsafe sex than those who are married.[6] It seems hard to believe intelligent people knowingly put their lives at risk. But they do. Often.

If you don't wake the neighbors, you're not enjoying yourself.

Some people scream their heads off at football games, others just wave a banner—that doesn't mean one's enjoying it more than the other. While it's great if your partner does make noise (it's good feedback), it really depends on their personality. For many women, reaching orgasm is a long, private process that involves intense concentration. She's battling to stay focused on the sensation so when she does climax, she isn't likely to blow all that hard work by announcing the fact to the entire world. Some men are also quiet achievers. To each his own.

It's not what you've got, it's how you use it.

Partly true, partly false. The saying should go, "It's not what you've got, it's how you compensate for it." If you're a half-inch or so under the average, chances are she hasn't noticed or cared. But if you're talking *really* little, you can "use it" (that is, thrust) all you like and it probably won't be the best penetration she's experienced. The small guy who has extraordinary oral sex and foreplay skills, however, won't have too many problems; the guy hung like a horse *will* if he relies exclusively on his penis.

> **!** *Opposites don't attract, similarity does. Couples who have the same values, attitudes, interests, and ways of looking at the world are more likely to say they've found "a soulmate" and more likely to stay together. On the other hand, hooking up with someone whose differences complement your own personality is a good idea. That's why worrier-relaxed and shy-outgoing combos work.*

Women are turned off by porn.

Both sexes are turned-on by pornography and erotica, just different kinds. Generally, men go for more explicit, hard-core stuff; women usually prefer erotic, soft images (and a plot, if it's at all possible). Women also often need to look at the people on the screen and think "I could/would like to do that" or they don't relate to it. But as for not enjoying it at all—nonsense. The recent boom in made-for-women-by-women flicks is evidence enough that if it's the right kind, we'll eat it up.

THE CUTTING EDGE: CIRCUMCISED VERSUS UNCIRCUMCISED

Circumcision—removing the foreskin of the penis—is commonly performed for "hygienic" or religious reasons. Even though many parents are now debating the value of this procedure, the vast majority of men in the United States are still circumcised because the medical community, including the American Academy of Pediatrics, upholds the theories that circumcision reduces the risk of penile cancer and infections of the foreskin (even though the research is in very early stages and not completely conclusive to date).[7] Chances are, however, many women will encounter both "cut" and "uncut" penises so let's challenge a few misconceptions right here and now.

Circumcised penises are prettier

This is a matter of personal taste and what you're used to. Take a look through some old photos and most of us will *cringe* at the getups we thought looked marvelous ten years ago. The fact is, they did—at the time. Fashions change and so does our perception of what looks good. If you've only slept with circumcised guys, an uncircumcised penis looks different and our natural reaction is to go "yuck." If everyone you've slept with is uncircumcised and you come across a circumcised one, it will look funny to you as well.

Uncircumcised men don't get as hard

Believe me, the blood pumps just as ferociously through an uncircumcised penis as it does a circumcised one. The reason it doesn't feel as hard around the glans (head), is that the extra skin "cushions" it slightly. Ever so slightly.

Uncircumcised ones are smelly

The uncircumcised guy *does* need to be scrupulous about his personal hygiene to avoid odor problems. But if he showers regularly and washes properly—gently pulling the foreskin back from the penis and washing underneath with mild soap—he'll smell (and taste) just as sweet as the next guy.

Uncircumcised guys are more sensitive

Quite true. Because the head of his penis is covered by skin, it's not exposed to things like rubbing against clothing. But this doesn't mean he'll come more quickly. Inside the vagina, the sensation's essentially the same and it's what he's used to, so if he blames premature ejaculation problems on being uncircumcised, he's putting you on. It's his brain, not his foreskin, that needs sorting out.

Which feels best for him?

Adrian was circumcised at twenty-four, so is in the unique position of having experienced both:

"I'm English and, as was the custom back then, not circumcised as a baby. A few girls commented that I was unusual, simply because most guys were, but I didn't think much about it until I was twenty-three and got a fibrous growth that caused thickening of the foreskin. It was incredibly painful. I couldn't pull the foreskin back to wash because it felt like my penis was being strangled. But I'd force it, it would tear, scab over, then form scar tissue and make the whole problem worse. I was too embarrassed to see a doctor but when it got to the point that sex was agony, I went.

> **❗ The biggest human penis ever recorded was 13 inches long. The smallest functioning penis was a tiny ⅝ inch long![8]**

"I felt quite humiliated getting circumcised at such an old age and it hurt like hell afterward. It felt like someone had put a red hot poker up my penis and it stung for days. I had to wear sarongs, much to the amusement of my girlfriend and her friends, and it took about two weeks to heal properly. Sex wasn't dramatically different—probably because I'd fooled around a bit even though I wasn't supposed to and got used to it. I felt more sensitive the first few times we had intercourse, but that quickly passed. As far as sensation and the time it took me to orgasm, there was no change whatsoever. But I'd probably say I prefer being circumcised. My penis is easier to care for (you don't have to mess around with the foreskin) and I think it looks cleaner and more attractive. If I had a child, I'd probably get him circumcised, simply because I'd hate him to have to go through the pain I endured if he also had problems at a later age."

ANSWERS TO SOME COMMON QUESTIONS

Am I normal (and is my partner)?

This is the most commonly asked question in sex therapy and the hardest to answer—"normal" is virtually impossible to define because we're all individuals. People ponder the question because they believe all the sex myths, know they don't apply to their own sex lives, don't realize they don't apply to other people's, either, and think everyone else is having a better time than they are. But not only is it unhealthy and inhibiting to aspire to be normal (not to mention boring—do you really want to be the quintessential Mr. and Mrs. Jones?), it's impossible. Read all the sex surveys you want but you still won't really know what other people do in bed because what people say and what people do are two totally different things.

Instead, steer toward another goal: developing a healthy, satisfying sex life where nothing is "kinky" or wrong provided both of you agree. Don't fall for the "but everyone else does it" argument and be pressured into doing things you don't want to, but consider trying things that sound reasonable at least once. If you're not sure if you're being narrow-minded, read a few good sex books to get an impression of whether what your partner is suggesting is standard sexual practice or listed with more unusual things (like sexual deviance). That will give you a good idea of whether your attitude to sex is prudish—or prudent.

My vagina sometimes makes noises during sex and it sounds like I'm breaking wind. Help!

Some positions of intercourse—particularly him entering from behind—force air into the vagina which is expelled (usually in a most unelegant fashion) after he withdraws. It's a totally normal bodily function which most couples ignore or giggle over. Tongues licking, mouths kissing, bodies slapping together—sex is noisy and this should add to the excitement rather than detract from it. The only way to stop your body from making noises is to stick exclusively to the missionary position and not get too carried away. Fun, eh?

My vagina's smelly—what should I do?

The French have a name for the smell of a woman's genitals—
cassolette—which means perfume box. Most men are turned-on
by your natural scent (even if you aren't) and that slightly acidic
smell is normal. If the smell has changed, become stronger, or a
discharge has appeared with it, see your doctor to make sure you
don't have an infection. Otherwise, wash with unscented soap,
wear cotton underwear, and steer clear of too much garlic (your
breath isn't the only place it turns up).

How much pubic hair is normal? I think I've got too much.

Yikes! There's that awful "normal" word again. Why is it some
people have curly hair and others perfectly straight? It's called
genes. If you feel Mom or Dad have been a little too generous in
the pubic department, trim, wax, shave, or have it removed by
electrolysis. Bear in mind though, some men love it!

A HIGHER LOVE

We've all heard the hype about how great sex is meant to be if
you've dropped ecstasy or are coked to the eyeballs. But what's the
reality? According to one young women's magazine survey, 25
percent of under twenty-five-year-olds take "party" drugs once a
month or less, 23 percent every weekend, and 18 percent every
day (with the average starting age being sixteen).[9] Faced with these
stats, I figured I'd better find out. You can guess the conclusion
by the fact that I've included it in this chapter—the one devoted
to debunking myths. The fact is, most of the extravagant claims
about the aphrodisiac effect of these drugs simply aren't true. And
even if you have had an out-of-this-world sex session after taking
them, there's a downside.

Some claims about drugs and sex *aren't* fiction. You *are* far
more likely to have sex without a condom, for instance, so your
chance of contracting an STI or HIV rises sharply if you indulge.
One-third of those surveyed in the magazine admitted they'd had

unsafe sex while on drugs; others "couldn't remember." Other truisms: you're far more likely to end up in bed with someone you wouldn't have been remotely interested in sober or straight; you're more likely to put yourself in dangerous situations; you'll have sex sooner than you usually would with a new partner. Illicit drugs also up your chances of becoming intimate with someone you hadn't planned on—the police.

I haven't included the numerous general health risks associated with recreational drugs, just the effect they may have on your sex life. I can generalize though: all are bad for you, all can cause long-term, serious health problems, all are addictive, and too much of some can kill you. All the information included here is provided by people who regularly use recreational drugs, as well as the health authorities who battle to clean up the not-so-fabulous side effects. I don't take illegal drugs. I hope you don't, either. No one's denying a few drinks can relax you and your inhibitions but *too* much alcohol and even small amounts of the other drugs I've covered here aren't safe and *won't improve your sex life long-term.* The best sex stimulants are your hands, your mouth, your genitals, your heart, and, most important, a clear, active, imaginative brain. No chemicals necessary. If you need drugs to enhance your enjoyment of *anything*, you've got problems.

Alcohol
Users claim
In small or moderate amounts, alcohol has psychological effects which can help us feel and be more sexy. A few drinks reduces our inhibitions and lends courage to those who are too shy to let loose sexually when sober. Alcohol makes us feel warm, fuzzy, and affectionate, making us more approachable and open to sexual advances.

The downside
Too much can make us a little too uninhibited—we're far more likely to have unsafe sex when drunk as well as sleep with someone we wouldn't have otherwise.

Drunk, some people become aggressive and violent, others sink into morbid moods.

Booze is also notorious for stopping him from getting an erection. In *Macbeth*, Shakespeare wrote that alcohol "provokes the desire, but takes away the performance." Clever boy, Shakespeare. Down more than the recommended two beers, spirits, or wines in an hour and hello impotence!

Because it's a depressant, alcohol chemically acts to slow down or stop the physical processes necessary for sexual arousal and orgasm. For men, this means either no erection or a semisoft one—and he'll have trouble coming to orgasm. It also affects arousal, lubrication, and ability to orgasm for women. Drink too much, and the only thing you'll do lying down is pass out.

If you're having a smoke along with that drink, your blood vessels will be narrowed. This reduces the blood flow into the penis (again, making for soft erections) and stops blood flow to the vaginal walls, decreasing lubrication. While 45 percent of people say alcohol enhances sex, 42 percent say it does quite the opposite.[10]

> **!** **Sobering news: The most popular aphrodisiac for men and women is alcohol.**

Real life

"Booze has landed me in bed with ex's, married men, and complete losers. They all look good when I've had a few too many and my morals go out the window. It's also made me sleep with guys I really do like way too early. They think I'm easy and I never see them again." *Jamie, 21, secretary*

Dope (marijuana or cannabis)

Users claim

When the young readers of a UK magazine were surveyed, 56 percent said they smoked it regularly and 63 percent said it enhances sex.[11]

Of all the party drugs, dope is the most sexually unpredictable of all. Some people swear it makes sex better, and chemically it just might. Dope increases blood levels of phenylethylamine, a neurotransmitter associated with love and lust.

Like alcohol, smoking a joint can help us overcome inhibitions and make us feel more relaxed, so it can increase the chances of female orgasm in someone who's normally too uptight to let go. It also increases awareness and sensitivity of our skin and genitals. Sex is lazier and more leisurely; and it seems to last longer because marijuana affects our perception of time.

The downside

The effects vary dramatically from one user to the next, and there's no way of telling which way you, or your partner, will go. Lots of people withdraw or become anxious and irritable rather than snuggly or sexy. It's a crapshoot. Habitual users eventually lose desire: it's an effort to drum up the motivation to *think* about sex, let alone *do* it.

Real life

"I love having sex while I'm stoned but only with a long-term lover. I did it once with a guy I'd just met and felt like he was raping me." *Tracey, 32, stylist*

"E" or ecstasy

Users claim

Eighty-three percent of users say it enhances sex.[12] Ecstasy is a chemical originally used as a diet pill. It was later rediscovered and introduced to partygoers as a drug that would boost desire and make sex better, along with feelings of intense happiness and affection (hence the name). Users say sex is amazing on E: they feel loving, skin feels soft and wonderful to touch, their bodies feel sensitive all over, and they spend longer on foreplay than usual.

❗ Regular coffee drinkers are considerably more sexually active than those who don't indulge in the brew. An undiscovered aphrodisiac? Nah! Researchers think it's simply because it keeps us awake long enough to have sex.[13]

The downside

It's incredibly dangerous, especially in impure forms, and since it's illegal, you have no idea what you're getting. Ecstasy alters our perceptions entirely: you "love" everyone (and end up in bed with more than a few) and you are full of the joys of humankind (you can't imagine that anyone could cause you harm so put yourself in dangerous situations). While ecstasy can make us feel more like sex, it makes us take longer to reach orgasm—if you can manage one at all.

Real life
"Everyone looks good on E. You're up on the dance floor and you think you're with the most gorgeous guy in the club. So you take him home and sleep with him. Sometimes, if I do it when I'm coming down, I suddenly become really lucid and think, *Who is this guy? What am I doing?* Once, I tried to get the guy to stop but he was so whacked, he couldn't comprehend what I was saying. The next day, you wake up beside guys you'd cross the street to avoid when you're straight. I stopped doing E for all those reasons."
Annie, 26, hairstylist

Coke (cocaine)
Users claim
Originally used as a local anesthetic, coke has had a reputation as an aphrodisiac for centuries. Fifty-nine percent of users agree it enhances their sex lives.[14] Coke makes people feel confident and exhilarated, and this increases their sense of desirability. In other words, they feel more attractive. Some people say it reduces their inhibitions while simultaneously increasing their libido and eroticism. The shy and insecure love coke because it helps them relate better to others and have more empathy. Advocates say it makes you "go all night" and you feel strong and full of energy, making sex seem more animalistic. It's less "touchy" than sex on an E and all your senses feel sharpened.

The downside
It's so addictive, improving your sex life becomes the least of your problems—funding your expensive habit is what you have to worry about. Heavy users find the intense experiences produced by coke impossible to

! The most common side effects of recreational drugs:
Mood swings—55 percent of users have them
Depression—46 percent
Frightening flashbacks—11 percent
Bad skin—26 percent
Lack of concentration—55 percent
Memory loss—44 percent[15]

replicate without it, so lose interest in sex if there's no "Charlie" on offer as well. Coke can either boost erections or severely reduce the chances of getting one. It has similarly varied effects on women: some find their desire and capacity for orgasm enhanced, lots say regular use makes them feel dead from the waist down and they couldn't come if their life depended on it. Habitual users (those whose life does depend on it) lose sexual desire completely. Many coke users find orgasms elusive, hovering on the brink but not able to actually have one. Crack is a refined form of coke, and has a similar—and even more addicting—effect on users.

Real life
"It's fantastic, sex on coke. Everyone should try it. You feel so alive and buzzing. My girlfriend and I don't even bother to have sex if we don't have any or can't afford enough to last all week. I guess we're both addicts but hey, we're young. We're supposed to be having fun." *Alan, 20, ad executive*

Speed (or uppers)
Users claim
Thirty-nine percent of young people use amphetamines like speed regularly.[16] It can stimulate sexual desire and lots take it to increase their stamina for sex because it gives an energy boost. Sex on it is "a rush," your senses are heightened, and your heart beats faster.

The downside
It's hard to orgasm, making sex decidedly frustrating. With regular use, desire fades completely. Speed can also make it difficult to get, and keep, an erection. Both sexes say they have trouble keeping their mind on the job, and they're eager to move on to something else.

Real life
"I'd been crazy about this girl for ages, and one night at a rave party, I took speed and she took an E. We went back to her place, had sex a few times and it felt fantastic, but then she got dressed and said we had to go back to the party. She didn't want her boyfriend to catch us—I didn't even know she had one. I felt really

let down and knew how girls felt when they've been used and abused. I haven't touched the stuff since." *Mel, 23, psychology student*

THREE IN A BED: THREE-SOMES, SWAPPING, AND GROUP SEX

"I must be the luckiest man alive," confided my friend James, three sheets to the wind. "My wife wants us to try a threesome with another woman."

"So, are you going to?" I asked him.

"Of *course!*" he sputtered. "God, what man in his right mind would knock the chance to sleep with two women at once?" There was a telling pause. "I mean, you'd have to be a real wimp to say no, wouldn't you . . . wouldn't you? It's every guy's dream . . . isn't it?"

"But not yours," I said, taking a guess.

"No," he admitted, embarrassed as hell. "Truth is, the idea frightens the hell out of me."

James isn't alone. While just about all of us have fantasized about threesomes and group sex, taking that leap to reality is something else. James was terrified he wouldn't be able to satisfy both women, that they'd think he was hopeless, that he'd be left out, and that his wife would turn gay and leave him.

"I'm also not entirely convinced I'll be able to handle watching someone I love getting it on with another person, male or female," he confessed sadly.

I'm with him. I'm far too jealous to share, but lots of people

"I was nineteen and had been going out with this guy for about a month. We had terrific sex but both of us knew that was all we had. We were fooling around with a girlfriend of mine who's really into sex as well and she French-kissed me as a joke, to see if he got jealous. He pretended to, so we hammed it up a bit and somewhere along the line, stopped laughing and started getting into it. It very naturally turned into a threesome and all of us enjoyed it but no one instigated a repeat performance. My girlfriend and I haven't mentioned it since."

Debbie, 31, receptionist

I know have had threesomes with varying results. Generalizing outrageously, I'd say the ones that it worked for were couples who hadn't been together long and didn't really mind their partner being with someone else. They had a trip, said it made great future fantasy material, but wouldn't rush to repeat it. For older, long-term couples, it was an emotional disaster. Even if they enjoyed it at the time, most said the fallout afterward was incredibly destructive. Jealousy, "broken" trust, paranoia that their partner secretly preferred the third person—three in a bed really is dicey stuff. Convinced your relationship could handle a *ménage à trois*? Read this first.

Why we want to do it

Often, threesomes appeal because we're too lazy to put the work in to boost a flagging sex life. We think a quicker, easier way to add spice is to introduce a third party—let them do the work. On the other hand, lots of us are aroused by the sight and sounds of others having sex—that's why we watch erotic videos. It can be instructive to watch other people's sexual techniques, it can make us feel desirable if there's more than one person enjoying our body, it undoubtedly adds variety and, of course, it's taboo. The thrill of doing something both naughty and novel is often a turn-on in itself.

Some like the idea of being the center of attention and the thought of all that pleasure—*two* tongues, *two* sets of hands, *two* penises or vaginas—sounds great. In our fantasy, many of us cast ourselves in the taking role. Generally, women are more aroused by the two women and a man combination than men are by two men and one woman.

Threesomes sometimes seem like a natural solution to couples who are bored with each other but don't want to leave or do something "behind their back." Doing it in front of their partner seems less of a betrayal and most imagine the third person as an enjoyable addition rather than a threat. The people I interviewed indulged with like-minded friends, placed or answered an ad in the personals, or went along to a massage parlor that catered to couples. Even if the experience was positive, in most cases, once was enough—they satisfied their curiosity but found one-on-one sex ultimately more fulfilling.

What can go wrong

Real life is very different from fantasy. Couples who love each other usually have a hard time seeing their partners with someone else and often the physical pleasure dulls because of the strong negative emotions threesomes throw up. Most of us are pretty territorial about relationships and our partners, and not used to sharing them so there's often jealousy (of the third person's body, technique, how your partner related to them). Three people in one bed is, by virtue of the fact that it's an uneven number, unequal— someone usually fancies someone else more and the attention seems to tilt that way.

After the thrill's worn off (and perhaps the alcohol—a few drinks can do wonders for turning us on physically and off mentally), lots of people feel guilty and resentful (particularly if they were talked into it), ashamed, "cheap," or disgusted with themselves. But the most common negative of all is feeling betrayed and that trust has disappeared. "I can't get the images out of my head" and "I'm scared they'll see them without me" were common comments from the people I surveyed. If your partner wants a repeat and you don't, you feel threatened. Sometimes wanting group sex is a sign of immaturity. It's all about instant gratification and it's far less personal than the one-on-one variety. It can also mean one or both of you have intimacy problems.

> "My boyfriend called his roommate in while we were having sex. I said nothing because I knew it was what my boyfriend wanted. When his friend said he was getting a hard-on, my boyfriend asked him to join us. They had a 'sandwich': My boyfriend penetrated me anally, the other guy vaginally. They'd obviously discussed it before. I felt like a whore."
>
> Judith, 22, promotions manager

In a sense, going along to an arranged sex party is more honest and less tricky than a threesome with a friend. Everyone knows what they're there for, there's little chance of a relationship developing because people swap around a lot and you're not likely to see each other again. "Swinging" or "swapping" usually means your partner's not in the same room or doing it in front

> **❗** *"If God had meant us to have group sex, I guess he'd have given us all more organs."—Malcolm Bradbury*

of you so there are no nasty images to replay in your head. Groups that organize swapping parties also usually enforce set rules about using condoms and stopping if one person isn't enjoying it.

If you are going to give it a whirl

If you decide to go ahead, here's what you should do:

- Have condoms ready.
- Talk through what will happen together: what's okay, what isn't. Is kissing allowed? What if one person wants to stop and the other doesn't? Spell out who's having sex with who. Seeing your boyfriend take another guy's penis into his mouth can be pretty shocking if it didn't occur to you the two men would have sex as well.
- As a couple, ask yourselves: Are we good at communicating, problem solving, and negotiating? You need all three skills to get through this one.
- Ask yourself: *Do* I feel comfortable having three-way sex? Do I feel comfortable about *my partner* having sex with someone else? If you're not 100 percent sure of either, don't do it.
- Examine your motives. Are you trying to hang on to someone by agreeing? Do you feel forced into it? Then don't do it.
- If you're intent on spicing up your sex life with other people, would you be better off agreeing on an open relationship, making a few rules like always using condoms, and then not talking about it? You don't have to have sex with someone new together.

11

Gay and Lesbian Sex

Am I? Is he? What now?

• •

The hostess ushers me into the living room. "This is Carrie and John," she says. Smiles all round. "And this is Peter and Mandy." Ditto. ". . . and Katie and Emma."

It's pretty obvious from the body language that Emma and Katie aren't linked together because they're roommates. Images whirl in my head: tongues plunging, mouths sucking, breasts colliding. I blink rapidly and wonder why the minute I realize a couple is gay or lesbian, I immediately imagine the two of them in bed. After all, the other couples also have sex—why don't I automatically think of them doing 69s? "You focus on it because that's the point of difference," a lesbian friend later explains patiently. "But isn't that wrong?" I ask, nervous I'm guilty of some sort of subconscious homophobia. "No," she says, "it's normal." Fiona's incredibly tolerant of my many questions about her sexuality, as are all of my gay and lesbian friends. Pity some members of society aren't as tolerant of them.

It always strikes me as odd that anyone should take exception to what people do behind closed doors. In classical Rome, ancient China, and precolonial America, homosexual sex was a part of everyday life. In Greece, it was common. Unfortunately, the liberal attitude was not always the popular opinion. Homosexuals have suffered under legal and social discrimination even in this century. But in 1969, in New York City's Greenwich Village, amid the rising tides of civil rights and antiwar movements, gay men had finally had enough of the persecution. As the police attempted to raid a small bar called Stonewall, the men took to the streets in protest. And discovered that men throughout the neighborhood were just as tired of having to keep their lives in the shadows. This one night of protest was the spark of a new era of activism, which has led to a greater acceptance of gay, lesbian, and bisexual lifestyles throughout North America.

But even with the major strides achieved since Stonewall, whispering, ostracism, and petty slights are dealt out to gay and lesbian people daily throughout the world. It's not easy being gay or lesbian. It's not easy being different from the majority in any sense. This chapter is not just for people who are confused about their sexuality or having difficulties coming to grips with being gay or lesbian, it's for "straights" as well, most particularly those who find the topic slightly distasteful. Do yourself a favor if this is you: read it. You just might learn something.

AM I GAY?

As the advice columnist for Australian *Cosmopolitan* magazine, I often receive letters from readers asking if they're gay. A simple enough question, they figure, but actually, it's not that easy to answer. As the psychologists, activists, counselors, and gay, lesbian, and bisexual people I spoke to verified, *all* of us have a male and a female side. Which part of *you* is going to be dominant for life is anyone's guess.

What do "gay" and "lesbian" mean?

If someone says they're gay or lesbian it usually means they have sexual relationships with the same sex and have adapted their lifestyle to suit. Terms like "gay" (men who have sexual relation-ships with men), "lesbian" (women who have sexual relationships with women), "straight" or "heterosexual" (people who have sex-ual relationships with the opposite sex), or "bi" (people who have same sex and opposite sex relationships) are society's way of sim-plifying sexuality. But while it's nice and easy to plunk people into simple categories, real life is a little different.

The fact is, our sexuality is fluid throughout our life. You may be "gay" for a period of months or years, then straight for the rest of your life, or vice versa. In prison, with no access to the opposite sex, some inmates become attracted to, fall in love with, or have sex with the same sex. Then, the minute they're out of jail, turn straight again. They're not the only ones who experiment. Lots of straight people have one or two sexual encounters with the same sex before deciding which sex suits them best. So a more apt definition might be, "I'm straight at the moment" or "I'm gay right now."

Some people identify with one group very early, are sure of their choice, and that's the end of the story. Toward the end of adolescence or in our early adult years, most of us have figured out which group we "belong" to, especially if we've decided we're straight. It's not quite so easy if we think we're gay. It may take a few more years before you accept that, and you may struggle with all the issues it throws up. Bisexual people are those who are quite comfortable with and equally attracted to both males and females. Some people consider them the most confused of all the groups. Others think, "How fabulous. They have the whole world to choose from!"

> ❗ *Gay students are five times more likely to skip school over fears of personal safety and four times more likely to have been threatened with a weapon while there. Not surprisingly, they have a 28 percent high school dropout rate.*[1]

What makes someone gay or lesbian?

Hundreds of thousands of studies have attempted to answer this question but, to date, there aren't any clear answers. Some tentative research points to a gay gene—that different structures of the brain may dictate our sexuality—but even that's not conclusive, and there's no concrete proof. The only thing scientists *are* reasonably certain of is this: if there *is* a biological factor at play, it will only be one factor of the complex events that shape our sexuality.

How can I tell if I'm sexually curious or seriously gay or lesbian?

One in four American men have had a sexual experience with another male during their teen or adult years.[2] That statistic includes everything from having a major crush on a same-sex teacher to actually having sex with the same sex. Of those who do experiment, the majority decide it's not for them after all. Others need to explore further before they decide. Some people stop having homosexual sex because they enjoy it with both sexes and it's less stressful and easier to be straight because that's what society accepts as normal. Others opt for casual sex with the same sex and relationships with the opposite for the same reason.

It's probably best if you don't try to fit yourself neatly into one box. Some people have always known they're either exclusively homosexual or heterosexual and never, ever waver. Lots of others aren't sure where they fit in. How can *you* tell? The closest I can get to a definite answer seems to be this: you'll know you're gay if it feels right for you and if you're *consistently* and *repeatedly* drawn to the same sex and rarely or never to the opposite. Try to be honest with yourself. Are you fighting being gay because you're scared of rejection if people find out? Some people feel gay but when they look out at the visible, public face of the gay community, either feel they don't fit in there either or don't want to. Ask yourself, what sort of relationship would satisfy me most *at the moment*? You don't have to make a decision for life.

As for finding out "for sure," start by working through your

> "I felt so isolated and didn't know any other lesbians. Eventually, I had to move to the city where I thought I'd be more accepted. I joined a support group immediately and was all set to attend my first meeting except I didn't go—I just couldn't walk in that front door. I called the people who ran the group the next day and told them, and they invited me to come into the office and have coffee. I did, got over my fears and my world changed from one of frustration and depression to feeling alive and good about myself."
>
> Fiona, 30, personal assistant

feelings and emotions. Seek counseling if you don't seem to be getting anywhere (most states have gay and lesbian counseling services). Two or three sessions might make things crystal clear. The counselor will focus on areas which may be holding you back from "admitting" you're gay (like how your family will react, concerns about not having children, etc.). Once these concerns are addressed, you'll be less anxious about the consequences and more likely to unearth your real inclination.

You may decide you need to sleep with the same sex, the opposite sex, or both before you can truly be sure. If you feel comfortable with that, go for it—just make sure you practice safe sex and don't get into dangerous situations. Know beforehand what you're prepared to do sexually and negotiate with your partner until you're sure they understand what you're hoping to get out of sex with them. Don't do it if it's going to get ugly with someone forcing you to continue if you don't want to. It's probably safer to meet someone through a support group and get to know them a little than it is to turn up at a gay or lesbian bar and take potluck. One word of warning for guys who are thinking of sleeping with another man: It's not a myth that gay males are a high-risk group for HIV. You

❗ Gay women have the best time in bed—at least that's the conclusion of a recent sex survey. Thirty-nine percent of lesbians surveyed said their last sex session lasted more than one hour, with only 15 percent of heterosexual women claiming the same. Only a fifth of the straight women had multiple orgasms compared to over a third of the lesbians. Gay men also clock up more orgasms per week than straight ones.[3]

❗ Fifty percent of gay and lesbian youth are rejected by their families, 80 percent report isolation problems, and 93 percent of all students—gay and straight—hear antigay or lesbian comments in school.[4]

must wear a condom during anal penetration. Oral sex is low risk but if you've got cuts or ulcers in your mouth, or he does on his penis, use a condom.

If I sleep with the same sex once, does that make me gay, lesbian, or bisexual? What about more than once?

One out of three men have had at least one sexual experience with another male since puberty. Three studies of gay men reported that between 62 and 79 percent had had intercourse with "straight" men.[5] For most, that was their only encounter and they were straight thereafter. So an isolated encounter probably means you're curious, not gay. More than one probably doesn't mean you're gay or lesbian either. Again, it's only when you're *consistently* attracted to the same sex and have *lots* of sexual encounters with them that you probably are more gay or lesbian than straight.

Should I tell people if I'm convinced I'm gay or lesbian? How do I tell my parents?

This is called "coming out" and whether it's wise to or not is something only you can decide. The upside: if everyone supports and accepts you, the relief is enormous. The downside: if they don't, your greatest fear is realized and you may be rejected, made fun of, or ostracized, perhaps lose dearly loved friends or family.

There's no rule that says once you decide you're gay you have to come out of the closet with a brass band. Be selective with who you tell and your timing. Some people don't need to know and you'll gain nothing by telling them. Here are some questions and issues you might want to consider.

- **How confident are you about your sexuality?** If you're confused or feel you might be passing through a phase, hold off.
- **Educate yourself about homosexuality.** Chances are, the people you tell will have some misconceptions about gays or lesbians. Prepare some answers to common questions like "Aren't you scared of getting AIDS?" and "It's Uncle John isn't it? He's turned you."
- **Choose your time.** Are things okay at home? If your family

is going through a stressful time—just moved, changed jobs, or dealing with sickness or death—hang on. And try not to blurt it out in the middle of a fight.

- **What are your reasons for telling them?** If it's to build a more open, loving, trusting, respectful relationship, fine. If it's to deliberately hurt them, it's not very constructive for anyone.

- **Accept that people may say things they don't mean and will need time to get used to your news.** Think about it. It took you years to get used to the idea of being gay or lesbian; it will take them a little time to readjust as well. If the person is extremely conservative or very religious, it will be hard for them to accept your decision no matter how much time you give them. Are you sure they need to know? Can you keep this part of your life separate and still maintain a good relationship?

- **Are you financially dependent on them?** If they reject you, can you take care of yourself?

- **Line up someone supportive to see afterward in case your friends or family react badly.** Call the GMHC (Gay Men's Health Crisis) in your state for the phone number of a gay and lesbian counseling service.

- **Make sure the decision to "come out" is _your decision_.** Ignore people who pressure you either way. Coming out will have a huge impact on your life—it could be positive, it could be negative. Make sure you've thought through the consequences before going ahead.

> "I decided to finally tell my mother I was gay and she was terrific. The only thing she was concerned about was AIDS. Once I assured her I was up on the facts and only had safe sex, she said, 'I'm honored you've told me and my only regret is that you didn't tell me earlier. This must have been hard for you.' It's no wonder I love her so much."
>
> Tim, 25, student

> **!** _Twice as many career women as homemakers admit to having a homosexual experience._[6]

The gay and lesbian bar scene doesn't appeal to me. Where else can I go to meet a partner?

Call a gay and lesbian counseling service for advice on what social groups operate in your area. There are gay and lesbian dance clubs, gay and lesbian basketball clubs; in other words, homosexual versions of lots of straight clubs. Some of them only mix within the gay community, others (like sport teams), play against straights. You could also try answering a personal ad but be careful. Arrange to meet in a public place and be aware that people often lie, not only about what they look like but what sort of relationship they're really after. Generally, the more gay people you know, the more gay people you'll meet. Cultivate friendships with people like you even if you don't romantically like them. We all need friends as well as lovers!

The thought of being gay or lesbian frightens the hell out of me. I don't want to be different. How will I cope?

It's hard being different in anything. We all like being individuals but we also try to be like everyone else. It feels uncomfortable being singled out, especially if you live in a rural community and feel like you're the only one who is different. But the fact is, you're not. Numerous studies have tried to pinpoint the number of homosexuals (people regularly having sex with the same sex) and the verdict appears to be about 10 percent of the population. So, there are lots of people like you, in your situation.

Instead of focusing on how different you are and whether you're gay or straight, shift to what you could do to lead a fulfilling and happy life. You might need to make some changes to achieve this: maybe change jobs, friends, or where you live. Moving to a city or neighborhood where homosexuality is more accepted could be a good idea. Once you meet other gay people and realize they're not only "normal" but everywhere, you'll feel more comfortable and be proud of who you are.

> **!** *Thirty-three percent of all teenage suicides are commited by gay and lesbian teenagers.[7]*

Having said that, I'm not pretending for a moment that it's

easy being in any minority group. Lots of people will judge you and many are prejudiced against homosexuals. The rewards for being "normal" are so great that those who can pass for straight often will. But trying to deny who you are and pretending you're not gay or lesbian isn't a terribly good idea, either. Those that do often suffer from low self-esteem and tend to distance themselves from family and friends (can't let anyone get too close in case they "find out"), and thus feel even more isolated and inferior. Their life is based on a lie so they never feel accepted.

It makes sense to surround yourself with people who accept you for who you are. If someone tells you you're sick, bad, or wrong often enough, you'll start believing it and stop looking after yourself. Studies show the gay and lesbian population has more drug and alcohol problems and unsafe sex than the straight population.[8] Suicide rates are also higher.

❗ Of all the sex groups, gay and bi women:
- **have the most sex — 59 percent have it two or three times a week**
- **are most likely to have sex with someone they didn't like, "just to be nice" — 27 percent**
- **masturbate the most — 38 percent do it once a day or more**
- **are most likely to have sex outdoors — 75 percent**
- **are most likely to use food to enhance masturbation — 22 percent**
- **are most likely to be involved in a relationship — 60 percent**

How do I deal with homophobes (people who hate or fear homosexuals)?

It's a crime in a number of states to ridicule or harm gays and lesbians, so in these states you are protected by legislation. Most city police stations have gay and lesbian liaison officers who will help you make a complaint and all states have antiviolence laws.

If we're talking about a muttered "fag" or "dyke" as you walk past some idiots in a bar, you're probably wise to ignore it (*especially* wise if you could end up hurt). Rise above the homophobes and recognize *they* are the ones with the problem. If you're the witty, articulate type, maybe you'll enjoy challenging them.

Who knows, if you present an intelligent argument, you might even change their perception. On the other hand, if they're going to behave like that in the first place, it's not likely.

I think my boyfriend/girlfriend is gay. How do I tell?

Ask them. Say why you think they might be gay and try to be open to what they have to say rather than accusing. Of course it's upsetting if you love them and fear they'll leave you, but at least try to put yourself in their shoes. They've probably been struggling with the issue for years and your support could be a lifeline. If they agree they might be, you need to discuss the implications for the relationship. Maybe you could agree to be friends for a while until they decide for sure. If you think your guy is having unprotected sex with men (or other women, for that matter) behind your back, get an HIV test, use condoms, and don't stop unless you're convinced you were just being paranoid.

> **What's the sign of a happy relationship?** Wearing a condom when you're sleeping with someone other than your partner. When live-in gay men are satisfied at home, they're more likely to practice safe sex when cheating. The findings mirror heterosexual relationships.[10]

I'm straight but my best friend's just told me they're gay/lesbian? What do I do now?

Nothing. Just because they're gay doesn't mean they want *you*. If you're worried about that, ask them. If they confess undying love, explain that you're straight and are sure of it. If they can accept a platonic relationship, the problem's solved; you might feel a bit funny for a little while, but that will pass. If they can't, maybe see them less often until they find a partner.

BUT I HEARD . . .

Lots of people, particularly straights, have certain misconceptions about gays and lesbians. Most aren't true and if there is a grain of truth under some piles of prejudice, the reasons behind the behavior aren't what you may assume.

Our new acceptance of gay and lesbian people will encourage confused teenagers to turn gay.

There is absolutely no evidence to support the "recruitment" theory that this thinking is based on. Equally untrue is the fear that if someone hangs around gay people, they'll be taken advantage of or turn gay themselves even if they're straight. They won't. The only thing they may turn into is tolerant, accepting, nonjudgmental people.

❗ *Should gay people have the legal right to marry? Fifty-two percent of straight men and 70 percent of straight women say yes.[11]*

Lesbians all use dildos because they secretly miss the "real thing."

Some straight couples use dildos, vibrators, and other sex toys to add variety to their sex life, some don't. Lesbians are no different. Some like penetration and use dildos, but I seriously doubt it's inspired by penis envy. Most are far too busy indulging in lots of mutual masturbation and oral sex to give it a thought. Lots of studies say gays and lesbians have more satisfying sex than straights. Certainly, they've got a distinct advantage: both partners have the same parts, so what usually feels good for them will feel good for their partner.

❗ *Forget vampy, lipstick lesbian chic— the new lesbian is just as likely to be a bluehaired bridge player. Psychologists now say women are increasingly likely to become lesbians in later life because of a shortage of men. There's already evidence of a radical change in the sexual habits of older women, revealing that many are turning to each other for love and sex.*

All gay men have anal sex.

Some gay men like being penetrated by a penis. Some gays only like doing it to their partner. Some gays don't like either doing it or receiving it, and some find it hurts. Like lesbians, gays usually have lots of oral sex and mutual masturbation or enjoy anal stimulation without penile penetration.

> "I was going out with this guy who had the most beautiful sister who was gay. I was fascinated by her and developed a massive crush. For a while there, I seriously toyed with the idea of switching camps—trouble was, I knew she wasn't interested in me. That was eight years ago. I've met a few women since who I've found attractive but know now I don't really want to act on it."
>
> Zara, 27, dentist

Gays are more promiscuous than straights.

If you think of the gay community as being the few thousand people who go to gay venues and parade around on Gay Pride Day, studies show it's possible they are more promiscuous than the average heterosexual. But that's like judging all straight people on those who go to bars and nightclubs. Neither group is representative of the majority. (By all accounts, even those gays and lesbians who frequent the clubs tire of the scene after a couple of years anyway.) Once involved in relationships, they're as likely, or unlikely, as the rest of us to play around on the side.

As with all sex studies, it's difficult to find out exactly what Mr. and Mr. or Ms. and Ms. Average are up to in day-to-day life. Even harder to survey when it's a minority group used to being persecuted.

If gays do become promiscuous, researchers say it's often a reaction to the treatment dished out by society. Those who accept the negative images of gays are more likely to adopt the "promiscuous" lifestyle society expects of them. Often, what seems like promiscuous behavior—having sex in parks and public toilets—may not be a choice, but the only means they have of exploring homosexuality. Unfortunately, it also ups their chances of contracting an STI or HIV. As for gays not caring if they catch AIDS, that's not far off the mark in *some isolated* instances. In one study, young gays who regularly practiced unsafe sex weren't on drugs, drunk, or particularly aroused, but were angry and depressed.[12] Why should they care if they get AIDS, they figured, if no one else does?

CHANGING CAMPS, SWITCHING BACK: REAL LIFE STORIES

Josh, 32, architect

Josh remained asexual for years until he came to terms with being gay.

"Looking back to elementary school, I can make the connection that I've always been gay. I had a huge crush on a male teacher in sixth grade and always communicated better with girls than I did guys, which I think's pretty typical of gays. But it was when everyone started pairing off with girls and I didn't want to pair off with anyone that it hit. I went out with girls to prove to myself I couldn't be gay—I even slept with a few—but it was pretty sad. It felt weird; I was going against what I was. I decided that wasn't for me and gave up on sex, didn't do anything.

"My first reaction to thinking I was gay was, 'Yuck! This can't be right. I don't want this.' I'm very religious and homosexuality was contrary to the church's teachings. (Interestingly, it's not written in the Bible that it's wrong. It was Queen Victoria, the stupid cow, that made the church say it was wrong.) I was in my early twenties before I decided I had to become a sexual person. I'd had a lot to struggle through, particularly working out how my religious and sexual sides could ever mesh. Adrian, the guy I'm with now, was the first guy I slept with and it wasn't until him that I came to terms with it totally. I was scared shitless the first time I slept with Adrian. It felt right and very comfortable but all that 'No, no, this is the wrong thing to do' stuff came up. Having sex with a man was the final thing: you're confronting it, you're doing it, you can't go back. The next morning I just got up and left. I was petrified! But the following day, there I was back and having lunch and I haven't looked back. Except then, of course, I had to decide whether to tell anyone or not.

"No one knew I was gay, and I briefly considered not telling anyone, thought maybe I could be celibate or get married and force myself to love a woman, but I'm so glad I didn't. I know so many people in that situation now and they've got kids but eventually it's going to come out and I think that's a horrible thing to do to the family. My boyfriend's sister has offered to have a baby for us but although Adrian wants kids, I'm not convinced it's fair on the child. It would have to be a girl. If it was a boy people would say, 'There's two queers who've got a little boy to play with.' Politically, I think gay couples should have kids, but in reality it can be cruel.

"I've never actually told my parents I'm gay though I think they know. They're pretty sheltered people and deeply religious and I don't want to throw it in their faces and say, 'Deal with it.' I'm breaking it to them by showing them. They know I live with Adrian, and they know there's only one bed. They love me, and they want whatever makes me happy, and I'm demonstrating to them I'm not a queen but the son they know.

"I was never the sort of guy who wanted to bang everything in sight. I think that's the way some guys come to terms with being gay. Sort of a 'Shit! Okay, I'd better just go and do it' reaction, so they sleep with as many people as possible to comfort themselves. They're the ones that don't want to fit into straight society: they stick to their own small community because they don't want to face the big picture. When people think 'gay,' that's who they think of—the queens that parade around. I'm quite proud of the fact that I'm not like that. You don't have to throw your sexuality in people's faces all the time, and people rarely pick me, or my partner, as being gay. Adrian and I have more straight friends than gay ones and are well integrated into 'normal' society. A lot of gay guys are in touch with their feminine sides but scared of the masculine. We're in touch with both and that makes it easier for us to get along with straight guys as well.

"People who say you choose to be gay, well, that's bullshit. I didn't have a choice and I believe in the gay chromosome theory. If you're not gay, there's no way you'd put yourself under all the emotional stress just to be fashionable. I mean, why would you do it? I know straight guys who've gotten drunk and ended up sleeping with another guy and their reaction is to wake up the next day and vomit. I think the hardest thing for me is, because I appear straight, girls come on to me a lot. I don't want to go around saying, 'Look honey, I'm gay' to everyone I meet, but there have been occasions where they find out and still persist. That annoys me. They're buying into that 'all you need is a good woman' theory.

"My advice to other guys who think they might be gay is this: There's only one way to find out and that's to experiment. Sleep with the opposite sex first, then meet some gay people, talk to them, and see if you connect. For God's sake, don't go to a gay bar if you're trying to find out: they're meat markets and you'll end up more screwed up than ever. The safest way is to contact a gay support group or gay counselor. Also remember, you're a person first, gay second. Don't define yourself by who you sleep with."

Amanda, 26, shop assistant

Amanda told her friends and family she was gay, then decided she wasn't.

"Sometimes I think my life sounds like a really bad script for a sitcom. Looking back, I actually think it's quite funny but it sure as hell wasn't at the time. I led a typical straight life up until I hit twenty-two—went out with guys, slept with them, the usual stuff. I'd had my share of bad boys but nothing none of my other girlfriends hadn't suffered through. I'd never thought much about being lesbian because it didn't seem relevant to me. I had a few girlfriends who were gay but what they did in bed was their business and I didn't think of them any differently from my straight girlfriends.

"Then I meet Darrell. She was introduced to me at a party, along with her boyfriend (who I thought was a complete jerk). She was amazing-looking and reminded me of a young colt: all legs, a long neck, and she held herself so proudly. I liked her and we chatted for ages when, much to my horror, I found myself flirting with her. I was a bit drunk but I couldn't stop looking at her lips and wondering what it would be like to kiss her. I felt strangely pissed when she left, arm-in-arm with her boyfriend, and thought, 'Wow! I was attracted to another woman.' That would have been that, except she got my phone number from the hostess and called me. We went out for coffee and dinner a few times and I thought we were just going to be friends. Except a few weeks later, she turned up on my doorstep sobbing because her boyfriend had dumped her. She said she didn't know many people in our town because she'd just moved there. I let her in, hugged her, and said she could stay with me. That night, she slept in my bed and we became lovers. She'd slept with other women before and said she was bi.

"I should have recognized it for what it was: experimentation and a fling. But, oh no, I had to take it all seriously. I bought some books on lesbians and didn't identify with any of what was written but still I wasn't deterred. I decided it wasn't fair on Darrell not to introduce her as my lover to my friends and family—so I did. I went around to my parents' house and made a dramatic announcement that I was a lesbian. They stared at me in absolute amazement and said, 'Are you sure, darling?' To their credit, they were wonderful about it. My parents are pretty cool and they didn't overreact and welcomed Darrell into our home. My friends, on the other hand, were either horrified or thought it extremely amusing. My best friend, who'd always said her favorite fantasy was sleeping with another woman, was more perceptive than most. 'Do you think you're lesbian or just have a thing about Darrell?' she said. 'Because if it's Darrell, you're going to end up hurt.' She was right, of course. I got up one morning and Darrell had split, leaving a beautiful letter saying she was a free spirit and thought I was getting in too deep, but it was a kiss-off all the same. The whole affair had lasted three months and I was devastated.

"I missed her desperately but as the weeks went on, gradually started to accept what had happened to me. Then, I was sitting in a bar with a girlfriend and the most gorgeous guy walked in and I became jelly. That was when I realized my best friend was right. I wasn't a lesbian, just attracted to one female. I now consider myself straight but it's taught me a lot about sexuality and I don't regret what happened for a minute. I don't even regret blabbing my business to everyone, even if my boss does think I'm a fruitcake now. Without exception, no one ridiculed me or insulted me, so I feel truly loved for whoever I am."

12

Everyday Couples, Exceptional Sex

I'm sorry, did you say monogamy
or monotony?

• •

When I was twenty-one, I got engaged to my childhood sweetheart. "Do you know," he said, gazing soulfully into my eyes, "I'll be the last person you'll ever have sex with for the rest of your life." It felt as though someone had kicked me in the stomach. I felt like a rabbit caught in the headlights of an approaching car. Like the jailers had just turned the key on the lock to my prison cell. My vision of marriage transformed from trendy career couple swilling wine while having wild sex on the back patio to polyester dresses, aprons, floury fingers, and twin single beds. The ring was off my finger within a week.

It wasn't that I hadn't thought about the sex side *or* that I wanted to do the entire male Olympic swim team (though I could think of worse ways to spend a week). It was the concept of one person being my first, my last, and one and only. I just couldn't do it. The word *monogamy* threw up frightening images of padded cells for years after that but somewhere along the line my attitude changed. I finally figured monogamy and monotony don't *have* to go together like peaches and cream. Here's how I look at it now . . .

Picture your favorite restaurant. Now imagine dining there *every single night for the rest of your life*. After a month, that greasy takeout Chinese food is looking appealing! Sex with the same person can be like that. Why would you crave a hamburger when you could have filet mignon? Simple. You're sick of filet mignon.

Okay. Now go back to the restaurant and imagine that each night you go there, something is different. One night, the music's soft and the lights are dimmed. The next, the stereo's blasting and they've cleared the tables to make a dance floor. One evening they serve French food, the next Italian, the following Thai. There's enough variety to order a different dish every night. The decor changes constantly: dark, gothic, and moody one night, bright, light and stainless steel the next. In winter, there's a fire, in summer the windows are flung open to catch the breeze and a view. Sometimes, you go alone and read a book. Other times, you and your lover solve the world's problems until the wee hours, or you're romantic and playful. The point is this: even if the place is the same, if you change the variables, it *seems* different. Ditto for monogamous sex.

You can make love to the same person for the rest of your life in a million different ways, places, and situations. Naked, half-naked, or clothed; clothes ripped off or stripped off. Sex can be slow and sensual, raw and wicked, intense and erotic; a two-hour marathon or a two-minute quickie up against the fridge. Dinner outside, dinner in—with dessert eaten off each other's bodies. Does monogamy *have* to be boring? In a word: no. Why then, do most people complain it is?

When pop gender-bender Boy George made headlines by admitting he'd prefer a cup of tea to sex most nights, thousands of couples secretly agreed with him. When Dr. Patricia Love released a book called *Hot Monogamy*, hordes of desperate couples deviated from their sacred Saturday, Starbucks/Ikea/Target circuit to head for the local bookstore. Eavesdrop on any cappuccino-fueled conversation between two females with kids and you'll hear, "Sex? God! I couldn't care less if I never did it again." Hell, neither would I if him on top, only on Sundays, and always in bed sex was all that was on offer. If that's monogamy, no wonder it's very,

very dull (if it was ever exciting in the first place). If slipping between the sheets and into the same sex ritual every time sums up *your* love life, two points for even mustering up enough enthusiasm to open this book!

But here are the words you've been waiting to hear: sex can get *better* as the years roll on. Not only that, it can improve RIGHT NOW. There's just one catch: you have to be prepared to put creativity and effort into your sex life ⌐ introduce the variety that's lacking. At first, if you're mind-numbingly bored by each other's bodies, this will be *a real drag*. One or two sessions later, it'll seem less like hard work. One month from that, you'll start grinning at each other whenever you think about last night. And two months from now? Your friends will be calling to say, "Where *were* you two last night? You never seem to go out much anymore . . ."

WHAT'S GREAT ABOUT MONOGAMY

- You can still have sex on "fat days"—you know he finds all of you sexy.
- You can relax a little—it doesn't matter if you don't get an erection, she knows it's a fluke.
- You don't have to use condoms—you've both had AIDS tests and don't want to have sex with other people.
- You can drop those inhibitions—you trust each other and know you won't be branded "weird," "slutty," or "perverted" if you confide a fantasy.
- You're pretty well guaranteed an orgasm—if you've taught each other well, you each know the right buttons to push.
- You enjoy all different types of sex, not just the lusty sort. Sometimes it's romantic and lazy, and it's always loving and intimate.
- You smile when you wake up together the morning after—rather than wonder how the hell you got there.

WHAT ISN'T

There are two major complaints about monogamy: sex can become routine and boring (try everything in this chapter, then get back to me on that one!) and the "newness" has gone. That's the number one beef of even happy couples. "I love X, but you just can't re-create that fabulously erotic feeling you get when it's someone you've *never* done it with before." Hmmm. I could lie and give you false hope. I could say, "Don't be silly, of course it's possible." But I honestly don't believe it is.

Playing games, acting out fantasies, introducing so much variety your head is spinning—all will help immeasurably. But it's still not the same as the very first time with someone new: that's the one downside of monogamy. But if it's the *only* bad thing, it's a small price to pay for all the pluses of being with someone you love. Cope with it by having sex with anyone you want—in your imagination. Fantasize wildly that she's the girl in your office or he's your best friend's boyfriend, but DON'T TAKE IT THROUGH TO REALITY even if you *can* get away with it.

> ❗ *According to a leading U.S. infidelity expert, many men who love their partners and enjoy good sex at home still never turn down an opportunity for sex on the side. Fifty-six percent of men who have affairs say their marriages are happy.*[1]

Every time you're tempted, work through this exercise. Imagine your partner's face if they found out (and it's amazing how most people do). Picture how hurt they would be. Remember that they, too, feel the odd urge to roam but don't, out of respect for you. Even if they never find out, you know you've betrayed them. You've broken that special bond and can never, ever look them in the eye honestly again. Then imagine your partner being so hurt and angry, they leave you. You've broken their heart, you've lost everything, you feel like a complete scumbag. Was that thrill, that one blissful moment of experiencing a new body, worth it? If you run all this through your mind and still consider it would be, get out of the relationship NOW. You don't just want sex on the side, you want to be single.

Some sex therapists say it's normal for each of you to have the odd sexual encounter during your lives together. What you don't know can't hurt you, etc. I don't agree. I've seen pointless they'll-*never*-find-out encounters destroy more than one otherwise blissfully happy couple. In all cases, the person who strayed counts it as the No. 1 Biggest Mistake of Their Life.

THEY'RE HOT, YOU'RE NOT

The third most common couple sex complaint is mismatched libidos: your partner wants sex more or less than you do. To a point, it's something you both have to learn to accept. Having said that, there's a hell of a lot you can do to even the scales.

Part of the turn-off of monogamous sex is that you've got sex on tap. It's *always* available. The single and sex-starved *crave* for someone to touch their genitals. Long-time lovers don't get a chance to build desire because it's always being satisfied. So, you start having sex when you don't really want to (because you feel you should), it becomes boring, and your brain starts to associate the two. Part of the solution is obviously variety (see "Foreplay for familiar lovers" on page 319), but you have to *want* to try the suggestions I've made—and if you don't feel like sex, why would you?

If your partner wants it more than you do

If you want sex less often than your partner, here are some tips from the experts for getting the urge back.

- **Put pen to paper.** Think back to the best sex you've had and work out what it was that made it so special. Who was your partner? Where were you? What led up to the experience? What did he do to you that made it so great? What did you do to him? Write down as many details as possible, then do the same for your worst sexual experiences, including the ho-hum ones. Compare the lists and use them to make another: list the significant things that make sex good for you and those that make it bad. Put them in order of importance and you should have a good idea of what you like, and what you don't. Regularly ask yourself: What would I like more of in bed? What would I like less of? What can I do to make it better?

> **More Please! Number of men who want more sex: 60 percent. Number of women who want more sex: 68.5 percent. The most sexually active age for men and women: between twenty-one and twenty-four.[2]**

- **Start keeping a diary.** Write down any sexy thoughts you have, any fantasies, how you felt when someone gave you a compliment. The aim is to remind yourself that you're a sexual person and find out what's stopping you from feeling sexy all the time. If you don't think of anything at all even related to sex and nothing happens, write that down, too. "Would rather have my fingernails pulled" is better than nothing. For every negative thought, try to write a reason why ("Because I'm so tired"). Keep the diary for at least three months. Rereading it will provide valuable insights into what's stopping those juices flowing.

- **Buy some erotic books.** By that I mean whatever turns *you* on. It doesn't matter if it's *Gardening by the Stars*, if that causes a pleasant little ache down below, read it.
- **Start masturbating.** Contrary to popular myth, masturbating while you're living with someone doesn't stop you from wanting "real" sex. The more you masturbate, the more your body gets used to having orgasms and starts craving sex on a regular basis.
- **Now involve your partner.** The better sex is, the more you'll want it. Both of you write down, being as specific as possible, what you do and don't like about your sex lives. Things like: Are you getting enough foreplay; what would you like more of, do the techniques suit you; are you happy with when, where, how often you have sex; what would you prefer; ideas on bringing back the "newness." Also include relationship issues: Are you generally happy, what's upsetting you, what do and don't you like about the relationship. Be as honest as you can be.
- **Talk about it.** Don't just hand over your lists—you'll both end up huffy. Instead, flip a coin to decide who goes first. You won? Okay, now go through your list and explain, point by point, as clearly as possible what you mean. Get your partner to repeat back to you, in their own words, what they think you've just said. This way, there's no room for misinterpretation. Then they get their turn and you sum-

> **❶** *Contrary to popular belief, a new study suggests women under forty are just as likely to cheat as men their own age.*[3]

marize each of their points. When you've both said your piece, you can then move into thinking up ideas of how to overcome any of the issues thrown up.

- **Do something about it.** Each of you write down five things you could do to make sex better for your partner based on what they've just told you. Schedule one day per week or two to do the things on the list (don't try to do them all at once). Make one small change each time you have sex. After a while, the new behavior will become second nature.

- **Have sex even if the urge is tiny.** The more you do it, the more you'll want to. Stimulate yourself. Turn *yourself* on, don't expect your partner to do it, and *make* time. If you're that busy, have a quickie.

- **Recharge your sex organs with the Sets of Nine.** This is a Taoist intercourse technique that "massages" the vagina and penis. Basically, he thrusts in a carefully sequenced order. 1. Only the head of the penis is inserted and withdrawn, nine times, then he thrusts the entire length in once. 2. Eight shallow strokes (penis head only), two deep strokes (with the entire length). 3. Seven of the shallow strokes, three deep ones. 4. Six shallow, four deep. 5. Five shallow, five deep. 6. Four shallow, six deep. 7. Three shallow, seven deep. 8. Two shallow, eight deep. 9. One shallow, nine deep.

If you're the one who wants it more

- **Try masturbating every second time you feel like sex.** It takes the pressure off both of you.

- **Make it very clear when you want sex and stop hassling if they say no.** "Tim *always* wants sex," says Sarah. "Every touch is sexual. Just once, I'd like him to touch me out of love and affection only." "I touch Sarah all the time and try to be as loving as possible," says Tim. "I make a real effort not to touch her only when I feel like sex, but it's still not working." Get the picture? If your partner's constantly feeling hassled, make it very clear when you are stroking them in an attempt to turn them on so that other times they'll interpret it as affection. Once they've said "no," leave it alone. You'll put them off even more if they feel harassed.

- **Make sex enjoyable.** Know your partner and what turns them on. Ask them, talk it through, do whatever it takes to make sex fun and something they look forward to. The better lover you are, the more they'll want to sleep with you. A massage works wonders for changing minds.

WHY SHOULD I HAVE SEX WITH HIM?

Here's a fact: You can't have a great sex life if your relationship isn't good. If you've barely spoken all day, glared at each other over the (deliberately) burnt toast, or are constantly flinging nasty, petty comments at each other, it's unlikely you're going to turn into a sex kitten and Sensitive New Age Lover once you hop into bed. If you're not relating out of bed, you won't relate in it. This means (groan!) your sex life isn't the only thing you have to work at.

The more educated you are, the more likely you are to enjoy oral sex—and the less likely you are to want children. Fear of being interrupted perhaps?[4]

If the only time you touch each other sexually is under the blankets, I guarantee you'll be bored silly—with sex and each other—within a year. Treat each other as desirable creatures *all* the time and you'll be surprised how much you'll want to act on it. Sex can't provide the intimacy that's missing elsewhere in your relationship.

- **Live life to the fullest.** People who love sex, love life and that attitude is attractive to everyone, not least of all their partners. Develop lots of passions, be energetic, get excited about new things and new people—don't just grab life with both hands, give it a big squeeze. Sexy is a state of mind. Hedonists are melt material.

- **Look sexy and keep fit.** Having dinner with a woman who only orders an appetizer and mineral water isn't fun. One who orders up big, eats with gusto, and appreciates a good wine is. The ability to let go, to stop counting calories is a turn-on— but not if you let go completely. Taking care of your appearance should be a priority. Yeah, yeah, I know it's what's inside that should count, but let's drop the politics and be realistic. Beer bellies, baggy tracksuits, greasy hair, butts straining to escape from too-tight jeans—they're not on *my* list of top turn-ons or yours. Exercise, eat well, get lots of sleep, and don't hit the booze too heavily, too often. The better you look, the better you'll feel about yourself, and the sexier you'll be to your partner. You need energy to throw yourself around that bedroom.

- **Touch each other as much as possible.** Do it all the time, in public, at home, always. "When I met Susan," says my friend Kevin, "the first thing I noticed was that she touched everyone. She couldn't help it. She hugged her best friend, smacked a huge kiss on her brother's cheek, threw her arms around the dog. I spent the whole night wishing she'd touch me and when she did, I was lost. Even now, three years later, I can't wait for her to make contact."

- **Have confidence.** Don't get dragged into those, "Oh, everyone plays around sooner or later" conversations. Ditto, any discussion that starts with, "Of course, sex dies after a while . . ." Refuse to believe your lover would want anyone else when he's already got you. Refuse to accept that sex isn't as good long-term—put the effort in and it'll get better and better and better and . . .

> ❗ *Always fighting and think the relationship is doomed? Not true if you're having good times, too. Stormy twosomes clock up more bad times than their passive peers, but they have more highs as well. Of 73 married couples studied, the happiest were those who maintained a 5:1 ratio of good to bad times.*[5]

- **Respect each other. Be polite.** Say "Thanks, that was great" for everything from a cup of coffee to a fabulous orgasm. Say "You look sensational. Thanks for going to so much effort" if she looks stunning when you go out. Take care of each other when you're sick; listen to each other's problems. Be *nice*.

- **Live your own life.** Spend too much time together, focus only on each other, and you'll fast become bored—and boring. What are you going to talk about if you do everything as a twosome?

- **Fight fair.** Argue about one issue at a time. If you find yourself saying, "And another thing . . ." stop. Ditto "This is so typical of you. It's like the time when you . . ."
- **Boost each other's egos.** "Hi, handsome." "Here she is—isn't she gorgeous?" Silly little compliments feel good and reinforce those "cozy couple" feelings.
- **Throw away your copy of *Mars and Venus*.** Forget all that men and women are aliens stuff and concentrate on the similarities. Men are taller, hairier, more oddly endowed versions of us. We're softer, curvier versions of them. He cries, you cry. He needs love, affection, and sex; so do you. There are more points of similarity between the sexes than differences. Refuse to wage war. Make a deal to be more like each other. You'll try to be more upfront sexually if they'll promise to be more romantic.

> ❶ *Number of couples who say they're very satisfied with their sex life: 58 percent. Twenty-seven percent of couples say an unwilling partner is to blame for their dissatisfaction.*[6]

- **Let him be him, let her be her.** Remember what first attracted you to them? Why are you trying to change it?

FIVE THINGS BOTH OF YOU SHOULD KNOW ABOUT SEX BY NOW

There's been a trillion sex surveys done and certain themes emerge frequently. The sex lives of long-term couples who consistently rate theirs as "excellent" all share the following characteristics.

1. You both know your way around your own and your partner's body. You know what you want in bed.

It's surprising how often people say, "I don't like my sex life but don't know what I need to make it better." You have to know what you want in order to get it. You each should have read at least three good sex books, masturbate regularly, and be able to bring yourself to orgasm without too much effort. If you don't know what your body requires to orgasm, how the hell is your partner expected to figure it out?

2. You talk about sex regularly to each other.

Imagine if your lover chose what books you read and what programs you watched. You'd be incensed, right? I mean, how could he possibly know what you feel like *at that exact moment* without asking you? Most people have no problem agreeing with this statement. Apply the same logic to the bedroom, however, and they become quite indignant. Sex should be spontaneous, instinctual, something that "just happens." Sex should all come naturally. Nice thought. Pity it doesn't work like that in real life.

Will someone please tell me why people say, "If you have to tell your lover what you want, it takes all the fun out of it"? Does cheesecake taste awful because we had to order it? Would it taste better if the waitress plunked it down in front of us because she got a telepathic signal that it's what we wanted? I don't think so. Lots of people expect their partners to be sexual mind readers. They think, "If he or she *really* loved me, they'd know exactly what to do in bed to make me happy." They don't. If there's one thing you can do to instantly improve your sex life, it's to talk to your lover about sex, as clearly and *specifically* as you can.

> **!** *Married couples enjoy better health, have more money and more satisfying sex lives than their single friends. Agree with the first two but can't quite believe the last? Psychologists say it's because you know each other's tastes better and can safely share your fantasies.[7]*

"I want you to kiss me more" isn't enough. Spell out where, how hard, what sort of kissing, and when during sex you'd like it to happen: "When we have intercourse, I'd love you to kiss me hard on the mouth just before I orgasm." Use phrases like "instead of" rather than "I don't like it when" and don't forget to say what you like as well as what you don't. If you're embarrassed, do whatever it takes to get over it. If you don't open your mouth at some point, your sex life (and relationship) really is destined for failure.

3. You plan for good sex and put thought into it.

These are the words just about all couples dread because they think (a) it means the lust has gone, (b) they must be *really* unhappy sexually to go to such extremes, and (c) it sounds like hard work. Wipe all three thoughts from your head. Accept that it's possible to put a little intellectual effort into your sex life without losing spontaneity.

Simmering is a technique that therapists often find quite successful. Every time you have an erotic thought during the day, write it down then use it as a jumping-off point. Develop a fantasy around the thought and tell your partner what it is and what you'd like to do with it *before you see them*. By the time you see each other, you're "simmering" with desire. Writing "10 P.M. Saturday" and sticking it on the fridge *won't* work. Simmering will. If you don't actively try to vary your sex life, you'll end up doing that fumbled first-thing-in-the-morning bleary stuff all the time.

> ❗ **Women are not only better at expressing emotion than men, they're better at knowing the emotions of others. Shown photos of people portraying different feelings, women far outscore men in guessing the correct emotion.[8]**

Hello monotonous monogamy.

4. You make your own rules and have stopped worrying about what other people are doing in bed.

There are two types of sex: manufactured sex and real sex. Manufactured sex is the sex that's dished up on TV, in erotic movies and books. Women orgasm after three good thrusts; men never, ever lose their erection from too many beers. Real sex isn't like that. You are both individuals with your own sexual desires and preferences and your sex life isn't going to be like Jake and Amanda's on *Melrose Place*—or the couple next door. There are no universal rules about what people should enjoy in bed and what they shouldn't. If she can only orgasm if you suck her right toe or he needs to wear a shower cap on his head, so what? Whatever makes both of you happy is fine. Don't be afraid to be different from the norm.

5. You're not embarrassed to let loose.

If it's your long-term lover, what have you got to be shy about? Be willing to experiment and take a few chances. Loosen up a little, laugh a lot, drop the inhibitions, and let your imagination run rampant.

FOREPLAY FOR FAMILIAR LOVERS (AND SOME GREAT IDEAS FOR JUST ABOUT ANYONE!)

Think back to when you met each other. The first few dates—particularly the ones before you've had intercourse—are one long, deliciously exciting foreplay session. Remember getting an erection by simply watching her walk across a room? Being told off by your friends for making out with him in hallways at parties? People chastising you for not being able to keep your hands off each other? This is what we're aiming to recapture. Sadly, that initial sell-your-mother-to-get-it type of lust that characterizes new relationships disappears all too quickly and sex gets relegated to a certain timeslot and place.

Sometimes this is not only sensible but necessary. If you've just started a new job, the last thing you're thinking about is

"Paul and I have been together about twelve years but, I have to say, sex lately has been better than ever. We went out to dinner recently and ended up reliving the best sex we'd had. By the time we got in the cab we were both drunk and went for it in the back. I spread my legs really wide and Paul slid his fingers in and out. It was extremely obvious what we were doing and I got off on the fact that the cab driver could see exactly what was going on. When we got out, he refused payment, said he'd 'enjoyed the show.' I slithered out, pushed Paul against the wall outside the elevator to his apartment, and gave him the best blow job he'd ever had, right there, in the fully lit foyer."

Pamela, 36, armed forces

whether the panties you put on that morning are sexy enough for him to peel off that night. If he's struggling with family problems, chances are he's not going to surprise you with a Chippendales-style strip before the 6 o'clock news. But the rest of the time—when you're simply coping with the usual hiccups of routine, run-of-the-mill life—give sex the priority it deserves.

Memorize the next three sentences. Our most erogenous zone is the brain. The most erotic tool you have at your disposal is your imagination. The biggest turn-on of all is anticipation. Repeat them one more time. Learn how to combine the three and *wham*!, you've just raised your sex life from ho-hum to horny. Most of us think of foreplay as genital touching and oral sex. Wrong. Foreplay can start at 6 A.M., continue while you're both at work, be drawn out through dinner, then, when you're both *begging* to touch each other, the physical part starts.

Skeptical anyone actually *does* the things I'm suggesting? You're absolutely right. Few people do—that's why everyone's madly doing everyone else behind each other's backs. It's easy to pick the couples who put effort into their sex lives. They are the two sixty-year-olds next door who hold hands when they're out perusing the roses. That devilish gleam in their eyes isn't put there from bingo. Ditto the couple you've always envied because sexual sparks seem to *fly* between them yet they've been together five years. Here's how they do it . . .

- **Combine romance with eroticism.** You feel great when he sends you flowers, why not return the favor? If you think they aren't quite his style, then try sending a bottle of expensive champagne, red wine, or scotch. Now turn that loving gesture into a sexy one. Enclose a note explaining in great detail exactly what he did to deserve such luxurious spoils. (No, not washing your car—the to-die-for oral sex he gave you last week. Got it?) Your postscript details what you're aching for him to do to you that night!

- **Become a bookworm.** Invest $100 in your love life by walking into any good bookstore and walking out with an armful of sex books. You've already bought this one, now branch out into areas that particularly tickle your fancy: Tantric sex, fantasies, how to have a dozen orgasms an hour. You don't have to read them cover to cover, just dip inside once in a while to keep things fresh and imaginative. While you're there, splurge on a racy, erotic novel. Find the good parts and read them to each other as a form of foreplay.

- **For the confident.** Use your vaginal juices as perfume. Yup, I'm not kidding. Slip your finger inside, then touch it around your throat, your breasts, on your lips. He won't know what it is but he won't be able to keep his hands off you.

- **Have a bed picnic.** Set up chilled wine and an ice bucket, foods you can eat with your

> ❗ *The most popular places to have sex outside the bedroom?*
> *The car: 73 percent of men and 68 percent of women*
> *Outside: 66 percent of men, 65 percent of women*
> *In their parents' bed: 45 percent of men, 36 percent of women*
> *In a public building: 30 percent of men, 26 percent of women[9]*

fingers (fresh fruit, chocolates); have an erotic movie playing in the background on the bedroom VCR.

- **Get snap happy.** Buy a Polaroid instant camera and take (flattering) shots of each other naked. Destroy the pics after you've had fun if either of you feel uncomfortable about having them around. Personally, I wouldn't keep any of the explicit shots, no matter how much I loved and knew my partner.

- **Once isn't always enough.** There's a lot of hype about women having more than one orgasm but he likes second helpings, too. Have sex in the morning on the weekend, then drag him back to bed an hour later.

- **Get wet.** Water does wonderful things: it makes us weightless and flexible and ensures every part of both of you tastes and smells wonderful. While I wouldn't recommend having intercourse in water (it dries up lubrication and forcing water up the vagina isn't recommended), the bathtub, a spa, a swimming pool, or the sea are great places to start off.

- **Be her sex slave for a day.** An especially good idea if you're broke and her birthday is looming. All you need to do is offer to devote one entire day to pleasuring her. She gets to order you around unashamedly—and whether it's serving her an erotic breakfast in bed, feeding her grapes and strawberries Roman-style, or spending the day dressed only in your Calvins, you're not allowed to utter even a *word* of complaint.

Love hurts: 44 percent of men and 41 percent of women like getting love bites.[10]

- **Take a tip from *The Story of O*.** The character in the novel is taught not to give all of herself each time she makes love. Use the same philosophy and instead of each sex session running the gauntlet from kissing to intercourse, concentrate on one activity at a time: kissing and fondling-only sessions (no tongues, no penises, just fingers), oral sex without intercourse, and intercourse without oral sex.

- **Flirt with each other**—even if you've been together years! Experts say flirting sends natural amphetamines and endorphins surging through the body, stimulating an instant emotional "high" not unlike orgasm. Pretend you've just met him and act as you did at the beginning. Dress sexily, look him straight in the eye when he's talking, twirl your hair around a finger. Be aware of your body when you move in front of him and chances are he'll sit up and take notice, too.

- **Send sexy notes.** The written word is extremely powerful. Plant notes everywhere (preferably not just before her mother comes to visit). In the fridge stuck to the juice, in her briefcase and makeup bag. Each one describes parts of her you find *so-o-o* sexy. The next time, make them ten things you'd love to do to her right that second.

- **Tease.** You've got friends over for dinner? Shove him up against the fridge, cup his penis with your hand, and give him a huge kiss while he's helping you in the kitchen. Chat innocently away to your guests while he hides out there, waiting for his erection to go down.

- **Go out without panties on.** This is one steamy idea even the least courageous of females can pull off. All you need to do is dress up for an evening out—and forget to put on your panties. You can either tell him about it, or "accidentally" show him by crossing your legs Sharon Stone style.

- **Feeling a little bored at her next office get-together?** Make things infinitely more interesting by feigning sickness, then take her with you to the bathroom. Emerge later feeling much better, thank you.

- **Be a voyeur.** Madonna's done it. So did Sabina in the erotic film *The Unbearable Lightness of Being*. We're talking mirrors and using them as sex props. Madonna and Sabina crawled and masturbated above mirrors laid flat on the floor. If yours is on the closet door, it's pretty difficult to follow their lead. Instead, try making love in front of any available mirror in the house (angled so you can see her rather than vice versa if she's shy).

- **Be his mistress.** If he's going to have an affair, make sure it's with you. Arrange to meet him at lunchtime in the bar of a plain but presentable hotel. Book a room, buy a bottle of champagne, and have forbidden, illicit, wild sex.

> "God knows what it was, but about three months ago, I went through a stage where all I could think about was sex. A lot of the time, I kept my mouth shut because we'd be over at Ian's mother's house or something. Then I started telling him about it and it built the sexual tension wonderfully. I called him at work one day and told him I was masturbating and he canceled a meeting, drove home, and we had the best sex ever. It hasn't been this good since the beginning."
>
> Helen, 32, mother

- **Get into the mood beforehand.** Masturbate several times during the day while you think about what the two of you will do that night—preferably telling her exactly what you're doing over the phone as you're doing it. Stop short of an orgasm, unless you're a premature ejaculator. If you are, masturbate an hour before you have sex—you'll last longer.

- **Remember kissing?** It's what you used to do when you first met. Many couples find that kissing stops once the relationship gets going or dwindles to a quick prelude before getting down to business. A long, passionate kiss can do more to turn both of you on than putting your hands straight down the front of his trousers. It's more intimate than intercourse (which is why many prostitutes won't do it).

- **Have intercourse with your clothes on.** Feel each other through your clothing, put your leg in between her thighs and let her gyrate against it.

- **Be pushy.** Bearing down with your vaginal muscles during intercourse seems to trigger orgasm for many women.

- **Keep your eyes open.** Watch what's going on when you have sex, look into their face, watch your genitals moving in and out. Stimulate the sense of sight, not just touch.

- **Be unpredictable.** Let's face it—you're not going to widen his eyes with astonishment if you suggest having sex on a Saturday night as you both climb into bed. But you will catch him unawares if you cuddle him from behind when he's washing the car, washing up, or reading a book. Start fondling him, bring him to the brink of orgasm, then refuse to follow through until later.

- **Bare all.** For a truly original Valentine's Day gift, shave your pubic hair into the shape of a heart or shave it off completely. The sight of your totally exposed genitals will make him jump to attention!

- **Turn her on in the most inappropriate places.** This is a tricky one. Done at the right time, it works fantastically, but it does have a tendency to backfire. Many sex books advise you whisper suggestive somethings into her ear while you're out to dinner with her boss, for instance. Sounds fabulously erotic but, in practice her boss is likely to think you're horribly rude, or that they have got something stuck between their teeth and you're making fun of them. Ditto the calling him at work bit. You want to get him hot and bothered but not so flustered he ends up blowing the deal of the century. By all

> **!** *Great Timing . . .*
> *When's the best time to have sex? In the morning. His testosterone levels peak around 9 A.M. and if you've been together a while, your cycle probably echoes his. An orgasm? Midway through your menstrual cycle. You're twice as likely to orgasm because your nerve endings are at their most sensitive.*

means try it—just check out the situation before you launch into your spiel.

- **Be anonymous.** Remember those silly masks you bought for the dress-up affair you both went to? Dig them out, put them on, laugh yourself stupid for five minutes, then have sex. Let your fantasies run wild and pretend you don't know each other.
- **Try Tantric.** It's the trendy thing to do. Basically, it's all about heightening and prolonging sexual arousal. To the newcomer, the most obvious thing about Tantric sex is that things progress very slowly (you'll do nothing but stroke each other for hours); often, it ends with neither of you having an orgasm. Sounds awful? I'm with you but couples who fully explore Tantric or the *Kama Sutra* swear the results are nothing short of spectacular.
- **Wake her up with the ultimate greeting**—licking her vagina. Do the same for him by licking his penis.
- **Make the move.** If your partner is always the one to initiate sex, the message you're sending is this: I do it to please you, not because I want to. This leaves both of you feeling cheated. The person who initiates sex feels sexier because they're taking control and giving themselves power. Surely you've watched enough movies by now to know that power's one of the biggest sexual turn-ons there is? Be the boss by suggesting sex and taking the lead role during lovemaking as well. Let them lie back while you do *all* the work.
- **Lie a little.** He's away on business? The next time he calls you late at night, skip the what-did-you-do-today stuff and tell him, in intimate detail, what you're wearing. No, not the truth—that Snoopy T-shirt and thick white socks are silky, black undies and a camisole. Move on to what you're going to do to him the

> **❗ What would you rather have in your life?**
> Great sex and an okay job: 59 percent
> Okay sex and a great job: 29 percent
> Awful sex and fame: 8 percent
> No sex and rule the world(!): 4 percent[11]

minute you get your hands on him. The juicier and more explicit the better.

- **Slide around on satin sheets.** So kitsch they're almost fashionable, you can't help but feel sensual with satin against bare skin. Great sex comes from indulging *all* the senses and satin sheets are one of a million ways to do it. Appeal to and vary one sense each time you make love and you'll never be bored again. Use music to stimulate his sense of hearing; talk to her while you're having sex, give a blow-by-blow description of how she's making you feel. Ignite his sense of smell by burning oils, wearing perfume, or letting him enjoy the naturally sweet scent your body emits when you're aroused. Touch is stimulated by different textures: use your hair, feathers, and scarves as well as fingertips. Use food, champagne, and all of your body parts to excite his taste buds.

- **Plan a dirty weekend.** More than one lackluster sex life has been saved by a spicy weekend bounding about on a king-size bed. Book the best hotel you can afford, pick her up from work on Friday night, and disappear into the sunset for a weekend she won't forget in a hurry.

- **Dress for success.** He adores red lipstick, black stockings, and high heels? You've got no excuse—any little black number can be spiced up with these elements. Make a night of it by playing the vamp, playing with your hair, playing with him under the table. She melts when you walk around the house in nothing but a pair of blue jeans, top button of the fly temptingly undone? Unless it's below freezing temperatures, indulge her on weekends.

- **Make a pact to try one new thing every two weeks.** If you're too shy to launch into my other suggestions, start off simple. Take a bath together,

> "I've been married nine years but I could watch Sally undress for bed a million times and never be bored. She's always so distracted, she doesn't notice me watching but I love her breasts and the way she always fluffs her hair up and pouts in the mirror when she's naked . . . even if the only thing she's craving is sleep."
>
> Calvin, 43, architect

give each other a foot massage, take off her top or his shirt without using your hands. Once you feel more comfortable, you can move into things like making love to them with their hands tied behind their back and (the real biggie) masturbating in front of each other. Get him to lick your fingers while you're masturbating yourself—you'll feel less embarrassed and both of you will find it a turn-on.

- **Turn undressing for bed into an art form.** It doesn't matter what you're wearing, it's how you take it off that counts. Unbutton tops slowly, stretch luxuriously as you pull that sweater over your head, put one leg up on the bed as you roll down your pantyhose. When you're naked, admire yourself for a minute in the mirror, running your hands over your breasts and hips. Not only will it keep him focused on your body and remove the familiarity of seeing you naked, it helps create a positive body image.

- **Suck each of his fingers as though it were a small penis.** Circle your tongue lazily around her palm to simulate oral sex.

- **Learn to love oral sex.** Don't just do it to please him or her, revel in it. Crave it, concentrate, make noises to show you're enjoying it as much as they are. Switch from intercourse to oral and back again for sensational contrasts.

- **If you're excited, show it.** The biggest turn-on of all is seeing how much you're exciting your partner. If he's driving you wild, show him—better still, say so.

Enough already! In the midst of all this lust, it's worth pointing out that no one can be a sexual dynamo all the time. If you don't feel like having sex, say so, and let him do the same. That way, it's guilt-free on both sides and it will save either of you from putting on lukewarm performances.

> **! What do most women do right after sex?**
> 43 percent take a shower
> 20 percent brush their teeth
> 30 percent roll over and go to sleep
> 7 percent smoke a cigarette[12]

SUGGESTIONS FROM THE SEXPERTS

Here, a sex therapist, relationship counselor, sex worker, erotica expert, and real people with really good sex lives share their secrets for keeping sex lusty long-term.

Dr. Janet Hall

Australian sex therapist, relationships counselor, author, and public speaker on sexuality, Dr. Janet Hall says:

- Put a magnet on the fridge that each of you moves to show how horny you're feeling. If it's high it means "You're in luck"; if it's low, it means "Don't bother asking." This takes away the anxiety of "Does he/she want it or don't they?" Both of you have the right to move the magnet around—or have two!

- Use a dirty weekend as a reward for something—one of you gets a pay raise, you've finished redecorating the house, etc. If a sexy weekend often follows a success or celebration, you'll condition yourself to enjoy them more because they're always associated with good times.

- Record your favorite fantasies and use the tapes as part of your sex warm-up. Have it playing as you sit down for dinner, slip one into her car tape deck and press play as you kiss her good-bye for work.

- Make a list of your current, favorite sex things (position, toy, lubricant, fantasy) and stick it on the bedroom mirror. Both do it and constantly update for surprise and variety.

- Schedule kissing sessions once a week. Take turns being the leader and the follower.

Amanda Dwyer

Owner/operator of Salon Kitty's in Sydney, Australia, which specializes in fulfilling fantasies and fetishes, Amanda says:

- You both have to be committed to the relationship. One-sided commitment isn't enough. You also have to trust each other. If you're suspicious, you'll always find something to doubt.

- Be honest about your sex life and never fake it. Tell the truth but use tact and sensitivity.

- Don't discuss former lovers in bed. If you must, do it some place else.

- Always practice safe sex until you're absolutely positive your lover is only involved with you.

- Look after your personal hygiene. Use deodorant, a mouthwash, and shower regularly. Don't clutter the bedroom or other places you make love in with smelly old gym shoes and clothes thrown all over the floor.

Jake Kubic

Jake is twenty-six and has been in a lusty, loving relationship for two years. He says:

- Keep each other on your toes and don't ever assume they'll never leave you. Recognize that you're both attractive to other people.
- Have common interests outside the bedroom. *Do* things together, not just shopping, going out to dinner, etc.
- Put some thought into your sex life. Think, "What can I do tonight to make it different?"
- Keep having sex even if you don't feel like it. It's a bit like exercise. Once you break the habit, it all becomes too hard.

Grant Brecht

Australian psychologist and relationships expert, author and media personality, Grant Brecht says:

- There's no such thing as too tired for sex. Have it *before* you get too tired or turn yourself on mentally and have a lazy session. You don't always have to be swinging off chandeliers.
- Keep up the romance. In the beginning, couples are always planning picnics, dinners out, days in bed—keep them going *throughout* the relationship.
- Ask, continually, what turns your partner on and off. Communication is so important—it's common sense to talk about sex but lots of people don't. Let your partner know you enjoy and value the lusty part of your intimacy. Don't just say, "I love you," say, "I think you're sexy."
- Look after the whole of the relationship. Make sure you've got a good balance in your life between work, play, time together, time alone.
- Tune in to the things you find sexy about your partner and use those thoughts and perceptions to turn yourself on when they're not around.

Di Palmer

Manager of Club Femme (Sydney), the biggest chain of women's erotica stores in Australia, Di Palmer says:

- Think erotically. Sensuality is learned. Constantly tell yourself, "I am sexually powerful and I love it, I am sensual and I love it." Don't give that power away to *anyone*, not even your partner. If your relationship isn't loving, caring, and trusting, ask yourself, What the hell am I doing in it?

- Be open-minded. Be prepared to experiment: what was a turn-off with your last partner might be a real turn-on with this one.

- Pull out all the stops and props when you really want to seduce each other. Light candles (they're flattering and great if you're body-conscious), wear lingerie or underwear that makes you *feel* as well as look sexy, experiment with body oils, try out some sex aids, play sexy music, watch an erotic video.

- Take him on a sex tour to find out what *really* turns men on. Go to a live peep show together, a strip show, or a club that has table-dancing. See how the female sex workers revel in their sexuality, unashamedly exposing their genitals. Learn from them. Men want to see your genitals spread: if you can reach that stage and be totally unembarrassed, he'll adore you.

- Wear duo-balls (balls you insert inside the vagina) while you're out to dinner. Tell him you've got them in; if the tablecloth's long enough for privacy, he can reach over and tug the string.

Cheryl Nobel

Cheryl, sixty-eight, is retired and has enjoyed a happy sex life for fifty-one years with her husband. She says:

- Look after your health. You need energy to enjoy good sex.
- Keep the memories strong. Look at old photos together, reminisce about the great sex you had in the past. Pinpoint what made those times special and try to re-create them.
- Splurge on sexy nightclothes. Whatever you wear to bed should be flattering.
- Stay young mentally. Be open to your partner's desires, find out what pleases them, then *do it*.
- Don't be unfaithful. If you find someone else attractive, weigh up

what you'll lose and what you'll gain. As you get older, the devil you know is a safer bet than the devil you don't.

- Don't get upset if you're not having regular sex. If it's only twice a month, fine. Go for quality not quantity by making that one night really special. Have dinner outside, dress up, make a wonderful meal, and make sex *outside* the dessert.

GOOD VIBRATIONS: SEX TOYS TRIED AND TESTED

Will sex aids send you to heaven or the nearest hospital? Are they a waste of time and money or a wickedly easy way to electrify your sex life? If the question is "Why use sex aids?" the answer has to be "Why not?" After all, they've been around for the last 2500 years and show no signs of disappearing! The ancient Egyptians used dildos, the Romans made candles in the shape of (rather enormous) penises, and the ancient Chinese invented the first cock ring by binding the base of the penis with silk. According to the erotica shops I canvassed, sex aids, particularly *female* sex toys, are selling as fast as Big Macs. While they'll never replace the real thing, say the managers, they put people in control of their own sexuality.

Today's toys are much more than playthings. The humble vibrator can be a lifeline for women who've had problems having an orgasm and many of the new aids are designed to improve vaginal muscle control. For every woman who squeals in horror at the mere mention of a sex toy, there's another who won't leave home without hers. Join the club. Don't just have a laugh during girls' night out, buy some of those strap-on dildos and balls that rattle noisily around inside. Men have more than a passing fascination with any type of sex toy, and the thought of your being even remotely interested in trying one will get him *very* excited.

Rather than waste valuable dollars on an expensive aid, buy a few cheaper items to start with. A lot of the time, it's the novelty factor that appeals. If you enjoy these, then it's worth making a larger investment. Don't know where to start? Take a tip from the people who bravely volunteered (well, were bribed) to tell all about their trip to toyland . . .

STA HARD Desensitising Spray

Cost: $12.50 (bought from a sex shop)

What is it? A spray-on potion designed to prolong his erection.

Tester: Peter, 32.

Satisfaction guaranteed? "A friend recommended it, so I thought I'd give it a try. I put a bit on the end of my penis and massaged it in but it did nothing the first time. The second time, I slathered it on and felt a weird tingling sensation but that time it did work. I stayed harder for longer. No complaints."

His rating: 7/10

Fun Tongue

Cost: $110 (bought from a women's erotica shop)

What is it? A bizarre, cylindrical contraption with a tongue protruding from one end. It's designed to simulate oral sex and devotees swear it's as good as the real thing—if you can stop laughing for long enough to take it seriously. Insert lubricant into a special compartment and set the (washable) tongue on one of five settings. It licks up and down, side to side, or moves in and out.

Tester: Susie, 40.

Satisfaction guaranteed? "I saw it in the window of a sex shop and thought, 'I've got to have it.' I tried it on my hand and it felt sensational. The first time, I put on some crotchless panties, dimmed the lights, and watched in a mirror, but it looked so ridiculous, I couldn't stop laughing. From then on, I closed my eyes. It's wild! It feels and licks like the real thing but it doesn't look the best. A friend of mine said he'd shoot it if he saw one lying on the side of the road."

Her rating: 9/10

Push Pearl Vibrator

Cost: $56.00 (bought through mail order)

What is it? It's one of Australia's most popular vibrators, with "pearls" in the shaft that rotate in dizzy circles and a clitoral stimulator that also vibrates.

Tester: Marie, 31.

Satisfaction guaranteed? "I saw a show on vibrators on TV and thought the clitoral attachment thing would make me orgasm

more often. I tried it inside and the rotating beads felt quite amazing but even though the clitoral stimulator was buzzing like crazy, nothing happened. Then I used it outside, pressed it against my clitoris and *wow!* The only problem is it makes orgasm so easy, you forget how to have one any other way."
Her rating: 9/10

Pink Pleasure Balls

Cost: $11.50 (bought from a sex shop)
What is it? Commonly known as duo balls, they're soft, prickly latex covered metal balls (the size of a golf ball), joined by a string. (Picture a kinky version of Click-Clacks that kids play with.) Inserted into the vagina they move around, supposedly making you feel sexy. Manufacturers also claim they help with muscle control.
Tester: Catherine, 23.
Satisfaction guaranteed? "They were a present and I unwrapped them in front of my mother—I almost killed the friend who gave them to me, but thought, 'Hey, I'll give it a try.' I slathered them with lubricant and inserted the first one, waited a bit, then put the second one in as well. A 'tampon' string hangs down to get them out again. I felt full up, like I was walking around with a big penis inside. I couldn't walk naturally and took them out after about three minutes. Boring!"
Her rating: 3/10

Fur Play

Cost: $92 (bought from a women's erotica shop)
What is it? Designed for slaves to fashion as well as light bondage, the fur-trimmed tie-me-up kit ensures you'll look trendy even when strapped to the bedposts.
Testers: Simon, 24, and Linda, 29.
Her satisfaction guaranteed? "Simon had been begging for ages to tie me up so I bought him the kit for his birthday. Boy, was he impressed! It's really easy to use, feels soft and comfortable and we both found it a hell of a turn-on. It's our favorite (if only) sex toy."
His satisfaction guaranteed? "The best present I've ever had."
His'n'her rating: 10/10

Double Dong Harness

Cost: $29.95 (bought from a sex shop)

What is it? It's a double "dong" or dildo on a white leather harness. The wearer penetrates herself, then uses the other dildo to penetrate her boyfriend anally or, if she's a lesbian, her girlfriend either anally or vaginally.

Testers: Nathan, 36, and Rachel, 24.

Her satisfaction guaranteed? "Nathan bought it—I hid around the corner. It didn't really appeal to me at all. He wanted to give it a go first and when he strapped it on I had to fight the urge to say "Ride 'em cowboy!" He used one dildo on me vaginally and it felt all rubbery and pinched a bit at first. But I got quite a kick out of penetrating myself and using it anally on him because I could experience what it's like to penetrate someone."

His satisfaction guaranteed? "Rachel wasn't into it that much and I was disappointed. But I think she got a kick out of playing 'the man.' Used with tons of lubricant, I quite enjoyed having it up my butt. Without lubricant, it hurts like hell."

Her rating: 2/10 on her; 9/10 using it on him.

His rating: 8/10

PORNOGRAPHY: WHY IT'S WORTH ANOTHER LOOK

Alex Comfort (in the infamous sex bible *The Joy of Sex*) says pornography is "the name given to any sexual literature somebody is trying to suppress." He goes on to say that "most normal people enjoy looking at sex books and reading sex fantasies—which is why abnormal people have to spend so much time and money attempting to suppress them."[13] I'm inclined to agree with him. I strongly believe that your standard porn mag and video (those not involving torture, violence, or children) should be available to the public. If *you* don't like them, don't buy or rent them. But you'd be surprised how many people—women included—do.

After numerous bizarre tests, which involved wiring people's genitals to machines, scientists have officially declared that women get as turned-on as men by reading or watching sexually explicit material. *Gosh*, we're amazed! The dispute has never really been that uninhibited, liberated women aren't turned-on by watching or reading sexy things. It's just that we're not really into that hard-core stuff. X-rated films are often dull, repetitive, and so unbelievable, we feel like laughing not screwing. Or they're so explicit, disturbing, and in-your-face, we feel like throwing up. But even if you have suffered through one of his flicks and vowed never to watch one again, here's some good news. Turn off your preconceptions and turn on that VCR because pornography has finally given birth to erotica—a much subtler, softer style of erotic material, often targeted specifically at women.

If he wants to watch an X-rated video, say yes, but you pick it. Select one made by women for women (they promote it heavily on the back—try any of the Candida Royalle range) and you won't be forced to watch degrading scenes or silly performances by perfectly formed females who orgasm just by looking at an erect penis. If you really don't feel comfortable or have extreme moral objections even to this new range, at least give an R-rated movie a try. Pick up an old classic (like *The Postman Always Rings Twice*) or opt for a film like *Damage*, *The Unbearable Lightness of Being*, or *9½ Weeks* as a compromise. For those who *do* want to use erotica and pornography as an adjunct to sex, keep the following points in mind.

Do:
- Try a few before dismissing adult films, magazines, or books totally. Take turns picking one and approve the decision with your partner. If you like one and they don't, watch it alone.
- Have it playing in the background. Often, they're too boring to watch all the way through, but looking up at the "good parts" can be fun.
- Laugh. And don't take them seriously. It's not real sex and there's lots of misinformation in them (like women don't need foreplay and enjoy penetration above all else).

Don't:
- Think it means your partner's not happy with you. It's just for fun, a way to spice things up, that's all.
- Feel guilty for feeling turned-on. It doesn't mean you're perverted, dirty, or sick; it means you're human.

- Force people to watch it if it does nothing for them or they're morally opposed. They're not a prude for not wanting to, and they're entitled to dislike it.
- Stop your partner indulging if you don't like pornography and they do. Just tell them you'd rather they watched/read it alone and kept it out of your sight. Unless it's extremely disturbing stuff (violent, a snuff film, or involving children, for instance), it's his or her business, not yours.
- Rely on pornography to turn you on. If the VCR is on every time you have sex, you're getting lazy.

THE TOP FIVE QUALITIES MEN LOOK FOR IN A SEX PARTNER

1. Personality
2. Beauty
3. Brains
4. Humor
5. Good body

THE TOP FIVE QUALITIES WOMEN LOOK FOR IN A SEX PARTNER

1. Personality
2. Humor
3. Sensitivity
4. Brains
5. Good body

13

Dear Diary, I Had Great Sex Today

Six people kiss, copulate—and keep a record

● ●

H e was this big."
"We had sex, nonstop, for twenty-four hours."
"I had twelve orgasms in a row."
Even if we are skeptical, claims like these make our own previously satisfying thrice-a-week-and-not-always-in-the-bedroom sex lives pale by comparison. It's unnerving to think everyone else has graduated to cybersex while we're still stuck with typewriter-sex, even if it is a sturdy, reliable old thing. Are they telling lies or could it really be true? Am I missing out on something?

To find out exactly what great sex means to each of us, I asked three women and three men to keep a month-long sex diary. Each person was chosen to represent different ages, sex drives, and stages in relationships. They were permitted to use false names but not allowed to alter or exaggerate any details and each diary is recorded in their own words. The result: a startlingly honest mishmash of appetites and activities ranging from one extreme to the other.

All the participants were shown the completed chapter, to see their reactions to what the rest of the team had recorded. There were snorts of disbelief ("She's copied a page from a Jackie Collins novel!") and disgust ("Ughh! If he's one of your friends, I don't want to meet him."). But there was also envy ("I wish I could swap lives") and all-round fascination. Most thought everyone else's sex life sounded more interesting than theirs. Emma wanted to "climax in one minute" like Maria could, Maria wanted Emma's freedom. David was desperately jealous of Robert's oral-sex-with-a-view encounter, Jane felt "utterly, depressingly" out of her league. Which all points pretty obviously to one general conclusion: comparing and trying to measure up to other people's sexual standards will do little else but leave you constantly dissatisfied. Read this to satisfy your curiosity but please yourself, not your friends.

THE SEX FILES: AN INTIMATE GLIMPSE INTO REAL-LIFE SEX LIVES
Emma
Emma, twenty-three, is single. She works in the media and is bisexual, though doesn't classify herself as such. She says she's simply "nondiscriminatory" when it comes to choosing a sex partner. Emma has had many lovers and several long-term relationships.

Week one
Ryan came over on Friday night and we went out to dinner then stayed up late talking. When we finally got to bed, it was already past 2 A.M. Ryan's a great friend and a wonderful lover—sensual, erotic, experienced, funny, relaxed. I love that controlled intensity of his. We fuck and it's good, but I don't come the first time, and he knows this so keeps touching me until I'm wet again. When he goes down on me, he knows exactly what he's doing and he enjoys doing it—an extra turn-on. He gets hard again and I put a condom on him using my mouth, which he finds very sexy. This time, when he makes love to me, I come and that makes him come, too. It's amazing. He sleeps over and when he finally leaves, I ask if he's got everything (he likes to leave his mark). Of course, he "forgets" a T-shirt that smells of his sweat and cologne and makes me horny, reminds me of him. I think about throwing it into the laundry with my stuff but end up sleeping with it under my pillow.

Later, I seduce myself, thinking about Ryan fucking me and

going down on me with that great oral technique of his. Actually, I fantasize about other things too but I always like to imagine someone I know once I start to get aroused. It makes it more intimate. I wonder how he'd feel if he knew. He'd probably like to know I was thinking about him.

Week two

I'm in Melbourne on business and I meet Mark, a smart, sexy lawyer, at a work function. There's an instant spark between us, one thing leads to another, and I end up back at his apartment, in his bed. (Normally, I would have waited, but I'm flying back to Sydney tomorrow and I just can't resist!) Like most men, he's a little impatient and a tad heavy-handed at first, but I manage to convey my base-level requirements for enjoyable arousal and he does a pretty good job of fulfilling them. We fuck—using a condom that he provides—and it's sexy, athletic, and abandoned. He goes down on me at one stage, quite expertly, and makes me extremely horny. Later, we do it doggie-style and by the time he comes (loudly, which is great—I like his lack of inhibition and sense of theatrics), I'm so turned-on that I only have to touch myself for thirty seconds or so and I also orgasm (not quite as loudly, which is probably just as well). We doze, cozily entwined, his hard body against my soft flesh. At seven, far too early, it's time to go. I leave him sleeping, again a stranger, creep into last night's clothes, and steal away, leaving nothing but a hastily penned phone number and a kiss.

Today I miss Stephen, my ex, once the Love of My Life. Back in Sydney, I go to see a film by myself and it makes me nostalgic and miss him more. I want a love with intensity. I want to feel that strongly again, to fuck someone I would die for, someone I'd want to get pregnant with. Someone I'd miss. My friend Max calls and he's sweet and concerned, but I don't feel passion for him. He's a darling, though, and it will be good to see him. I could use some steadying. I could use some more sex, too.

Week three

I'm at work and a big bouquet of tiny pink roses arrives from Mark. I call to thank him, and we arrange to catch up next time I'm in town. He's great on the phone—he's got a really sexy English accent—but I shouldn't think this way when I'm in the office. I can't wait to go to Melbourne again.

I have spent the last twenty-four hours on a hot date at home. Max came over and we cooked Italian, drank a bottle of good red wine, and watched a steamy video. It was quite good but I lost attention halfway through when Max took his shirt off. It was a shameless bid for my attention—and it worked. Great body. He used to have a hairy back and a white, pasty torso that reminded me of uncooked bread. But he waxes now, works out, and goes to the tanning salon. He's too young but utterly charming and seductive, witty, quick, manually dextrous, and great around the house. Kind of a nice package, don't you think? I was quite happy to go along with everything he suggested (again). I didn't like anal sex much before Max but he uses his fingers and tongue-fucks my anus and for the first time, I actually contemplated having his penis inside my rectum. It's very addictive, what he does. Ryan called on my machine as Max was licking me and that was such a turn-on: hearing one guy on my machine saying how much he wanted me while another gives me the licking of my life. Max doesn't want me as his; we're just friends who fuck. He didn't put his shirt back on until 8:30 the *following* evening. Yum.

Ryan calls, just for a chat. We arrange to go out together next week and easily slip into friendship mode. He's the perfect escort—polite, sociable, good-looking, and he wears fantastic designer clothes. There's no guarantee we'll end up in bed together after our date and even if we do, we'll probably just cuddle and go to sleep. We're more friends than lovers, really. Both of us know we're not soulmates, but we're extremely fond of each other, and I can imagine us being friends for life. If only more men were like him—most want to own you or run away.

Week four
I feel really horny tonight—it's that time of the month. I get out the trusty vibrator, read some porn to get off, go for quantity rather than quality. It's fun even though it's tacky. At least it stops me climbing the walls, gets the circulation going, and I wake up satisfied. Guys—who needs them?

I've always slept with women and can't really imagine why anyone would write off half the population sexually just because they're the same sex. So when Natasha and I stay in, cooking dinner, dancing to the stereo, trying on clothes, it's natural that I start to feel horny. She comes up and starts stroking me and it feels sensual, comfortable, and at the same time, very exciting. Girls having sex is still such a taboo it always gives me an illicit thrill. We kiss and her mouth is so soft, it couldn't possibly be a man. Both of us are horny but we take it slowly, like two sleepy cats. Going down on her is warm and erotic. As always, it makes me understand how guys feel—it isn't easy to give good head to a girl! I stop before she comes and she kisses me everywhere. We end up with our legs entwined and come that way. It's wild and wonderful and the best thing is, when it's over, we got back to being two girlfriends having a cozy evening. No pressure. No intimacy. I like girls, they have their own special charm, but I don't fall in love with them.

It's morning and I'm in Melbourne for the week. I'm at Mark's, trying to write this, and he's being very provocative. Later, maybe—or maybe really soon. He's shaping up rather nicely—lived up to the few phone calls we've had and we haven't stopped having sex since I got here. It's weird, the more sex I have, the more I need it and the less it seems to matter who it's with.

My sex life is . . . Exciting and satisfying—although I have my disappointments like everyone else. I know this diary makes me sound like I always have fantastic sex but I think you just caught me at a wild, wonderful time in my life. I guess you would say I'm promiscuous if you counted the number of lovers I've had but I don't think I sleep around at all. I pick my lovers very carefully because sex is extremely, extremely important to me. It's one of the most important things in my life and I put a great deal of energy into it. I'm definitely in tune with my body and my needs. Some of my friends say they envy my sex life but I think anyone can have great sex if they just learn to let go, relax, and really listen to what their body is telling them. They seem so hung up on what their lovers will think if they do this or that. I say, forget the lovers, satisfy yourself first!

Jane

Jane, thirty-two, has been seeing Brad, twenty-seven, for the past ten months. Jane finds it difficult to trust men and has not had a relationship that's lasted more than three months since she was eighteen. Brad's clocked up four long-term lovers. They describe their relationship as "shaky at best."

Week one

I resigned from my job yesterday which was pretty nerve-racking because I'd been working there for five years. During the day, while I was waiting to see my boss, I made half a dozen phone calls to Brad so he could reassure me about what I was doing. He's very good at boosting my self-confidence. When I finally called to tell him I'd done it, he told me he'd booked us into a five-star hotel for the night. We spent the night drinking champagne, eating room service food, and making love. Brad's also very good at that. He's the only one who's ever been able to make me orgasm.

I don't know why, but I've always been uptight about sex. In my wild days, I used to hang around with a few girlfriends who I guess were quite promiscuous and I started to take a more recreational view of sex. It was probably quite good for me, but I started having one-night stands like they did and they hurt too much and put me off sex again. My friends were seriously into it for the sex but I only wanted the affection. I fell in love all the time.

Week two

My stress level's cranked up to maximum. I'm worried about whether I've done the right thing switching jobs, I've got work projects due, and I'm paranoid about the weight I've put on since I gave up smoking. All of which means I don't feel particularly desirable or desiring of sex. Brad always says he doesn't want me to feel as though I have to make love but sometimes, like Thursday, I do even when I don't feel like it. It felt awful. I was so dry he couldn't have enjoyed it, but I don't think he should pay just because I'm having a bad week.

Week three

This week was the worst on record. I start a new job then get the flu. Unfortunately, it's a bad week for Brad, too. I want attention, he wants attention. So we both get it by arguing with each other—constantly. The end result is we haven't made love in eight days. Even though I'm not that excited about sex, it makes me feel close to him. It's like the chicken and the egg thing: I can't feel close to him until we have sex but we can't because I don't feel close. Figure that out.

Week four

All we've done is take turns at ending the relationship. One day we argue and I call it off. Then he backpedals and it's on again. The next day, it's his turn to end it and I do the apologizing. Last night, I told him I wanted him to sleep in the spare room. That's because I can deceive myself very easily when I'm asleep or half-asleep and pretend everything is okay. Ever since we started sharing a bed, we've been a very cuddly couple. In the middle of the night, I'll sometimes wake up and Brad is putting his arms around me and telling me he loves me. Even when we're fighting, I'll wake up to discover I'm wrapped around him and I forget about being angry. We did end up sleeping together in the end but that's all we did. I don't think we touched each other all night and then, this morning, he just got up and left. I'm scared. Where do we go now?

My sex life is . . . Sadly over for the moment! We're definitely over and I have no hope it will be okay again. It's a shame because this was the best sex I'd ever had in terms of physical sensations. The touchy-feely side of the relationship was pretty good, too. But we really are different personalities: he's laid-back and easygoing, I'm someone whose button is permanently stuck on fast-forward. I always wanted to move forward, he wanted to stop and smell the roses. Perhaps that's why he was so good in bed and I'm not.

Maria

Maria, forty, has been married to Ian, thirty-nine, for a year. She works as a receptionist at a large community health center. She is highly sexed and frustrated by her husband's lack of interest. She has just started having an affair with a married friend of theirs.

Week one

Had coffee with a girlfriend and we started talking about sex. I was going through one of my horny-as-hell times and trying to explain to her what it felt like. I told her I'm attracted to lots and lots of different kinds of men—often the main attraction is simply that they're new and I haven't conquered them yet. Unless a guy's really unattractive, I can usually find something about him that makes me want him. He might look at me in a way that I know means he wants to sleep with me and that's enough to get the juices flowing. Sometimes, I'll look at his hands and imagine them dipping in and out of me. Once, I was at a barbeque and there was a guy there who was a complete jerk but he had the best body. At one stage, he took off his shirt to show us a scar and he had these fabulous back muscles and brown, gorgeous skin. I felt hot and flushed and if I could have, would have had him there and then. I think I've got more male hormones than female because men understand my feelings about sex totally. (Well, apart from my husband.) When I talk about sex with women they look at me like I'm crazy. But then, most of them don't like sex. I rarely act on my fantasies—though I would if I could get away with it.

Had another erotic dream last night about an old boyfriend. I often have dreams about guys I've dumped who want me back again. In my dreams, I'm sneaking around corners to see them, go back, then get bored again. I'm not that different in real life—once the game is over, I leave. I never should have gotten married, because I miss the chase so much. When you're in the middle of someone pursuing you, you're so aware of your body, it feels like it's on fire. I'm like a dog in heat and if the person I'm lusting after comes near me, my body involuntarily arches toward them. That's what I miss about being married. I'm not supposed to have those thoughts anymore, I have to put a tight rein on my natural feelings.

It's funny how when Ian and I have had sex for a few nights running, it's assumed we won't do it for the next three. I looked over at him last night, all tucked in, peacefully asleep, and I wondered if he really cared whether I was satisfied after sex or only interested in getting his own rocks off. Sex with Ian is fine, but that's the problem— it's just so totally, predictably, annoyingly okay.

Week two
It's now been five days since I last had sex. I've masturbated a billion times but want "the real thing," not just me and a copy of Nancy Friday. Went to a party last night and flirted with Gary, this really old friend of ours. He's good-looking and always eyes me, and I think it's obvious we're both attracted to each other. Neither Ian or Gary's wife seem to notice, which is typical: if you're not in tune with sex, I guess you don't pick up vibes between other people either. I bet Gary would be more open to new things than Ian is. I heard a story once that he got caught fucking his secretary in the bathroom at work. His wife was devastated, but I was turned-on. Anyone who screws someone in the bathroom is into sex big time. Gary got married really young and his wife is now pregnant. I feel sorry for him. If I get that bored with Ian I can leave. He can't.

From my conversations with other people it seems to me that everyone is bored with their sex life. It's because we're all trying to be monogamous. The other day someone was saying how amazing it was that the boyfriend of this famous celebrity was caught playing around with another woman who wasn't half as attractive. I don't think it's amazing at all. Looks don't come into it: He just wanted someone new. Someone whose every move he didn't know by heart.

I don't believe in PMS because I don't get it, but I do believe in biorhythms. Sometimes, I can imagine being faithful to Ian, other times it seems impossible. It's a Jekyll and Hyde thing. Reading what I've written so far now seems alien to me because I'm going through a happy-to-be-married period. Today I feel righteous and in love with Ian. We even talked about having kids. All I want to do is have slow, gentle sex with him. What a loony I am!

Week three

I'm still in my "couldn't care less if I never got it again" mood. Had sex on Friday night but it was really frustrating because Ian was giving me oral sex and I was just about to come, then he did something and the delicious orgasm went and I was just left with the mechanics of it, the contractions minus the pleasure. I told Ian and he said male orgasms are always like that, that the intense, pleasurable part lasts less than a second. Men are even more stupid than I thought. If their orgasm is so short, why are they in such a hurry to get to it? Why aren't they more into foreplay?

Ian was away on business for two days but the "unsexy" period is coming to a close. I can feel the first stirrings of lust slowly uncoiling in my belly. It sounds dramatic, but that's what it feels like. Sometimes I feel controlled by my body because desire takes over and I do things I regret later. It's like this big monster is about to take over my life again —the sheer force of my sexual urges frightens me. I really do love Ian but at those moments, I'd risk it all just to satisfy them.

Week four

I feel really nervous committing this to paper. Remember Gary? The very-very-married-with-pregnant-wife guy I fancied? Well, I slept with him. Ian and I were at their house on Sunday and we were all dipping into the champagne and swimming in their pool. Ian went off to the liquor store to buy some booze and munchies and the minute he left, Gary's wife said she wanted to pop over and see a friend who was sick. I mean, they asked for it! I felt quite embarrassed at first because it was just Gary and I in the pool. But we started chatting and flirting and next thing, he kissed me. A long, sexy, erotic French kiss. I think I knew it was coming but I was still startled. I laughingly tried to stop him but he kept kissing my neck and it was getting dark and I got so hot I didn't care anymore. He slipped his fingers inside my swimsuit and I was gone. The next minute we were frantically fucking on the side of the pool—and I mean *fucking*—and I climaxed in about one minute flat. I got up quickly afterward and was drying myself off when poor Ian came back, laden with booze, food, and cigarettes. I felt guilty and sad. I've now betrayed him in reality, not just in my head.

Gary called me at work today and said he was sorry. I didn't want him to be sorry, I wanted more, and I told him so. I still feel guilty but now that I've thought about it, I've decided to see Gary again. Ian knows I need more from our sex life than he's giving me and yet he still doesn't make an effort. If he's not going to satisfy me, he can't expect me to be faithful. I feel bad about Gary's wife but she's never been a huge fan of mine anyway, and I'm not taking him away from her permanently, just borrowing him for a few hours now and again.

My sex life is . . . Guilt-ridden. On the one hand, sex gives me the very best moments of my life and I couldn't live without it; on the other, my urges get me in a lot of trouble—like the situation I'm in now. I do love Ian and would like to make it work, but the "bad girl" so often beats the "good girl" side of me. I also feel resentful that we've slipped into "married sex" even though we've only been married for a year. I have no idea what will happen now that I'm having an affair, but at least Gary's good in bed. Actually, it's not Gary, it's the forbidden part that appeals. In terms of technique, Ian's better.

Robert
Robert, thirty-five, separated from his wife three years ago. He works as an account executive for a finance firm and describes his sex life as "active but selective."

Week one
I'm making love to Sarah but it's not really Sarah, it's Linda. Linda was a married woman I had an affair with over a year ago but she still haunts me. I met her through a mutual work friend at a function and we ended up getting drunk together and smooching on the balcony. Her husband was working. She was so beautiful and so unattainable, I

thought that was it. But she called me soon after I met her and asked if she could drop in for coffee. So we started meeting and kissing and cuddling, then one day she came over and stripped right down to her underwear before snuggling up to me. I knew she wanted sex but I didn't want to push it. I mean, she was married and on this massive guilt-trip. We had intercourse but it felt like she wouldn't give herself fully although she had no trouble orgasming. I did—I was nervous as hell. For some reason, she didn't want much foreplay. It was like kissing, touching, then *bam*! she wanted penetration. I felt like I was starting halfway through. I'm not the sort of guy who can just drop my duds and get into it. She ended the affair soon after that so we only had intercourse three times. I knew the score. I knew she would end it, but I've never forgotten her. I'd love to go out with someone as good-looking as her again and have other guys check out my girl. It's a huge ego-boost.

Sarah's probably a better fuck, if truth be told, and she gives an amazing blow job. She's the opposite of Linda: she wants a relationship and gives her all. The first time I slept with Sarah, we had sex with her six-month-old son asleep beside us. I thought it was a bit outrageous but the kid was fast asleep. It didn't turn me on at all—I actually felt quite uncomfortable and couldn't look at the child—but I admired Sarah for going for what she wanted. I'm the guilty one now. Sarah loves me, and I love her, but I make love to Linda whenever I touch her.

Week two

Sarah's gone away for a week with her folks so I meet some friends down at the bar. There's a girl there who's exotic and very horny. We talk and I give her my phone number. She's called Cristina and is from South America. That was on Friday. On Tuesday, she called me at 11:30 P.M., said she was lonely and would I like to come over. I was in bed but she said she was down, so off I went. Cristina lived in a penthouse apartment overlooking the city and her roommates were out. She answered the door wearing a see-through lace teddy, led me to the couch, pushed me back, and just went for it. Then she led me to the balcony and within five minutes of walking in the door, I was standing there, pants around my ankles, getting a blow job while overlooking the harbor! She took me into her room and she had this mirror that she loved to watch herself in. She wanted it doggie-style and kept on saying, "Fuck me, fuck me like an animal." I felt like I should write in to *Penthouse*. It was like one of those letters you read and never believe. I took her phone number but it was pretty obvious she only got off on someone new. I don't think I ever approach any sex session as just a fuck. I guess I hope they'll all lead to something. I told the guys at the bar what had happened. One of them said, "Dude, that must have been the best sex of your life." I guess it was because it was so unexpected but the best is always the last one you've had, really. I thought my wife gave the best blow job, then I thought Linda did, then Sarah. Now Cristina's in front.

Week three
Sarah's back. I expected her to be relaxed, tanned, and hot for sex; instead, she's irritable and worn out because she had a shitty time. Sex is awful because she's not responsive. I hate that more than anything. The worst sex I ever had was with a girl who led me from the living room to the bedroom by my penis. She instigated it all and I thought I was in for the ride of my life. But when I penetrated her, she lay there like a dead fish. I don't know if she was really drunk and it hit her then or what. She couldn't have been bored because we'd just started! Anyway, it goes down as the absolute worst sex of all and I think it's a worry that sex with Sarah reminded me of it. Sarah wants a commitment but I'm not sure I want to. I'm feeling incredibly pressured and also not sure I want to take on someone else's child. I've already got two of my own.

Week four
Cristina called and Sarah answered the phone. Neither were terribly impressed and even I wouldn't have believed the story I made up to try and get out of it. For some weird reason, Cristina was upset that I hadn't told her about Sarah. A bit much when she had her mouth wrapped around my penis before I'd even had a chance to speak! I feel guilty but pissed off for feeling like that. I've never promised Sarah a monogamous relationship—she just took it for granted—and Cristina was obviously just in it for the sex. My month ends where it started: with fantasies about Linda. Even though she was married, at least I knew where I stood.

My sex life is . . . A hell of a lot more interesting than it was when I was married. My wife was pretty conservative, and missionary was about it. I didn't have much experience before I got married so I'm making up for it now but aiming for quality, not quantity. I find women so much more liberated and in touch with their sexuality than the first time around. Sometimes it freaks me a little bit, and I worry I'm not going to be able to satisfy them. I think that's why I'm so into foreplay; I feel more confident with my oral sex skills. Besides, intercourse is intercourse and most women's vaginas feel pretty much the same. There's only one girl who's stood out from the pack and she had a vice for a vagina. Her grip was incredible!

David

David, twenty-one, admits he's "as promiscuous as he possibly can be" and uninterested in a long-term monogamous relationship right now. He manages a gym.

Week one

Last night I was out at my usual club and made instant eye contact with a girl that oozed "fuck me." I got close to her and tried to pick up if the vibes were positive or negative, though even if they're negative, I'll still go for it. She started dancing so I danced with her and without speaking a word, we started kissing. I took her out to the back of my four-wheel-drive and we had sex. Immediately it was over, I thought, "Why did I bother?" I should have whacked-off—it would have been much more pleasurable. The sluts never live up to expectations. There's no challenge. This girl left me, went back inside and I saw her leave to do the same thing with another guy within half an hour. When I say slut, I mean slut.

I went out with Diane tonight, a "nice girl" I met through some friends. We had dinner and she's pretty, though pretty stupid as well. She came back to my place and it was obvious she expected sex which is weird. She comes from a well-to-do family and I thought she'd be different. I obliged but she freaked out because I couldn't come with a condom on. I never can. I have to almost get there, then pull out, take it off, and finish myself off with my hand. Eighty percent of girls don't mind but some react badly. They always think it's their fault. I can always get it up and going but ejaculating isn't the automatic process girls think it is. It goes back to when I was seventeen. I was with this girl and we had a wild weekend of sex and I came twenty-one times in three days. I don't know if it's psychological but since then, I've been pushing to come twice in a weekend. I remember feeling so drained and worn-out afterward, I felt physically sick. It doesn't bother me though. Sex feels great even if I don't ejaculate.

Week two

Trish was at the club last night and I'm wondering if she's still a virgin. My best friend and I had a threesome with this girl a month ago. We met her at a party and took her outside, in full view of anyone who wanted to watch, but she'd only do oral. No penetration whatsoever. She said it was because she was a virgin and I was like, "Yeah, right," but she loved sucking penises and she swallowed every drop. (It's a big thing, swallowing. The only thing that's better is if she swallows most of it but some sperm's trickling out of her mouth. That is so hot!) I didn't for a minute believe Trish but her best friend swears it's true. She really is a virgin.

I've just had the worst sex experience of my life. I went to go down on this girl and I was hit by a cloud of odor that turned my stomach. I literally dry-retched. The girl must have had a yeast infection because no one could smell like that naturally. I still feel sick just thinking about it.

Week three

I watched a girl for two hours last night and she was something else. So beautiful and fresh. I didn't want to have sex with her; I knew I wanted a relationship just by looking at her. I blundered my way through a conversation but she's already got a boyfriend. Bummer. Despite what I sound like, I do think it's feasible to have sex with one person for the rest of your life. You'd have to love them incredibly and she'd have to be adventurous, open to new ideas, and interested in doing the things I like, but it's possible. Every guy checks out other women but I think you'd be surprised how many stay faithful when they really love their wives or girlfriends. In one sense, I'm relieved that girl had a boyfriend. I would have fallen for her for sure.

Week four

Writing this diary has made me think about my sex life. I counted up how many women I've slept with over the past year and didn't know whether to boast or be horrified. I go through periods where I'm picking up two to three girls a week for three to four months. Then I start feeling really dirty and think, "Slow down. You're hurting people." You fuck girls once and they want you to call them, so I usually take them out one more time. But then, they want more and say "Didn't that mean anything to you?" How do you tell them, "No, the sex didn't and you didn't"? I don't mean to hurt them, but I know I do.

My sex life is . . . Totally wild and depraved. I don't think I'll ever get sick of seeing a girl naked; I don't think men ever get over it even if they've been with the same woman for years. Single sex is better than the sex I had with a three-year live-in girlfriend. When she said no to sex, I used to feel very disheartened. I'd think, "I'm losing it. She doesn't want me" and I'd never be sure if she was doing it to wield power over me, like "I've got what you want but you can't have it." I'd love to have sex several times a day—it doesn't matter that I couldn't ejaculate most of the time. My worst nightmare would be to fall in love with some girl who only wanted missionary-style sex. I hate it. I like doing it doggie-style because that's the only chance I have of coming.

Stephen

Stephen, twenty-eight, has been married for two years. He's a stockbroker and says he loves his wife more now than when they first got married.

Week one

I arrive home from a fourteen-hour work day and Jess is in a panic, running around with her underwear on because she's late meeting a girlfriend. I try to talk her into a quickie because she looks so sexy but no way. She won't even laugh with me. I get out a porn video (Jess hates them) and jerk off instead. When she comes home, she's tipsy and sits on my lap and gives me a deep kiss, using her tongue. Ironically, now it's me who can't be bothered. The day's caught up with me.

The next morning I wake up "pee-proud" (my grandmother's term for a morning erection). I wake Jess by stroking and licking her back but she's hungover and not interested. I try really hard not to act pissed off but she knows I am and gets shitty herself. Somehow, this turns into a huge fight and ruins the weekend.

Week two

The three-day war is over and Jess finally lets me have sex with her. She's really wet and I have to think about football to stop orgasming within a second. It's funny, even though she's really lubricated I get the feeling she's not really into it. Afterward, we watch TV and she's asleep within two minutes. I guess she was tired.

Jess's best friend has the best body I've ever seen in the flesh. She knows it and always wears the shortest skirts. Tanya was bending over at a lunch and she's got the most fabulous legs: no lumps, just smooth flesh. Jess caught me watching, leaned over, and felt to see if I had an erection. It was certainly getting there. She was Not Impressed and announced to the whole table what had happened. I laughed it off but was totally pissed off. We had a huge fight when we got home, so—no sex *again*.

Week three

Jess's sexual calendar is so predictable, I could literally circle the days when she'll feel like it and when she won't. The week before her period she turns into this intense nympho and screws really seriously, closes her eyes and concentrates like this is the last time ever. Jess also likes sex during her period, and I have to pretend I do, too. Actually, I hate it, but Jess is a real feminist and if I dared to admit I'm turned off by menstrual blood I'd never hear the end of it.

My boss has just gotten a new secretary. She flirted with me today and asked me to go to lunch. I said fine, I like having women as friends, but made it very clear I was married and very happily so. Her behavior changed after that—she wasn't interested in getting to know me as a person, just a potential Mr. Right. Stupid woman. It really annoyed me.

Week four

I'm raring to go and so is Jess—a rare moment in our household. She pulls on this amazing two-piece underwear thing, all white and virginal, which she knows I love. She gives me a massage and I'm so tense and it feels so good, I almost lose the urge and just want to sleep. But then her tongue flicks over my penis and it responds, though not as quick as my brain does, so I move down on her. I love giving Jess oral sex. I love the smell of her. If I could bottle her vaginal juices I would. Sometimes, if she's really turned-on and climaxes loudly, I'll almost come without any stimulation of my genitals at all. This session is so good, I feel really vulnerable afterward. I bury my nose in her hair and pray to God she'll never leave me.

My sex life is . . . Up and down but satisfying. I guess it reflects our relationship. We argue a lot, which stops us having sex as often as I'd like but that's okay; I like Jess's spirit and married a passionate woman. I have no desire for sex with anyone else. Jess turns me on as much now as she did when I first met her and I don't see why her appeal would ever wear off. We're experimenting more now and she's not backward in coming forward about her desires. I think I scored lucky!

Appendix:
A Sex Dictionary

"Those G-spot things sound great—
where do you buy one?"
Read this and you won't be the one who says it

••

abortion: Prematurely ending a pregnancy, usually through an operation called a termination.

AIDS (acquired immune deficiency syndrome): A condition caused by the human immunodeficiency virus (HIV) where the body loses its ability to defend itself against illness. The most feared sexually transmitted infection of all, but avoided by using condoms and practicing safe sex.

anal intercourse: When a man inserts his penis into his partner's anus. Some people's idea of heaven, others' of hell.

aphrodisiac: Any substance believed to stimulate or enhance sexual desire. Everything from oysters and champagne to ground-up goat's toenails has been touted as one. Some work psychologically, few actually do anything.

areola: The pinky-brown ring surrounding the nipple.

arousal: Getting excited or turned-on. The physiological and mental changes that happen to our body when someone we like touches us in all the right places.

A-spot: The "anterior fornex erogenous," an extremely sensitive section of the front vaginal wall, about one-third of the way down from the cervix. The G-spot's neighbor.

bestiality: If your neighbors confess to it, lock up your dog. It means they enjoy sex with animals.

bisexual: Being attracted to both John and Jane—and not really minding which one you end up with.

blow job: The everyday term for her giving him oral sex. The official term is "fellatio."

bondage: Tying someone up before having your wicked way with them or vice versa.

breasts: Two, frequently ogled, mounds of flesh found at chest level on women. Breasts come in all different shapes and sizes and you can buy a new pair if you don't like your own.

buttocks: The fleshy, muscular cheeks of our butts that frequently dictate our jean size.

casual sex: Short-term affairs spent mostly in the bedroom.

CAT (Coital Alignment Technique): A new way to have intercourse that involves rolling rather than thrusting.

celibacy: Voluntarily abstaining from sex for reasons the rest of us can't fathom.

cervix: The neck of the uterus that connects it to the vagina. Otherwise known as the part that hurts when hit by an overenthusiastic, long penis.

chemistry: The X-factor, the I-don't-know-why-I-like-him-I-just-do thing. Chemistry is God's way of ensuring we all don't like the same person, since a healthy dose of it can make an ugly duckling seem like a swan to someone who's tuned in to their vibes.

circumcision: Removal of the foreskin of the penis, usually done at birth for religious or hygienic reasons.

climax: Orgasm, coming, getting off. The point during sex when someone could cut your big toe off and you wouldn't notice.

clitoris: A little, pea-sized organ at the top of a woman's vulva which becomes erect when stimulated. Plays a huge part in the process that leads to orgasm. Find hers, treat it with respect, and she's yours forever.

come: Slang for the semen he ejaculates on orgasm. "Coming" is slang for orgasm.

come out: A short form for "coming out of the closet" or openly admitting you're gay—when you realize all that bending over with a low-cut top on was totally wasted on your best friend's roommate.

compatibility: Sharing the same interest and outlook on life as your partner. *Dick and Dora are very compatible because they both like dressing up in latex.*

condom: A thin rubber sheath designed to stop sperm and nasty germs from entering the vagina. Unfortunately, they don't work unless you take them out of the packet and place them over an erect penis before having intercourse.

contraception: Things you swallow, insert, or put on to avoid getting pregnant.

crotch: The genital area that both sexes emphasize with tight, body-hugging clothing if they think they've got something worth advertising.

cunnilingus: Giving her head, going down on her. The correct term for oral sex that no one uses because they either can't pronounce it or think it's gross.

deep throat: A term inspired by the bottomless-mouthed porn queen, Linda Lovelace. She was able to take the entire length of the penis into her mouth and throat without gagging. The rest of us find our tonsils get in the way.

deviation: Any form of sexual activity considered to be abnormal by the majority of the population.

dildo: An artificial erect penis used for masturbation.

douche: A device for squirting water or other liquid into the vagina to cleanse it. Totally useless and quite harmful since the liquid often messes up the natural pH level in the vagina.

ejaculation: Shooting your load, coming. The ejection of semen from the penis through a series of pleasurable muscle contractions.

erection: Getting a hard-on, or a stiffy. The swelling and stiffening of the penis (or clitoris or nipples) during sexual stimulation.

erogenous zones: Parts of the body especially sensitive to sexual stimulation, differing dramatically from person to person and the situation. His forehead may turn into an erogenous zone if Pamela Anderson's the one touching it.

erotica: Something (usually a book, magazine, video, or sex aid) that tastefully turns us on and makes us feel like having sex. (We call tasteless turn-ons pornography.)

erotic massage: Specific massage techniques that concentrate on the genitals.

ESO (Extended Sexual Orgasms) technique: A long and involved (but worth trying) series of techniques designed to make your orgasms last longer.

exhibitionist: A sexual show-off. Someone who likes others watching them. Having sex on your dining table with the blinds open in full view of the neighbors innocently watching *The Simpsons* is exhibitionistic behavior.

family planning clinic: A special clinic that provides information and advice about contraception and all sex-related matters. (*See* Planned Parenthood, index.)

fantasy: Imagining sexual situations or events involving real or imaginary people. The official term for those X-rated daydreams you amuse yourself with on the bus.

fellatio: Blow job, sucking him off. Using your tongue and mouth to excite his penis.

fertile: Being able to get pregnant or capable of making someone pregnant.

fetish: A sexual behavior where the handling of a specific, often inanimate object (like rubber clothing or preworn panties) is necessary for sexual satisfaction. If he can only orgasm if you wear your high heels to bed, he's got a shoe fetish.

fidelity: Resisting going home with the best-looking guy at the party because you'd upset the one you already have. Staying faithful.

foreplay: Petting, feeling each other up, playing with each other. The stuff most people do before intercourse but should do during and after as well.

foreskin: The retractable fold of skin covering the tip of the penis on uncircumcised men that hurts if you yank it back too quickly.

frenulum: The string of particularly sensitive skin where the head of the penis meets the shaft. It's on the underside (the side closest to his testicles) and well worth introducing yourself to.

frigid: An outdated, Victorian term used to describe women who aren't interested in sex. Only used today by drunk men in bars to explain why the woman they attempted to screw wasn't interested.

gay: Homosexual, camp. This used to be a blanket term for all homosexuals but is now mainly used to describe men who are attracted to or have sexual relations with other men. Female homosexuals generally prefer being called "lesbian."

genitals: The external sex organs—a man's penis and testicles, a woman's labia, clitoris, and vagina.

group sex: More than two people having sex with each other at the same time. Works great in fantasies, has a tendency to backfire in reality.

G-spot: A hot spot discovered by the German physician Dr. Ernst Grafenberg. It's a small, slightly raised, sensitive area about 2.5 inches inside the vagina on the front wall.

hard-on: *See* erection.

head (of the penis): The mushroom-shaped bit at the top of the penis that's softer than a baby's bottom.

heterosexual: People who are only sexually attracted to the opposite sex. If you're female and can't have John, you wouldn't even consider Jane.

HIV (human immunodeficiency virus): The virus that causes AIDS.

homophobes: People who are incredibly rude to and about

homosexuals because they have psychological hang-ups about them.

homosexual: People who are attracted to people of the same sex.

hormone: A chemical substance produced by the endocrine gland which plays an important part in sexual and reproductive functions and alters moods. Why one day you feel like being Annie Sprinkle, the next Mother Theresa.

hymen: A thin membrane that partly covers the entrance to the vagina before a woman first has intercourse. The hymen used to be considered proof that a woman was a virgin. These days, tampons and physical exercise break it more often than penises do.

impotence: Not being able to get it up, the inability to achieve an erection.

inhibitions: Thoughts, morals, or feelings that stop you from letting loose and enjoying sex to the fullest.

***Kama Sutra*:** Possibly the world's first sex manual and a literary classic. Written by Vatsyana in the fourth to fifth centuries A.D.

Kegels: Exercises designed to strengthen the pubococcygeal muscle (PC), which controls the size and grip of the vagina. Men also have a PC muscle and should also exercise it.

kinky: Something sexual you do that others would love to but don't have the courage.

Kinsey (the Kinsey Institute): World-respected American sexperts.

K-Y jelly: The brand name of a popular water-based lubricant.

labia: The lips of the female genitals. The small ones are called the "labia minora," the larger outer ones the "labia majora."

lesbian: A woman who has sexual relations with another woman.

libido: The desire or urge to have sex, your "sex drive."

love: A very strong feeling of attachment or desire to someone or something. Often confused with "lust" (*see below*).

lubrication: Oils, creams, or gels that are used to add moisture to the genital area to reduce friction and make sex more comfortable. Any couple who is serious about sex has some in their bathroom or bedside cabinet. K-Y jelly and Astroglide are lubricants.

lust: A strong desire to have sex with someone. The havoc-wreaking emotion that makes us go for the hunk on the Harley over the sensible accountant our mother wants us to date.

making love: Having sex with someone you're happy to wake up with in the morning as opposed to simply having sex.

masochist: Someone who gets pleasure from pain.

Masters and Johnson: Pioneer sex researchers.

masturbation: Playing with yourself. Stimulating your own genitals to achieve orgasm. Mutual masturbation is when you and your partner stimulate each other's genitals.

ménage à trois: The French term for a threesome.

menstruation: Period. The monthly discharge of blood that takes place if no eggs are fertilized.

missionary: The most famous, most used position for intercourse. He lies on top of her.

monogamy: Only having sex with one person over a specific period of time.

mons pubis or mound of Venus: The soft, mound-shaped pad of fat, covered in hair, that cushions the woman's pubic bone so it doesn't hurt when he's on top.

Morning After Pill (MAP): A pill containing a high dose of estrogen that can prevent pregnancy if taken seventy-two hours after unprotected intercourse.

necrophiliacs: Seriously weird people who want to have sex with dead bodies.

nipple: The tip of the breast that becomes erect if sexually stimulated (or it's really freezing).

Nonoxynol-9: A chemical present in most spermicides. It kills the HIV virus in laboratories, but unfortunately doesn't appear to be as successful in real life.

normal: Like everyone else, average, not different. The most commonly asked sex question in relation to any behavior is

"Am I normal?" Somehow, being "normal" makes people feel better. Strange, when normal often equates to boring.

nymphomaniac: A woman who wants lots of sex or sex with more than one man. Commonly used by men to describe a girlfriend who wants it more than they feel like providing.

oral sex: Using the mouth to stimulate the genitals. *See also* cunnilingus, fellatio.

orgasm: Climax, coming. The peak of sexual excitement usually accompanied by muscle contractions.

orgy: A wild, abandoned group sex experience usually involving excessive drinking and drugs. A favorite in Roman times and really bad R-rated movies. Good luck finding one outside Hollywood.

ovaries: The two female sex glands on either side of the uterus.

ovulation: The monthly release of an ovum (egg) from an ovary.

Pap test: A smear test used to screen against cancer, particularly cancer of the cervix. If you're over sixteen, sexually active, and female, you should be having them regularly.

PC muscle: *See* Kegels.

penetration: Putting something inside something, him "entering" you. Usually used to describe the insertion of his penis into a vagina or anus.

penis: The erectile male sex organ. The long, hard thing that pokes you in the back while you're trying to sleep.

perineum: In women, the area between the vagina and the anus; in men, the area between the scrotum and the anus. In both, a highly charged sexual area.

period: *See* menstruation.

pervert: Anyone who gets sexual satisfaction from doing something unusual. Definitions of "perverted" behavior vary depending on who's using the word. To a ninety-six-year-old virgin, tongue-kissing may be seen as perverted. To a twenty-one-year-old male, smearing chocolate sauce all over his girlfriend's body and licking it off while she's tied to the fridge isn't.

petting: Feeling each other up. *See also* foreplay.

pheromones: Substances secreted by the body, with an often undetectable odor, that stimulate sexual desire in others. Perfumes attempt to simulate the effect of natural pheromones; some are more successful than others.

Pill, the: A tiny tablet that turned a set of sexual mores upside down. Taken daily and correctly, it's an oral contraceptive that stops women from getting pregnant.

platonic relationship: A close relationship between two people that doesn't involve sex. Liking but not lusting after someone.

pornography: Material designed to stimulate sexual exitement that's rarely left on people's coffee tables. Hard-core porn is explicit, nothing-left-to-the-imagination stuff. Soft-core porn doesn't require any imagination either but you don't get to see any pink parts.

precome or preejaculatory fluid: The stuff that comes out of his penis before the real whoosh. Mother Nature thoughtfully provided it so the penis slips easily into the vagina.

pregnant: Knocked up, having a bun in the oven, about to have a baby. A time of great joy or desperation depending on the woman it happens to and what's happening in her life.

premarital sex: Sex between two people who aren't married. What just about everyone under the age of twenty-five is doing. Extramarital sex is sex between two people when one, or both, are already married to someone else. What lots of people over the age of twenty-five are doing.

premature ejaculation: When he ejaculates before his partner or he is finished with his erect penis. This could be before he's even penetrated, three thrusts in, or an hour later—it all depends on what the couple's definition of "too early" is.

promiscuity: Sleeping with lots of people on a casual basis. Promiscuous to one person might mean three partners a year, another might define it as more than three a week.

prostate gland: The male gland that surrounds the neck of the bladder and the urethra. The male G-spot (found in his rectum).

prostitute: Someone who gets paid for having sex. Women or men who marry purely for money aren't called prostitutes but they technically fit the definition.

quickie: Sex in a hurry, usually when both of you are so hot you don't need foreplay and want penetration NOW!

rape or sexual abuse: To force someone, either with violence or verbal threats, to have any type of sexual contact against their will.

rear entry: Him penetrating her from behind.

rubber: Slang for condom.

sadism: When a person gains pleasure from inflicting pain or "disciplining" another. S and M is short for "sadism and masochism," getting turned-on by inflicting and/or receiving pain.

safe period: The stage in a woman's menstrual cycle when she's least likely to get pregnant.

safe sex: Sex that carries a relatively low risk of contracting STIs or HIV, like kissing, mutual masturbation, or using a condom during other activities.

scrotum: The pouch of loose, wrinkled skin that contains a man's testicles.

semen: The mixture of sperm and seminal fluid ejaculated from a man's penis during orgasm. We usually say "sperm" but the correct term is "semen."

sex aid or toy: Any object used to generate or enhance sexual arousal and/or orgasm. If a jar of peanut butter puts a twinkle in your eye when used in a certain way, it's a sex aid.

sex drive: *See* libido.

sex therapist: A psychologist who is specially trained to solve your sexual problems. A good one is worth his or her weight in gold.

shaft: The length of the penis.

69: Two people simultaneously giving each other oral sex. The position they adopt—head to toe—resembles the number 69 when viewed from certain angles.

sleeping with someone: A euphemism usually meaning you did everything but.

smegma: A smelly, cheeselike substance that accumulates under the foreskin of an uncircumcised male or under the hood of a woman's clitoris because of poor hygiene. Capable of putting either sex off oral sex for good.

sodomy: Anal intercourse.

sperm: The male reproductive cell. Millions of sperm are produced in the testicles and mixed with seminal fluid before being ejaculated from the penis.

spermicide: A substance placed in the vagina or used with condoms or diaphragms to kill the hardy little buggers.

squeeze technique: A method of curing premature ejaculation where a man or his partner squeezes the head of the penis before he reaches the point where ejaculation is inevitable.

STD: *See* STI. STD is the old term for STI. They dropped "disease" and replaced it with "infection" because it sounds less offputting.

STI (sexually transmitted infection): Infections that are passed from one person to another during some form of sex. Not high on anyone's wish list.

straight: *See* heterosexual.

stripping: Removing your clothes provocatively rather than yanking them off willy-nilly and leaving them in a pile at the end of the bed.

swinging: Partner swapping with other singles or couples. Dangerous stuff.

testicles: Balls, nuts, testes. The two male sex glands carried in the scrotum that manufacture sperm and produce sex hormones. Extremely sensitive, they produce a pain quite unlike any other if knocked or kicked.

testosterone: The primary male sex hormone responsible for the male sex drive. Women also produce it and it's responsible for our sex drive as well.

thrusting: The act of him pushing his penis in and out of a vagina or anus.

transsexual: A man or woman who feels they are really a member of the opposite sex trapped in the wrong body. Many undergo sex change operations.

transvestite: A man (sometimes a woman) who has a compulsion to cross-dress (i.e., dress in the clothes of the opposite sex).

Him throwing on your robe to get you both a cup of coffee on a cold morning doesn't make him a transvestite.

uncut: An uncut penis is one that is uncircumcised.

unprotected sex: Sex without a condom which puts you at risk of pregnancy and STIs.

urethra: The tube through which urine is passed from the bladder. In men, it's also the tube through which semen is ejaculated.

uterus: The womb. A tranquil place where the baby lives until it's ready to face the world. Not surprisingly, most refuse to budge and have to be pushed out.

vagina: The soft, short passage that leads from a woman's vulva to her cervix. Also the part where he puts his penis during intercourse.

vas deferens: Either of the two tubes that carry sperm from the testicles.

vasectomy: A male sterilization procedure that cuts or seals the vas deferens so sperm can't pass into the semen.

VD (venereal disease): An old-fashioned term for STIs.

vibrator: Battery or electrically powered device, often penis-shaped, that's used to stimulate the genitals. Guaranteed to fall out of a closet when your mother-in-law visits.

virgin: Any person who has not had sexual intercourse.

voyeur: Peeping Tom. Someone who enjoys watching others have sex (often more than doing it themselves).

vulva: The external sex organs of a woman. Everything you can see.

water sports: Playing polo or volleyball in water, skiing on top of it—or having sex that somehow involves urination.

wet dreams: Previously used to describe a nocturnal experience that made men involuntarily ejaculate in their sleep and the sheets stick together. Now, sexperts believe women have wet dreams, too (though they're a lot less messy). Any dream where either sex is so turned-on, they have an orgasm in their sleep or wake during the throes of one.

withdrawal method: A somewhat risky method of contraception where he agrees to remove his penis from the vagina just when he's enjoying being in there the most.

Xmas: The time of the year when no one has sex very much because they're either (a) too drunk, (b) too full, or (c) too broke to go out and get some.

Endnotes

CHAPTER 1

1. June M. Reinisch, Ph.D., and Ruth Beasley, M.L.S., *The Kinsey Institute New Report on Sex* (New York: St. Martin's Press, 1990), pp. 96, 278.
2. Jared Diamond, *Why is Sex Fun? The Evolution of Human Sexuality* (New York: Basic Books, 1998), p. 33.
3. "1997 College Sex Survey," *Details* magazine (May 1997), p. 161. Poll of 20,000 college-student graduates by marketing research firm Willard & Shullman.
4. Susan Quilliam, *Women on Sex* (London: Smith Gryphon Limited, 1994), p. 87.
5. *Ibid.*, p. 88.
6. *Ibid.*, p. 88.
7. Samuel S. Janus, Ph.D., and Cynthia L. Janus, M.D., *The Janus Report on Sexual Behavior* (New York: John Wiley & Sons, Inc., 1993), p. 295.
8. Reinisch and Beasley, p. 96.
9. *Ibid.*, p. 92.
10. *Ibid.*, p. 98.

CHAPTER 2

1. Susan Quilliam, *Women on Sex* (London: Smith Gryphon Limited, 1994), p. 117.
2. *UK for Women* magazine (December 1996), p. 69.
3. Quilliam, p. 43.
4. Samuel S. Janus, Ph.D., and Cynthia L. Janus, M.D., *The Janus Report on Sexual Behavior* (New York: John Wiley & Sons, Inc., 1993), pp. 53, 98.
5. Quilliam, p. 59.

CHAPTER 3

1. Alex Comfort, M.B., D.Sc., *The Joy of Sex* (London: Mitchell Beazley, 1996), p. 82.
   June Reinisch, Ph.D., and Ruth Beasley, M.L.S., *The Kinsey Institute New Report on Sex* (New York: St. Martin's Press, 1990), p. 124.
2. *Ibid.*, p. 123. Magazine survey by *UK Options* magazine (February 1996), p. 51.

3. Susan Crain Bakos, *Dear Superlady of Sex* (New York: St. Martin's Press, 1990), p. 113.

4. Jared Diamond, *Why Is Sex Fun?* (New York: Basic Books, 1998), pp. 8, 89.

5. Doreen E. Massey, *The Lover's Guide Encyclopedia* (London: Bloomsbury, 1996), p. 26.

6. Bakos, pp. 118, 119.

7. Susan Quilliam, *Women on Sex* (London: Smith Gryphon Limited, 1994), pp. 134, 142, 151.

8. Edward W. Eichel (contrib.) and Philip Nobile, *The Perfect Fit: How to Achieve Mutual Fulfillment and Monogamous Passion Through the New Intercourse* (New York: Signet, 1993), p. 11.

CHAPTER 4

1. Rodney Brennan, Principal of Nature Care College, Sydney, Australia, author interview, 1998.

2. Durex Condoms, *Durex Global Sex Survey,* 1997, p. 11. Survey covered fourteen countries, questioning almost 10,000 adults.

3. June Reinisch, Ph.D., and Ruth Beasley, M.L.S., *The Kinsey Institute New Report on Sex* (New York: St. Martin's Press, 1990), p. 89.

4. *Ibid.,* p. 82. Dr. Miriam Stoppard, *The Magic of Sex* (London: Allen & Unwin, 1991), p. 31.

5. Susan Crain Bakos, *Dear Superlady of Sex* (New York: St. Martin's Press, 1990), p. 131.

6. John Gottman, *Why Marriages Succeed or Fail* (London: Bloomsbury, 1997), p. 95.

7. Bakos, p. 114.

8. Reinisch and Beasley, p. 128. Susan Quilliam, *Women on Sex* (London: Smith Gryphon Limited, 1994), p. 142.

9. Stoppard, p. 97.

10. Samuel S. Janus, Ph.D., and Cynthia L. Janus, M.D., *The Janus Report on Sexual Behavior* (New York: John Wiley & Sons, Inc., 1993), p. 53.

11. As reported in "Hit the A-spot" by Lisa Sussman, Australian *Cosmopolitan* (June 1996), p. 90.

12. Bakos, p. 151.

13. Reinisch and Beasley, p. 203.

14. Quilliam, p. 116. Bakos, p. 107.

CHAPTER 5

1. Durex Condoms, *Durex Global Sex Survey,* 1997, p. 6.

2. Shere Hite, *Women and Love: The New Hite Report* (London: Viking, 1988), pp. 804, 849, 850, 856.

3. "1997 College Sex Survey," *Details* magazine (May 1997), p. 162.
4. Durex Condoms, pp. 6, 7.
5. John Gottman, *Why Marriages Succeed or Fail* (London: Bloomsbury, 1997), p. 128.
6. Samuel S. Janus, Ph.D., and Cynthia L. Janus, M.D., *The Janus Report on Sexual Behavior* (New York: John Wiley & Sons, Inc., 1993), p. 295.
7. *Details* magazine college survey, p. 160.
8. Based on research by David Quadagno, Ph.D., professor of biology, Florida State University.
9. Hite, pp. 815, 820.

CHAPTER 6

1. Condomania corporate office, Los Angeles, and Condomania on-line, www.condomania.com.
2. June Reinisch, Ph.D., and Ruth Beasley, M.L.S., *The Kinsey Institute New Report on Sex* (New York: St. Martin's Press, 1990), p. 11.
3. AIDS Council of New South Wales (ACON), "So When Do We Stop Using Condoms?" December 1995, p. 2.
4. Powerhouse Museum, eds., *Taking Precautions: The Story of Contraception* (Sydney: Bloxham & Chambers, 1995), p. 3.
5. James Trussell, Jennifer Strickler, and Barbara Vaughan, "Contraceptive Efficacy of the Diaphragm, the Sponge, and the Cervical Cap," *Family Planning Perspectives* 25, no. 3 (May/June 1993): 100.
6. "Understanding IUDs," available from PPFA Web site (www.plannedparenthood.org) © 1998, Planned Parenthood® Federation of America, Inc. (cited 14 September 1998), p. 3.
7. Based on a study of 364 women, aged 18–26 by San Francisco State University by Norma McCoy. "Of Birth Control: Pills'n'-thrills," *Psychology Today* (September/October 1996), p. 22.
8. Susan Quilliam, *Women on Sex* (London: Smith Gryphon Limited, 1994), p. 155.
9. Powerhouse Museum, p. 7.
10. "The Fight to Make RU486 Legal," available from The Feminist Majority Web site (www.feminist.org) © 1996, The Feminist Majority and New Media Publishing, Inc. (cited 14 September 1998), pp. 1–3.
11. "Sexually Transmitted Infections: Herpes: Questions and Answers," available from PPFA Web site (www.plannedparenthood.org) © 1998, Planned Parenthood® Federation of America, Inc. (cited 14 September 1998), p. 3.

12. Edith Weisberg, "52 Different Types of Wart Virus," *Options* (Family Planning, New South Wales, Australia), Special Autumn Issue 1993, p. 7.

13. *Ibid*.

14. "Sexually Transmitted Infections: Chlamydia: Questions and Answers," available from PPFA Web site (www.plannedparent hood.org) © 1998, Planned Parenthood® Federation of America, Inc. (cited 14 September 1998), p. 2.

15. Dr. Jane Macquarie, *Below the Belt: An Owner's Guide to Gynaecology* (Melbourne: The Text Publishing Company, 1994), p. 165.

16. "GMHC Facts & Statistics," available from the GMHC Web site (www.gmhc.org) © 1998 GMHC, Inc. (cited 10 July 1998), p. 3. Statistics from UNAIDS/WHO, June 1996; CDC, December 1996.

17. Quilliam, p. 155.

18. Martin E. Wilkie, Michael K. Almond, and Frank P. Marsh, "Diagnosis and Management of Urinary Tract Infections in Adults," *British Medical Journal* 305, no. 6862 (November 7, 1992): 1137.

CHAPTER 7

1. June Reinisch, Ph.D., and Ruth Beasley, M.L.S., *The Kinsey Institute New Report on Sex* (New York: St. Martin's Press, 1990), p. 16.

2. *Ibid.*, p. 129.

3. Dr. Miriam Stoppard, *The Magic of Sex* (London: Allyn and Unwin, 1991), p. 209.

4. "Declining Sperm Counts," *British Medical Journal* 312, no. 7029 (February 24, 1996): 457.
   Stewart Irvine, Elizabeth Cawood, David Richardson, Eileen MacDonald, and John Aitken, "Evidence of Deteriorating Semen Quality in the United Kingdom; Birth Cohort Study in 577 Men in Scotland Over 11 Years," *British Medical Journal* 312, no. 7029 (February 24, 1996): 467.
   "Worldwide Decline in Semen Quality Might Be Due to Smoking," *British Medical Journal* 312, no. 7029 (February 24, 1996): 506.

5. Reinisch and Beasley, p. 203. Stoppard, p. 200.

6. Dr. Janet Hall, sex therapist. Author interview, 1998.

7. William Axinn, Ph.D., and Jennifer Barber, Ph.D., Penn State, "Not married—and Not Interested," *Psychology Today* (March/April 1998), p. 19.

8. Barbara De Angelis, *Ask Barbara: The 100 Most-Asked Questions About Love, Sex, and Relationships* (New York: Delacorte Press, 1997), pp. 29, 30.

9. "The Sex Files: *Sky*'s Sex Survey 1996," *Sky* magazine (December 1996), p. 84. Reader survey (polled in July by *Sky* magazine).

10. Tracey Cox, "Sex Report," Australian *Cosmopolitan* (April 1997), p. 47.

11. Robert Epstein, Ph.D., "Folk Wisdom: Was Your Grandmother Right?" *Psychology Today* (November/December 1997), p. 76.

CHAPTER 8

1. Dr. Jane Macquarie, *Below the Belt: An Owner's Guide to Gynaecology* (Melbourne: The Text Publishing Company, 1994), p. 114.
   "Abortion: Fact Sheets," available from PPFA Web site (www.plannedparenthood.org) © 1998, Planned Parenthood® Federation of America, Inc. (cited 14 September 1998), p. 1.

2. Opinion of Fiona Lecren, Australian Birth Control, a termination center in Sydney, Australia. Author interview, 1998.

3. Lisa Tolin, "The Effects of Abortion," *Psychology Today* (August 1997), p. 12.

4. Samuel S. Janus, Ph.D., and Cynthia L. Janus, M.D., *The Janus Report on Sexual Behavior* (New York: John Wiley & Sons Inc., 1993), p. 72.

5. Statistics from the Department of Health and Human Services, Administration for Children and Families, Child Maltreatment, from the RAINN Web site (www.rainn.org), (cited 10 July 1998), p. 2.

6. Statistics from the National Crime Victimization Survey, Bureau of Justice Statistics, U.S. Department of Justice, 1997, from the RAINN Web site (www.rainn.org), (cited 10 July 1998), p. 2.

7. Statistics from the National Crime Victimization Survey, Bureau of Justice Statistics, U.S. Department of Justice, 1996, from the RAINN Web site (www.rainn.org), (cited 10 July 1998), pp. 1, 3.

8. Statistics from the Response to Rape, Senate Judiciary Report, 1993, from the Sexual Assault Response Team Web site (www.uww.wdu/stdRsces/SART/AssaultFacts.htm), (cited 11 January 1999), p. 1.

CHAPTER 9

1. Susan Quilliam, *Women on Sex* (London: Smith Gryphon Limited, 1994), p. 164.
2. *Ibid.*, p. 65.
3. Statistics from a survey conducted by the EROS Foundation of Australia (representing sex workers) on behalf of the author, February 1997.
4. Dr. Andrew Stanway, *The Joy of Sexual Fantasy* (London: Headline Book Publishing, 1994), p. 23.
5. Quilliam, p. 164. Stanway, pp. 28, 29.
6. "1997 College Sex Survey," *Details* magazine (May 1997), p. 163.

CHAPTER 10

1. "The Ups and Downs of Testosterone," *Psychology Today* (November/December 1997), p. 18.
2. Nadia Hohn and Annie Paul, "Does Fate Make Mates?" *Psychology Today* (July/August 1998), p. 16.
3. Durex Condoms, *Durex Global Sex Survey,* 1997, pp. 18–19.
4. *Ibid.*
5. Study of 670 couples by John Gottman, University of Washington, Seattle. Hara Estroff Marano, "Another Round, Honey?" *Psychology Today* (September/October 1997), p. 20.
6. Kay Wellings, Julia Field, Anne Johnson, and Jane Wadsworth, with Sally Bradshaw, *Sexual Behavior in Britain: The National Survey of Sexual Attitudes and Lifestyles* (London: Penguin Books, 1994), p. 365.
7. Steven P. Shelov, *Your Baby's First Year* (New York: Bantam Books, 1998), p. 24.
8. "Durex Scientific," available from the Durex Web site (www.durex.com), © 1998 London International Group PLC (cited 14 September, 1998). June M. Reinisch, Ph.D., and Ruth Beasley, M.L.S., *The Kinsey Institute New Report on Sex* (New York: St. Martin's Press, 1990), p. 47.
9. Debbie Atwell, "Drugs and You," *UK Company* (July 1997), p. 92. Results of a drug survey published in March 1997 issue of *UK Company.* More than 1000 readers responded.
10. Michael Castleman, "Recipes for Lust," *Psychology Today* (July/August 1997), p. 54.
11. Atwell, p. 92.
12. "1997 College Sex Survey," *Details* magazine (May 1997), p. 163.
13. "Safe Sex?" *Psychology Today* (July/August 1997), p. 22.

14. *Details,* p. 163.
15. Atwell, p. 92.
16. *Ibid.*

CHAPTER 11

1. Statistics from the *Journal of Pediatrics* in "About Project YES," available from the Project YES Web site (www.projectyes.org), © 1998 Project YES (cited 15 September, 1998).
2. June M. Reinisch, Ph.D., and Ruth Beasley, M.L.S., *The Kinsey Institute New Report on Sex* (New York: St. Martin's Press, 1990), p. 13.
3. "1997 College Sex Survey," *Details* magazine (May 1997), p. 161.
4. Statistics from the *Journal of Pediatrics* in "About Project YES," available from the Project YES Web site (www.projectyes.org), © 1998 Project YES (cited 15 September, 1998).
5. Reinisch and Beasley, p. 466.
6. Samuel S. Janus, Ph.D., and Cynthia L. Janus, M.D., *The Janus Report on Sexual Behavior* (New York: John Wiley & Sons, Inc., 1993), p. 53.
7. Statistics from the *Journal of Pediatrics* in "About Project YES," available from the Project YES Web site (www.projectyes.org), © 1998 Project YES (cited 15 September, 1998).
8. Research provided by The Positive Fun & Self-Esteem Group, run through the AIDS Council of New South Wales, Australia.
9. *Details* college survey, p. 161.
10. University of Quebec study published in *Psychology Today* (July/August 1996), p. 22.
11. *Details* college survey, p. 163.
12. Doreen A. Rosenthal and Helen Shepherd, "HIV/AIDS Knowledge and Attitudes to Condoms," *Journal of Community and Applied Social Psychology* 3 (1993): 53–65.

CHAPTER 12

1. Shirley Glass, Ph.D., "Shattered Vows," *Psychology Today* (August 1998), p. 36.
2. Susan Quilliam, *Women on Sex* (London: Smith Gryphon Limited, 1994), p. 196.
3. Ball State University, Indiana, 1996 survey of 884 men and 1288 women.
4. Samuel S. Janus, Ph.D., and Cynthia L. Janus, M.D., *The Janus Report on Sexual Behavior* (New York: John Wiley & Sons, Inc., 1993), p. 295.

5. John Gottman, *Why Marriages Succeed or Fail* (London: Bloomsbury, 1997), p. 57.
6. "1997 College Sex Survey," *Details* magazine (May 1997), p. 159.
7. Hara Estroff Marano, "A New Focus on Family Values," *Psychology Today,* (November/December 1997), p. 54.
8. Cris Evatt, *He & She: 60 Significant Differences Between Men and Women* (Berkeley, CA: Conari Press), p. 29.
9. *Details,* p. 160.
10. June M. Reinisch, Ph.D., and Ruth Beasley, M.L.S., *The Kinsey Institute New Report on Sex* (New York: St. Martin's Press, 1990), p. 111.
11. "The Sex Files: *Sky*'s Sex Survey 1996," *Sky* magazine (December 1996), p. 80. Reader survey (polled in July, by *Sky* magazine).
12. Magazine survey by *UK Options* magazine (February 1996), p. 51.
13. Alex Comfort, M.B., D.Sc., *The Joy of Sex* (London: Mitchell Beazley, 1996), p. 156.

About the Author

Tracey Cox is Australia's foremost sex and relationships writer and has a degree in psychology. A former associate editor of Australian *Cosmopolitan*, she writes for leading women's magazines both at home and abroad, has her own weekly radio show, and regularly appears on television as a "sexpert." She lives in New South Wales, Australia, and is currently working on her next book, *Hot Relationships: How to Have One*, and a novel.

Index

woman-on-top position for, 64–66

intrauterine device (IUD), 157–60, 233
see also contraception

Kama Sutra, 32, 61, 325, 360

Kegel exercises, 15, 26, 86, 110, 111, 360

kinky, 218–19, 259, 360

Kinsey (the Kinsey Institute), 2, 98, 103, 202, 273, 360

Kubic, Jake, 329

K-Y jelly, 360, 361
see also lubricants, personal

labia majora, 7, 360
see also genitals (female)

labia minora, 7, 360
see also genitals (female)

lesbian, 360
see also gays and lesbians

libido, 360
lack of desire in men, 204–5
lack of desire in women, 208–10
mismatched, 204, 311–14

love, 225, 360
fate and, 274
at first sight, 272

lubricants, personal, 9, 10, 12, 21, 72, 85, 86–87, 212, 217, 360–61

lubrication, natural, 7, 72, 85, 110, 212, 217

lust, 225, 361

making love, 361

marijuana (dope), 283–84
see also drugs

marriage, 317
attitudes toward, 134, 215
gay, 301
see also monogamy

masochist, 361

masochistic fantasies, 257

massages, 30–37
erotic, 32–37, 358
sensual, 31–32

Masters and Johnson, 75, 361

masturbation, 1–28, 110, 112, 323, 361
anatomy and, 3–9
in becoming a better lover, 25–27
dealing with hangups about, 10–12
fantasies about, 28, 256
female, orgasm in, 10, 13, 15, 16, 17, 18, 25–26, 115
in foreplay, 40, 41, 43–48
in front of each other, 27–28, 220–21
good reasons for, 18–19
guide for her, 9–19
guide for him, 19–25
in learning how to orgasm, 115–17
male, orgasm in, 22, 23–24, 25, 26–27
mutual, 30, 43–48, 361
orgasms from, 102–3
premature ejaculation and, 25, 26–27, 87–88, 203

ménage à trois, 361
see also group sex

menstruation, 361
sex during, 223

Mifepristone (RU486), 170

Mini Pill, 162–64
see also contraception

missionary position, 62–64, 72, 75, 361
see also intercourse

monogamy, 307–36, 361
affairs and, 310
characteristics of couples with excellent sex lives, 316–19

vasectomy, 169–70, 366
VD (venereal disease), 366
  see also sexually transmitted
    infections
vibrators, 15–17, 25–26, 115–16,
    331, 332–33, 366
  see also sex toys (sex aids)
virgin, 366
virginity, losing, 70–74
voyeur, 256, 323, 366
vulva, 7, 366
  see also genitals (female)

warts (human papilloma virus),
    123, 173, 182–83

  see also sexually transmitted
    infections
water sports, 366
wet dreams, 94, 366–67
wet spot, 217
withdrawal method, 147–48, 171,
    367
  see also contraception
woman-on-top position, 64–66
  see also intercourse

yeast infection (candida), 192–93,
    212